ORTHOPAEDIC TESTING

A Rational Approach to Diagnosis

ORTHOPAEDIC TESTING

A Rational Approach to Diagnosis

Janet A. Gerard, D.A.B.C.O.

Clinician, Department of Clinical Sciences, Levittown Outpatient Health Center,
Division of New York Chiropractic College, Levittown, New York;
Faculty Instructor, Postgraduate Education: Orthopedic Diplomate Program,
New York Chiropractic College Centre for Postgraduate and Continuing Education,
Syracuse, New York

Steven L. Kleinfield, D.A.B.C.O.

Associate Professor, Department of Clinical Sciences, University of Bridgeport
College of Chiropractic, Bridgeport, Connecticut; Former Associate Clinical
Director, Levittown Outpatient Health Center, Division of New York Chiropractic
College, Levittown, New York; President and Founder of Dual County
Chiropractors, P.C., Huntington Station, New York

Churchill Livingstone
A Harcourt Health Sciences Company
New York, Edinburgh, London, Philadelphia, Tokyo

CHURCHILL LIVINGSTONE
A Harcourt Health Sciences Company

Library of Congress Cataloging-in-Publication Data

Gerard, Janet A.
    Orthopaedic testing/Janet A. Gerard, Steven L. Kleinfield.
       p.   cm.
    Includes bibliographical references.
    ISBN 0-443-08876-4
    1. Physical orthopedic tests. I. Kleinfield, Steven L.
II. Title.
    [DNLM: 1. Orthopedic—methods—handbooks. 2. Musculoskeletal
Diseases—diagnosis—handbooks. WE 39 G3560 1993]
    RD734.5.P58G47   1993
    617.3'0028—dc20
    DNLM/DLC

                                              93-19306

Acquisitions Editor: *Leslie Burgess*
Copy Editor: *Bridgett Dickinson*
Production Supervisor: *Jeanine Furino*

Printed in the United States of America

First published in 1993   9 8 7 6 5 4 3

I am especially appreciative of my family and friends, whose patience and understanding have been limitless in respecting my absence while this text was in progress.

To my dear friend Judy: Your undaunted confidence in me has been my inspiration. A special thank you to Theresa who has helped me through my most trying times. Your love has been my strength.

I am grateful to my brother Eric and his wife Yvette, who allowed their son Alec Richard Gerard to model for the pediatric tests and to my Goddaughter Michelle Leigh Wright, for permission to photograph her feet for use in this text.

This book is dedicated to my nephew, Daniel, afflicted by Batten's disease. I hope you will find as much comfort and support in family and friends as I have when difficult times approach. I love you.

Janet A. Gerard

I thank my wife Lori and my three sons, Ian, Sean, and Michael, for giving me the support needed in preparing the manuscript of this book. There were many times when normal family life was disrupted, but they gave me the time so that I could remain focused in my desire to create this text.

Steven L. Kleinfield

Foreword

Often in modern clinical practice too much emphasis is placed on complex imaging techniques and not enough on careful thorough physical examination and history taking. Patients quite commonly complain that physicians, chiropractors, and other health care professionals do not spend sufficient time listening to or discussing their problems with them. This leads to patient dissatisfaction and sometimes to delayed diagnosis or misdiagnosis. It is also a common cause of malpractice suits.

Orthopaedic Testing goes far to correct our perspective of where the emphasis should be placed in beginning the diagnostic process. The authors are well aware of the void that exists in the approach clinicians use to decide on a working diagnosis and believe this book will provide the knowledge needed to undertake the appropriate orthopaedic examinations.

Orthopaedic Testing has been prepared with the clinician and the student in mind. It will be of help not only to chiropractors but equally to orthopaedic surgeons and neurosurgeons, physical therapists, and others. It describes the tests used in the examination of the neuromusculoskeletal system of the body from neck to foot. It is written attractively, clearly, and concisely. Numerous illustrations are included, all of which are quite excellent and give the whole text its outstanding value. It should be available to every health care professional who tackles problems of the neuromusculoskeletal system and in the library of every clinic and hospital where such conditions are being treated.

I recommend this book highly and believe it will become the classic text on this subject.

William H. Kirkaldy-Willis, M.A., M.D., F.R.C.S.(Edin)
(C), F.A.C.S., F.I.C.C.(Hon)
Emeritus Professor, Department
of Orthopaedic Surgery, University
of Saskatchewan College of
Medicine; Former Orthopaedic
Surgeon, Department of Orthopaedics,
Royal University Hospital,
Saskatoon, Saskatchewan, Canada

Preface

Orthopaedic Testing is a reference text for use by both the health care practitioner and health care student alike. Orthopaedic testing is designed to re-create the patient's complaint by introducing a mechanical disadvantage or external stress into the area being tested. Although classically the patient's response to such testing is designated as positive or negative, clinically the interpretation of patient's response is not always clear-cut. This can lead to misinterpretation. Reliance on classical findings alone for diagnosis, while disregarding nonclassical findings, can lead to a wrong diagnosis and ultimately to a delay in proper treatment. Thus, the most important aspects of the clinical evaluation are (1) a thorough history of the patient with a proper review of systems pertinent to the patient's symptom complex (which will determine the initial clinical finding); and (2) a thorough orthopaedic examination to finalize the diagnosis.

Each chapter in *Orthopaedic Testing* is centered on a specific part of the body and brings into one place the tests most often used in that area. An outline of the tests is provided below the respective chapter title for ease in locating a specific test; these are also included in the table of contents. The tests are in alphabetical order and are numbered. All but two chapters have a flowchart at the beginning of the chapter diagraming the pathways through differential diagnoses. Range of motion studies are included in appropriate chapters and are the first test discussed in those chapters. The figures in the range of motion studies are directly below the description of the movement. The text discussion of each test describes the Procedure (how to perform the test), the Classical Signficance (positive findings), and the Clinical Significance (other important but atypical findings). The Rationale of each test is also given. The final section is the Follow-up, which lists at least two tests to use to confirm or narrow down the diagnosis, and referrals to other specialties when necessary.

It is our hope that this text will help the reader understand that a patient's response is not simply positive or negative. In the interest of better health it is important *not* to disregard patient findings that do not fit the classical mold. The more accurate the diagnosis, the more effective the treatment and, ultimately, the more rewarding the prognosis of recovery.

Janet A. Gerard, D.A.B.C.O.
Steven L. Kleinfield, D.A.B.C.O.

Acknowledgments

We thank Clifford Haymes, D.C. of Hackensack, New Jersey for his expertise in taking the modeled photographs and John J. Spano M.S., D.C., Assistant Clinical Professor, New York Chiropractic College, who was responsible for the photography of some of the radiographic plates used in this text. The plates are from the New York Chiropractic College X-Ray Library.

A special thank you to Cybex in Ronkonkoma, New York for the use of the EDI-320 and also to Camp International, Inc. in Jackson, Michigan for their donation of a Jamar P5030J1 Adjustable Hand Dynamometer for use in *Orthopaedic Testing*.

We acknowledge Jil-Crest Color Laboratories in Massapequa, New York for their work in producing the patient photographs used in this text.

Contents

— own

9 Sacroiliac Testing 397

Permissions

Note: the first number of each figure number corresponds to the chapter number; the second number corresponds to the test number.

Figure 4-10F
Modified from Rowe CR: The Shoulder. Churchill Livingstone, New York, 1988, p. 106

Figures 4-26C, 6-4F, 6-12E, 6-20D, 6-21D, 6-22F, 6-24E, 6-24F, 6-25E, and 6-29E
From Walther DS: Applied Kinesiology: The Advanced Approach in Chiropractic. Systems DC, Pueblo, CO, 1976, pp. 102, 113, 114, 115, 288

Figures 3-2B and 3-6A
From Turek SL: Orthopaedics: Principles and Their Applications. Vol. 2. 4th Ed. JB Lippincott, Philadelphia, 1984, p. 900

Figure 11-2F
From Tria AJ Jr, Klein KS: An Illustrated Guide to the Knee. Churchill Livingstone, New York, 1992, p 15

Figure 11-7E
Modified from Tria AJ Jr, Klein KS: An Illustrated Guide to the Knee. Churchill Livingstone, New York, 1992, p. 134

Figures 11-2E and 11-20E
From Insall JN, Kelly MA: Anatomy. p. 1. In Insall JN, Scott NW, Windsor RE et al (eds): Surgery of the Knee. 2nd Ed. Churchill Livingstone, New York, 1993

Figures 12-3E and 12-8D
From Anderson KJ, LeCocq JF, LeCocq EA: Recurrent anterior subluxation of the ankle joint. A report of two cases and an experimental study. J Bone Joint Surg 34A:853, 1952

Figure 12-11E
From Elstrom JA, Pankovich AM: Muscle and Tendon Surgery of the Leg. In Evarts CM (ed): Surgery of the Musculoskeletal System. Vol. 4. 2nd Ed. Churchill Livingstone, 1990, p. 3938

Figure 12-17E
From Harkless LB, Krych SM: Handbook of Common Foot Problems. Churchill Livingstone, New York, 1990, p. 24

Figures 2-17F, 5-11E, 6-4F, 6-7E, 6-10E, 6-27F, 8-2B, 10-20F, 11-46E, 11-47E, and 12-6F
From Rich EA: Atlas of Clinical Roentgenology. 3rd Ed. Texas Chiropractic College, Pasadena, TX, 1975, pp. 12, 33, 34, 37, 46, 66, 92, 96, 112, 186, 236

Orientation and Vestibular Testing

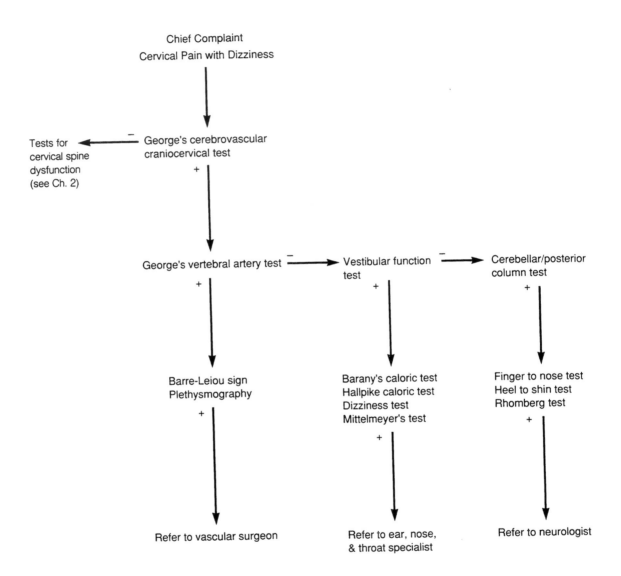

Chief Complaint
Cervical Pain with Dizziness

Tests for
cervical spine
dysfunction
(see Ch. 2)

George's cerebrovascular
craniocervical test

George's vertebral artery test

Vestibular function
test

Cerebellar/posterior
column test

Barre-Leiou sign
Plethysmography

Barany's caloric test
Hallpike caloric test
Dizziness test
Mittelmeyer's test

Finger to nose test
Heel to shin test
Rhomberg test

Refer to vascular surgeon

Refer to ear, nose,
& throat specialist

Refer to neurologist

1 | *Orthopaedic Testing Orientation*

Before performing orthopaedic tests in the cervical spine one must establish that (1) the vertebral arteries are not compromised, (2) the vestibular system is intact, and (3) the cerebellar/posterior columns are intact. To this end, one must perform several tests, the first of which is George's cerebrovascular craniocervical test. All test results should be recorded.

High-Risk Profile Identification

First, one must review the patient's history to determine whether predisposing risks for vascular disease are present. Risks include transient ischemic attack, arteriosclerosis, hypertension, cerebrovascular disease, diabetes, cervical arthrosis, neck sprain injury, medication (especially the use of oral contraceptives or coumedin), a family history of stroke, and a history of cigarette smoking.

Hypertensive Patient and Subclavian Vessel Evaluation

Evaluate the hypertensive patient by first taking the bilateral blood pressures. Next, determine which side has the lower value of systolic pressure, as well as the difference between the systolic values. The difference should not be more than 10 mmHg. A difference greater than 10 mmHg indicates a possible stenosis in the subclavian vessel on the side with the lower systolic pressure. Third, palpate the pulse on the low side to determine whether the radial artery is normal, feeble, or absent. Finally, auscultate the subclavian arteries for audible bruits, while the patient holds the breath for several seconds.

Carotid Vessel Evaluation

Palpate the left and right carotid vessels at the level of C4 to determine whether the pulse is normal, feeble, or absent. Next, auscultate the carotid vessels for bruits.

Vertebrobasilar Artery Functional Maneuvers

The patient is seated. To test for ischemic reactions, ask the patient to turn the head as far as possible to one side and then to hyperextend the head and neck for 3 to 5 seconds. Some authors suggest that the patient's head should stay in this provocative position for 40 to 60 seconds; however, George indicates that if the test is positive, the reactions will occur within 10 seconds. Ischemic reactions include vertigo, dizziness, or light-headedness; visual dysfunction, double vision, blurring, or photophobia; nausea or vomiting; headache or sudden occipital pain; numbness, paresthesia, or coldness; ataxia, falling to one side, or difficulty maintaining balance; slurred speech or hoarseness; tinnitus; and dysphagia.

Often the patient complains of vertigo, a disturbance for which one has a subjective impression of movement in space or of an object moving around one, with a resultant loss of equilibrium. True vertigo must be distinguished from faintness, light-headedness, or other forms of dizziness that result from a disturbance in the equilibratory apparatus (vestibular system), cranial nerve VIII, vestibular nuclei in the brain stem, or other central nervous system (CNS) connections. Nystagmus, pastpointing, inability to tandem walk, and persistent deviation to one side often indicate a problem in the vestibular system or CNS. The source of the vertigo will be either peripheral (vestibulum, vestibular system) or central (vestibular nuclei, CNS lesion). This must be determined. If the source is peripheral, episodes of normalcy with paroxysmal vertigo, unilateral nerve deafness, tinnitus (cochlear nerve), and intense symptoms (vestibular system) of the above will be present. If the source is central, persistent vertigo, gait disturbance, and a vertical/rotary component of the nystagmus will be present.

Procedures

2 | George's Vertebral Artery Test With Klyne's Maneuver

Procedure: Take the patient's history, specifically for hypertension. Palpate the bilateral pulses and take the bilateral blood pressures. Auscultate the subclavian and carotid vessels for bruits. *Do not proceed* if the results of any two of the above are abnormal. If none of the above is problematic proceed with the test. The patient is seated and rotates the head completely to one side and hyperextends the neck (Figs. A–F).

Rationale: Occlusion of the vertebral artery compromises the blood supply to the brain as it passes through the transverse foramen.

Classical Significance: If a problem exists, the patient will have a feeling of dizziness or nystagmus, or both. The patient may also note a feeling of fullness in the head.

Clinical Significance: A positive result may be a determining factor in whether to adjust the cervical spine, and is a warning of impending stroke because an obstruction in the blood supply to the brain may be present. Perform lateral flexion adjustment only.

Follow-up: Refer the patient for arteriography or plethysmography.

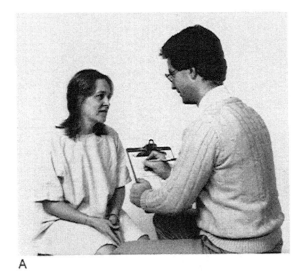

A

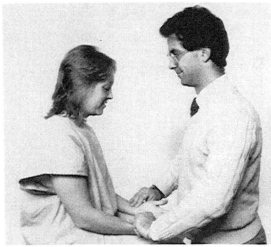

B

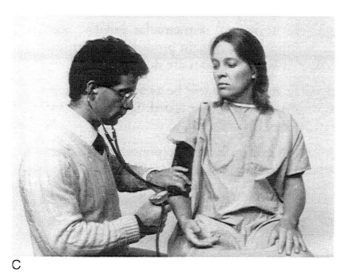

C

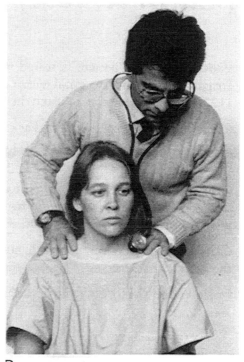

D

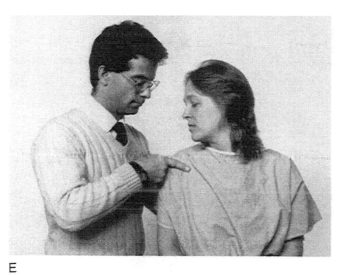

E

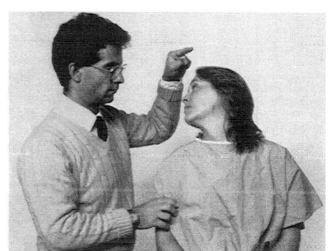

F

3 | *Barany's Caloric Test (Caloric Test)*

Procedure: The patient is seated with eyes open and extends the neck 30 degrees. Irrigate the external ear canal with 3 to 4 oz of 60°F water. Repeat the procedure using 112°F water. Remember to catch the water in a basin placed under the ear (Figs. A–C).

Rationale: Tilting the head back aligns the horizontal semicircular canal in the vertical plane. Artificial stimulation of the vestibular component produces nystagmus along with the autonomic response of emesis. These responses are normal.

Classical Significance: Using the cold water, nystagmus will be away from the ear tested. Using the warm water, nystagmus will be toward the ear tested. The nystagmus will be horizontal in the direction indicated (Figs. D & E).

Clinical Significance: Acoustic neuromas will cause a lack of response using either the warm or cold water. The neuroma results in a canal paresis (Fig. F).

Follow-up: Perform the Hallpike caloric test, Mittelmeyer's test, or the dizziness test.

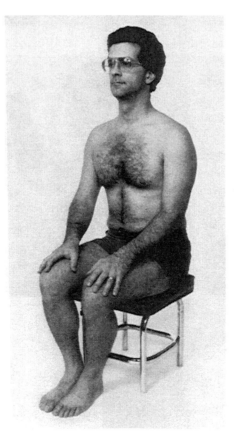 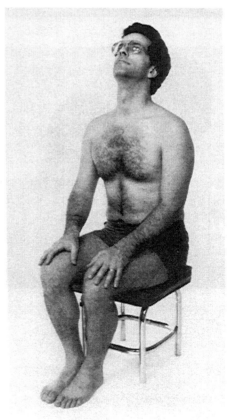

A   B

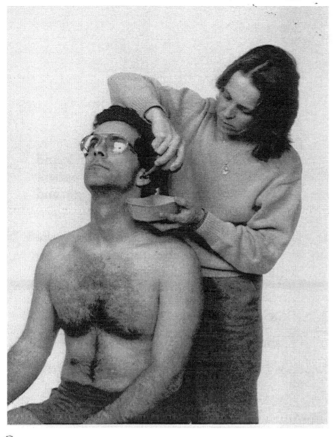

C

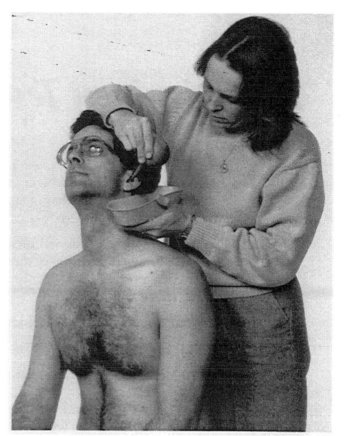

D

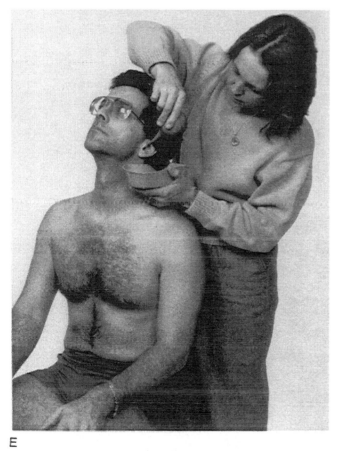

E

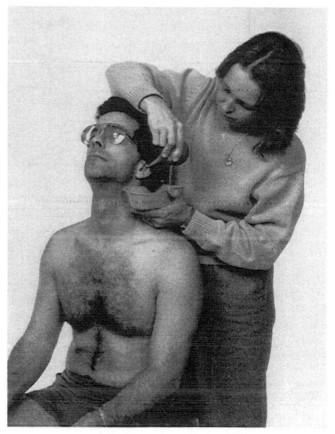

F

4 | *Dizziness Test*

Procedure: The patient is seated. Rotate the patient's head as far right as possible and then as far left as possible. Next, hold the patient's head centered with the patient looking directly ahead and have the patient actively rotate the shoulders as far right and left as possible (Figs. A–E).

Rationale: Active rotation of the head causes a torque on the vertebral artery at the transverse foramen. Rotation of the trunk with the head still causes the same effect on the vertebral artery. If dizziness occurs only with head rotation consider vestibular, not cervical spinal, dysfunction.

Classical Significance: If dizziness occurs the test is positive.

Clinical Significance: See Classical Significance.

Follow-up: Perform Barany's caloric test, the Hallpike caloric test, or Mittelmeyer's test.

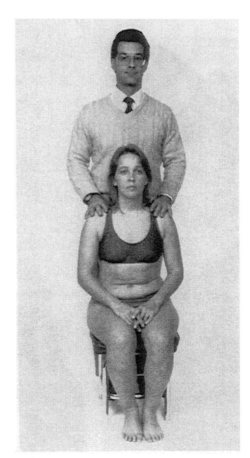

A

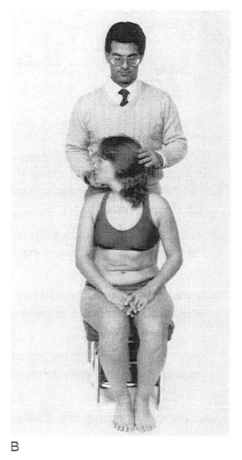

B

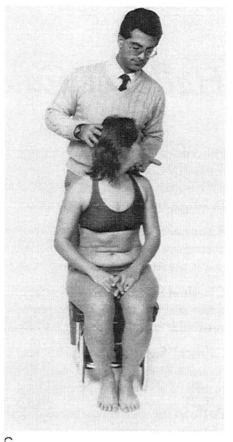

C

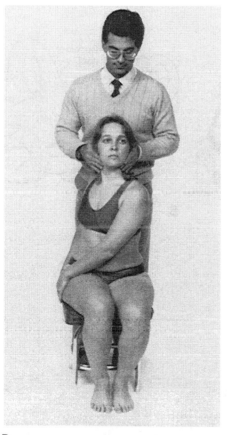

D

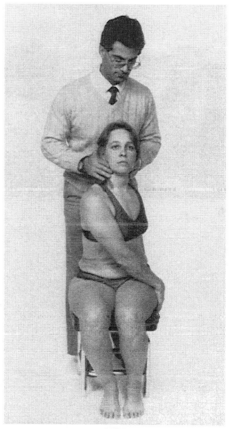

E

5 | *Hallpike Caloric Test*

Procedure: The patient is supine with the head elevated about 30 degrees; this aligns the horizontal semicircular canal to the vertical plane. Irrigate the external canal with 60°F water and then with 111.2°F to 112.0°F water. Allow the water to accumulate in an irrigation basin. Perform this test bilaterally (Figs. A & B).

Rationale: Artificial stimulation of the vestibular apparatus is known to produce a nystagmus as well as the autonomic response of emesis. Since dizziness may occur, this test is preferred over Barany's caloric test.

Classical Significance: Nystagmus will be away from the ear tested when using cold water and toward the ear tested when using warm water. This is a normal response to vestibular stimulation (Figs. C & D).

Clinical Significance: This test is an accurate measure of vestibular sensitivity. In patients with end-organ pathology or an acoustic neuroma, paresis may set in and results in abnormal findings (Figs. E & F).

Follow-up: Perform Barany's caloric test, cerebellar testing, the dizziness test, or Mittelmeyer's test.

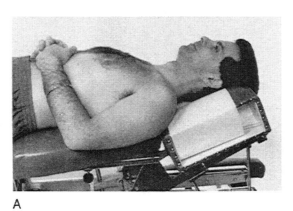

A

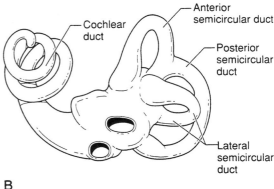

B

Cochlear duct

Anterior semicircular duct

Posterior semicircular duct

Lateral semicircular duct

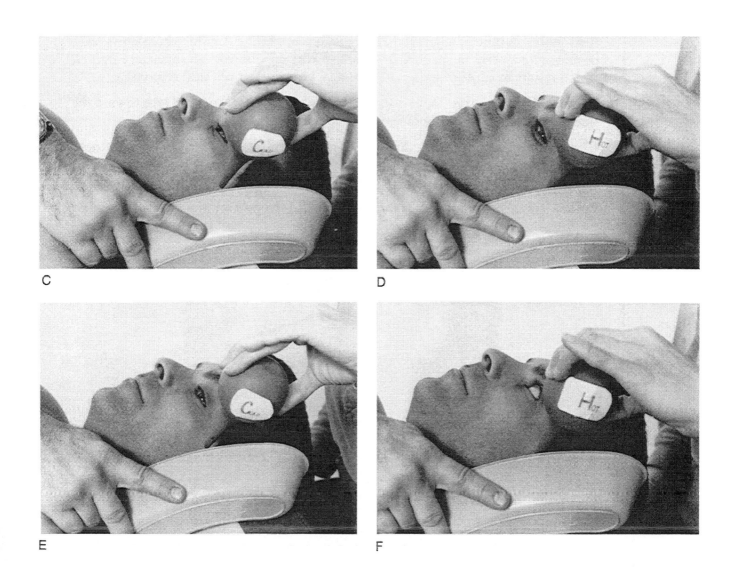

C

D

E

F

6 | *Mittelmeyer's Test*

Procedure: Instruct the patient to march in place first with eyes open and then with eyes closed (Figs. A–C).

Rationale: A functional vestibular apparatus is needed bilaterally to keep one's body positioned properly in space. If a problem exists on one side, an imbalance occurs, which results in a loss of sensorial input and, ultimately, a physical response.

Classical Significance: Patients with a vestibular deficit will usually turn toward the side of the lesion while marching (Fig. D).

Clinical Significance: With the eyes closed the problem is exacerbated and thus more pronounced. If the patient turns while marching with open eyes as well as with closed eyes, expect a cerebellar dysfunction, as this is an ataxic response (Figs. E & F).

Follow-up: Perform the Hallpike caloric test or the temperature test, or both.

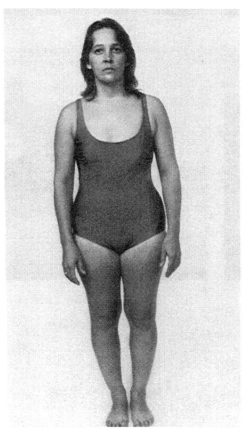

A

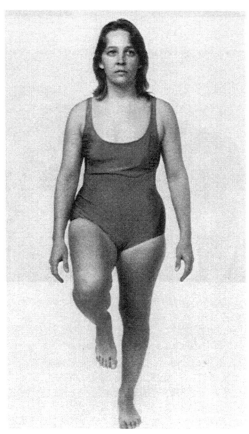

B

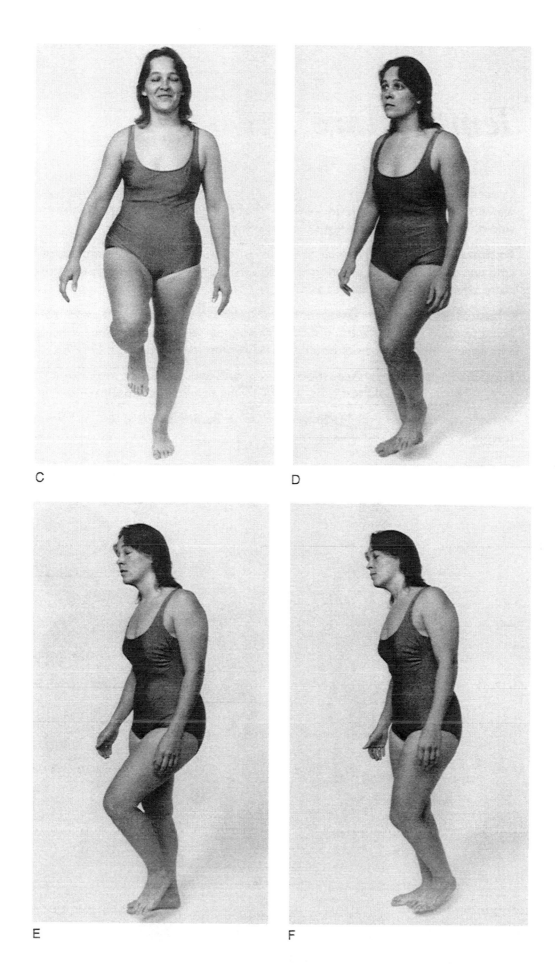

C

D

E

F

7 | *Temperature Test*

Procedure: The patient is seated. Alternately apply test tubes filled with hot and cold water, respectively, on each side of the head at the mastoid area. Perform the test on one side of the head at a time (Figs. A–C).

Rationale: This test is similar to Barany's caloric test. The alternate use of hot and cold test tubes creates an autonomic response of vertigo because the changes of temperature affect the semicircular canals.

Classical Significance: Using the cold test tube, nystagmus will be away from the ear being tested. Using the warm test tube, nystagmus will be toward the ear being tested. The nystagmus will be horizontal in the direction indicated (Figs. D & E).

Clinical Significance: Acoustic neuromas will cause a lack of response when using either the warm or cold test tube. The neuroma results in a canal paresis (Fig. F).

Follow-up: Perform the Hallpike caloric test, Barany's caloric test, or Mittelmeyer's test.

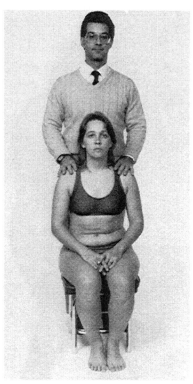

A

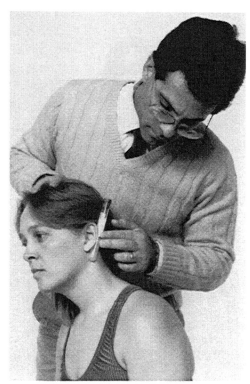

B

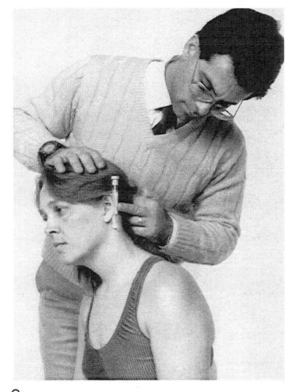

C

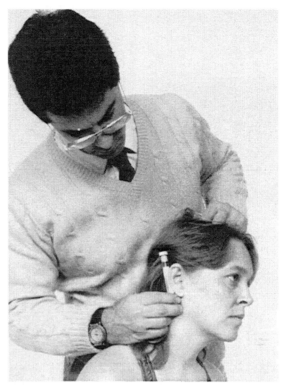

D

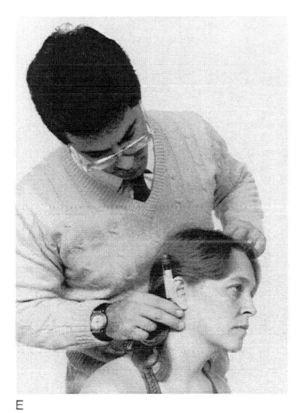

E

F

Cervical Testing

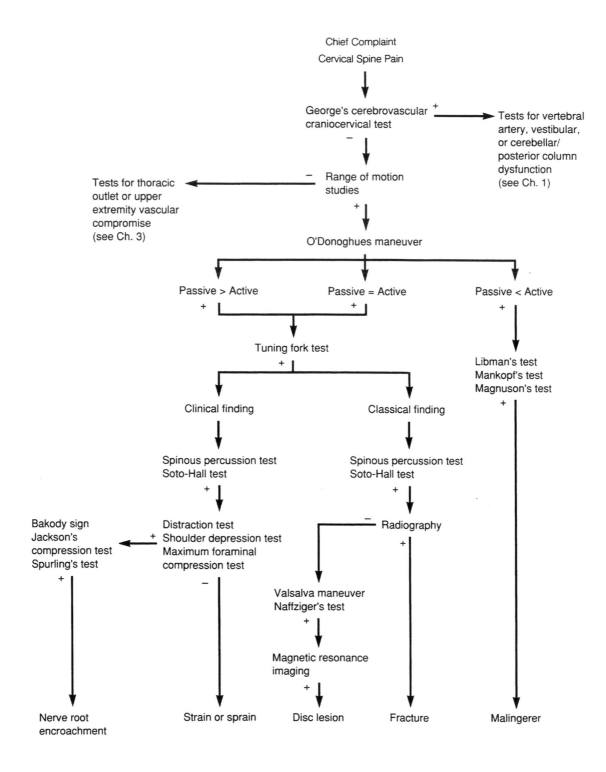

Chief Complaint
Cervical Spine Pain

George's cerebrovascular craniocervical test
+ → Tests for vertebral artery, vestibular, or cerebellar/ posterior column dysfunction (see Ch. 1)

−

Range of motion studies

− → Tests for thoracic outlet or upper extremity vascular compromise (see Ch. 3)

+

O'Donoghues maneuver

Passive > Active   Passive = Active   Passive < Active
+   +   +

Tuning fork test
+

Clinical finding   Classical finding

Spinous percussion test   Spinous percussion test
Soto-Hall test   Soto-Hall test
+   +

Bakody sign
Jackson's compression test
Spurling's test   + ← Distraction test
                       Shoulder depression test
                       Maximum foraminal compression test
+   −

Libman's test
Mankopf's test
Magnuson's test
+

− Radiography
+

Valsalva maneuver
Naffziger's test
+

Magnetic resonance imaging
+

Nerve root encroachment   Strain or sprain   Disc lesion   Fracture   Malingerer

1 | *Range of Motion Studies*

When performing range of motion studies, it is important to use either an arthrodial protractor or an inclinometer. The *American Medical Association Guides for Impairment Ratings* now recommend the use of the inclinometer exclusively.

Flexion: Have the patient try to touch the chin to the chest. Normal flexion is 30 to 45 degrees. As a quick check ask the patient to place the index and middle fingers on the chest and to bring the chin to the fingers. If the patient can touch the fingers with the chin then flexion is normal.

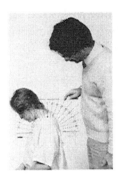 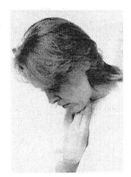

Extension: Instruct the patient to bring the head back as far as possible. Normal extension is 30 to 45 degrees. As a quick check ask the patient to bring the head back as far as possible. Look at the tip of the nose and the level of the frontal bones. If they are parallel with the plane of the floor, then extension is normal.

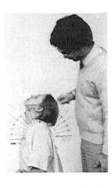 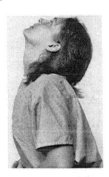

Rotation: Have the patient turn the head from side to side; note the degrees of rotation bilaterally. Normal rotation is 60 to 80 degrees.

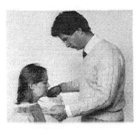 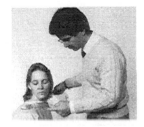

Lateral Flexion: Instruct the patient to try and touch the ear to the shoulder, bilaterally. Normal lateral flexion is 30 to 45 degrees.

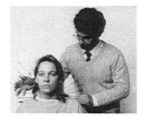 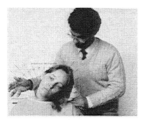

Classical Significance: The patient's ranges of motion should be within the normal ranges and the values should be equal bilaterally.

Clinical Significance: Acute or chronic injury may restrict ranges of motion bilaterally. If the ranges of motion are still within normal limits this is not normal. It is imperative to have good baseline ranges of motion on all patients.

Note: Active ranges of motion are largely a function of volition. An area that is strained is reactively guarded and any attempt to move will be restricted and discomforting. If the patient allows passive ranges of motion, they will be achieved to a greater degree and with less pain than with the active ranges of motion.

Procedures

2 | *Bakody Sign (Shoulder Abduction Test)*

Procedure: The patient is seated. Raise the patient's arm on the side of the complaint to a level above the head. Alternatively, have the patient actively elevate the arm above the head (Figs. A–C).

Rationale: If the pain is relieved when the patient's arm is raised, the Bakody sign is positive. This is because the nerve root irritation is caused by cervical tractioning of the roots when the arm hangs freely at the patient's side.

Classical Significance: Relief of pain when the arm is elevated above the level of the head is a positive result (Figs. D & E).

Clinical Significance: Exacerbation of pain when performing this test indicates thoracic outlet syndrome or compression of a nerve root at the intervertebral foramen as the weight of the hand on the head creates axial loading of the disc (Fig. F).

Follow-up: Perform the foraminal compression test, the costoclavicular test, or the elevated arm stress test (EAST) (see Ch. 3 for the latter two).

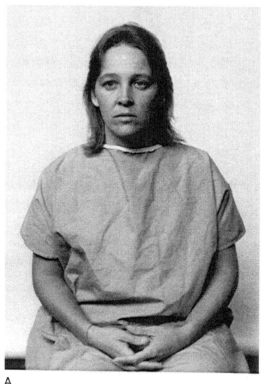

A

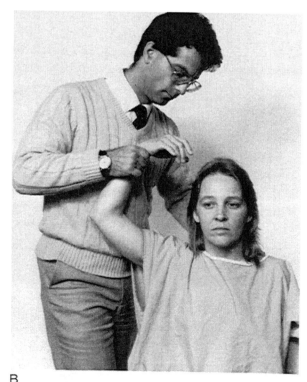

B

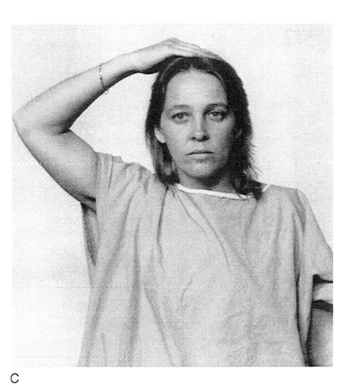

C

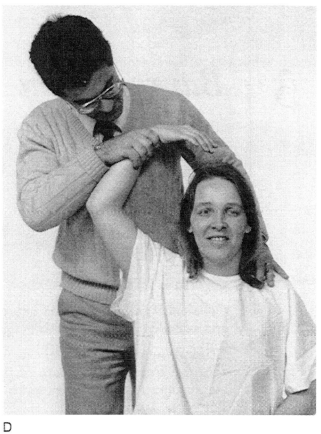

D

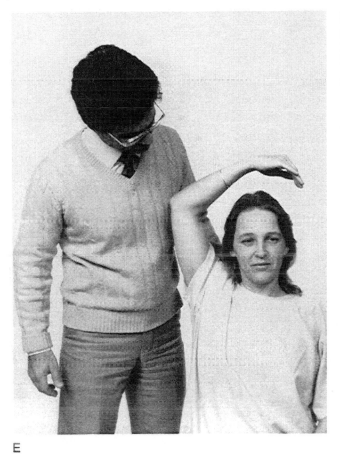

E

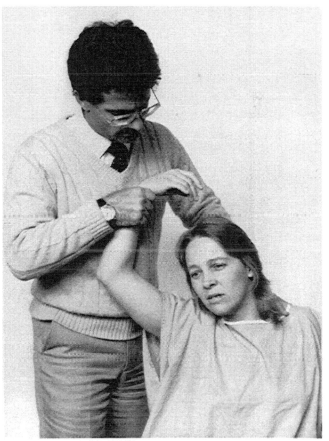

F

3 | *Barre-Leiou Sign*

Procedure: The patient is seated and turns the head actively in both directions slowly. To determine whether the symptoms are being produced by vertebral artery compression or from stimulation of the sympathetics, further instruct the patient to flex and extend the head (Figs. A–D).

Rationale: Vasoconstriction of the arteries supplying the basilar pons area of the brain occurs with rotation as well as flexion and extension. The vertebral arteries are only compromised when the head is rotated 30 to 45 degrees and are not affected when the head is flexed and extended.

Classical Significance: Reproduction of an ischemic reaction with the head flexed and extended is a positive result (Figs. E & F).

Clinical Significance: Adequate function of the vessels must be established so that excessive force is not introduced to a compromised area by high velocity rotation adjustments (Keck maneuver, forced posterior to anterior thrusts), which create extension of the neck.

Follow-up: Perform George's vertebral artery test (see Ch. 1).

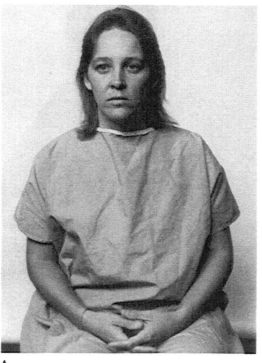

A

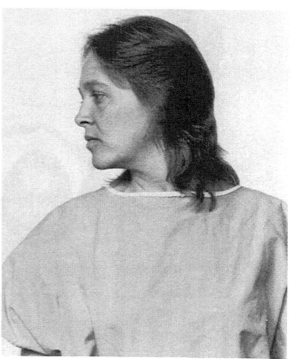

B

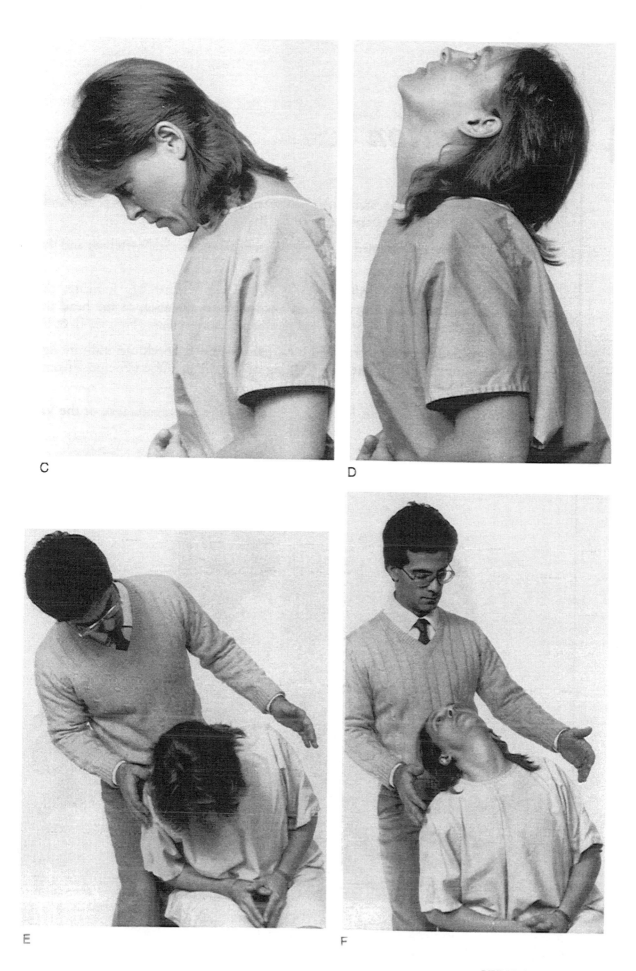

C

D

E

F

4 | *Distraction Test*

Procedure: The patient is seated with the head neutral. Cup your hands gently under the jaw and the base of the occiput and gently lift up (Figs. A & B).

Rationale: This test is designed to reduce pressure on the cervical vertebrae and thus on the affected disc.

Classical Significance: A reduction in radicular symptomatology indicates that pressure was on the disc or nerve roots, or both. Passive rotation of the head that increases with distraction indicates relief from nerve root pressure (Figs. C, E, & F).

Clinical Significance: An increase in local pain within the neck can indicate ligamentous or muscular injury due to stretching or tearing of these structures from a traumatic incident (Fig. D).

Follow-up: Perform the Soto-Hall test, the foraminal compression test, or the Valsalva maneuver.

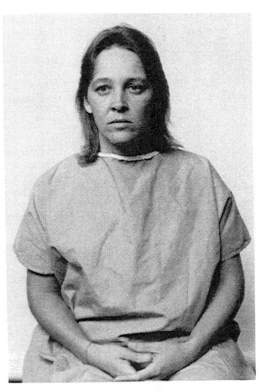

A

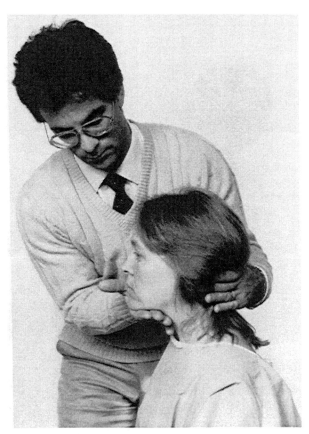

B

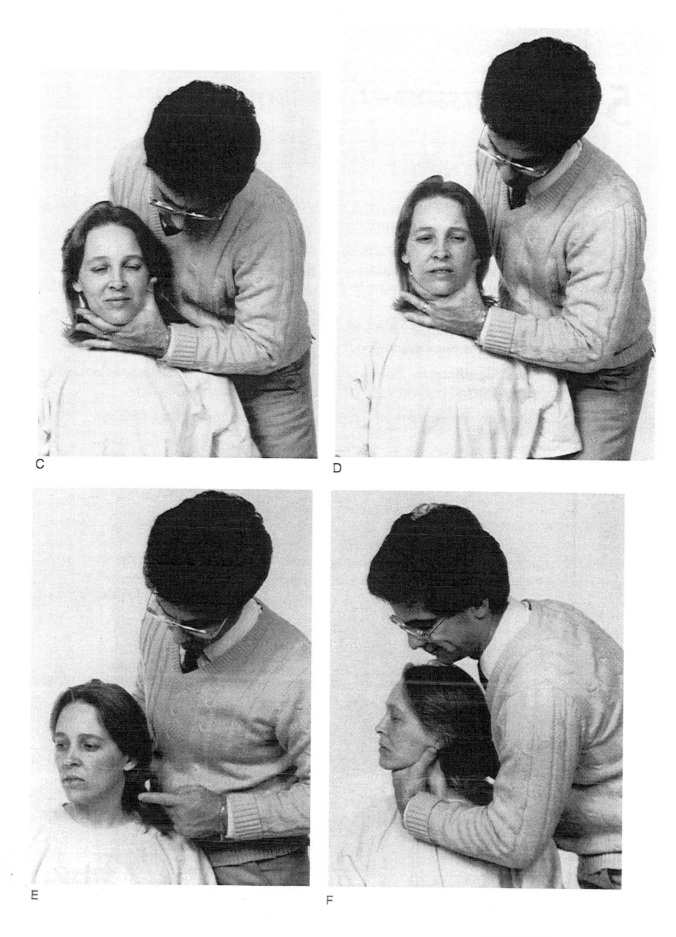

5 | *Extension – Compression Test*

Procedure: The patient is seated. Ask the patient to extend the head about 30 degrees. Then, gently press down on the head (Figs. A–C).

Rationale: This procedure is good for testing discal integrity. If a posterolateral bulge is present with the annulus intact, pushing the disc more anterior can actually decrease the symptomatology. Irritation of the posterior apophyseal joints can result from this test as well.

Classical Significance: Reduction of radicular symptomatology may indicate the presence of a cervical disc lesion (Fig. D).

Clinical Significance: An increase in peripheral ill-defined pain may indicate scleratogenous referral from irritated posterior apophyseal joints (Fig. E).

Follow-up: Perform the flexion–compression test or the distraction test.

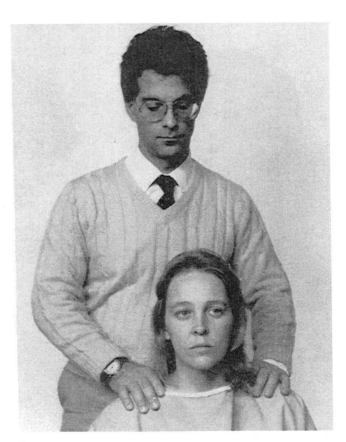

A

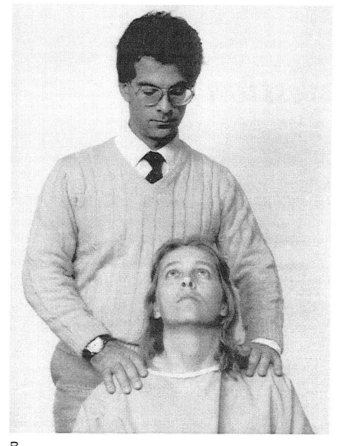

B

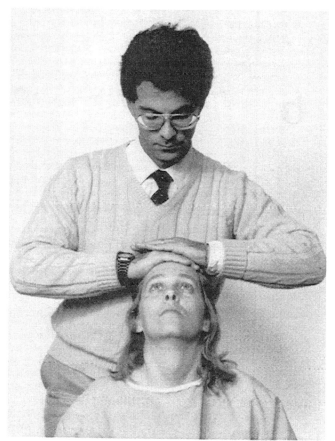

C

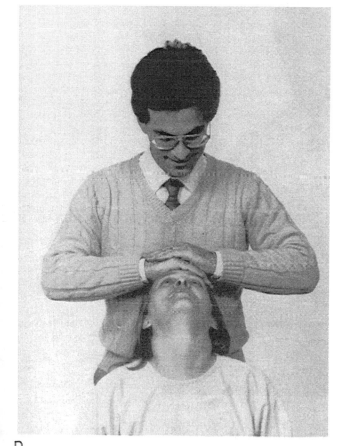

D

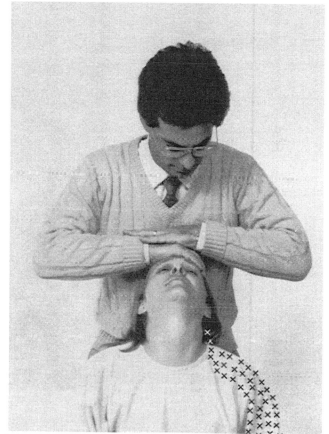

E

6 | *Flexion–Compression Test*

Procedure: The patient is seated. Ask the patient to flex the head. Then, gently press downward on the top of the head (Figs. A–C).

Rationale: This is a good test for discal integrity. If a posterolateral disc bulge is present, forcing the head into flexion will cause the disc to bulge more posteriorly. Compression of the head will augment the above.

Classical Significance: An increase in radicular symptomatology can indicate the presence of a posterolateral disc lesion (Fig. D).

Clinical Significance: Flexion of the head removes the strain on the posterior joints and may lessen scleratogenous pain. Increased pain may indicate injury to the posterior holding elements (Fig. E).

Follow-up: Perform the distraction test or the Soto-Hall test, or both.

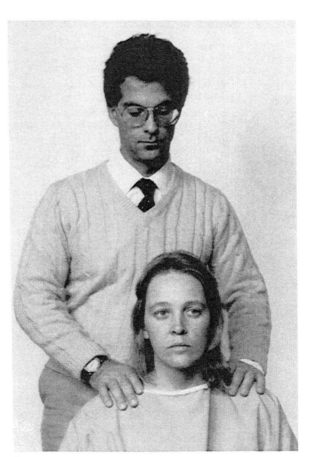

A

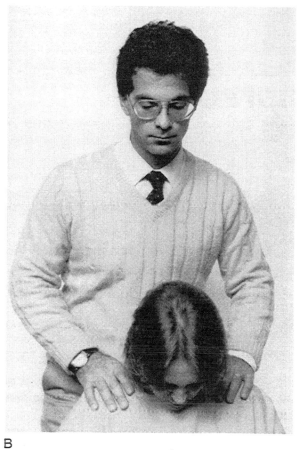

B

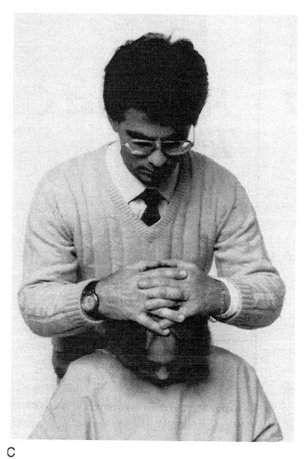

C

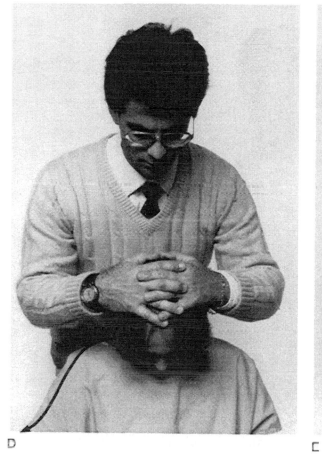

D

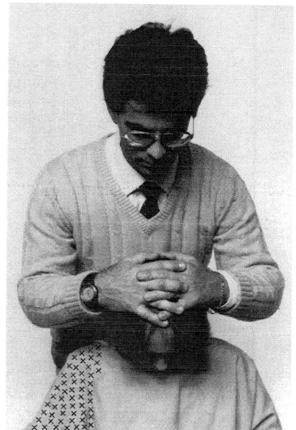

E

7 | Foraminal Compression Test

Procedure: The patient is seated. Place both hands on top of the patient's head and then press downward (Figs. A & B).

Rationale: This test places extra stress on the discs and also puts pressure on the apophyseal joints. The intervertebral foramina are also compromised.

Classical Significance: Radicular symptomatology along a specific dermatome indicates nerve root compression (Fig. C).

Clinical Significance: Ill-defined peripheral symptomatology can indicate scleratogenous referral from the apophyseal joint. Local pain in the cervical spine is not truly significant (Figs. D & E).

Follow-up: Perform Jackson's compression test, the Valsalva maneuver, or the distraction test.

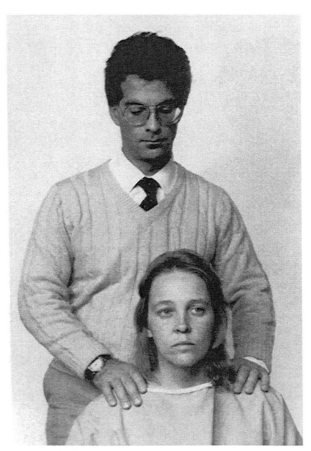

A

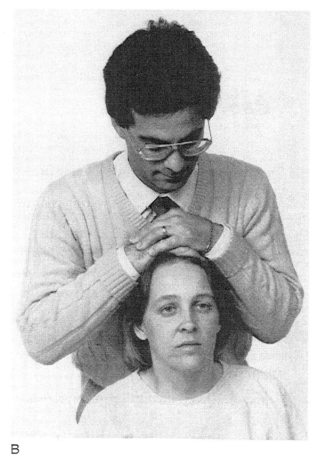

B

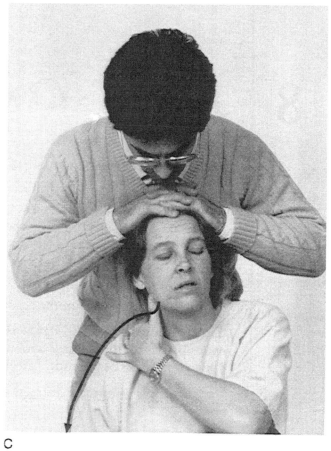

C

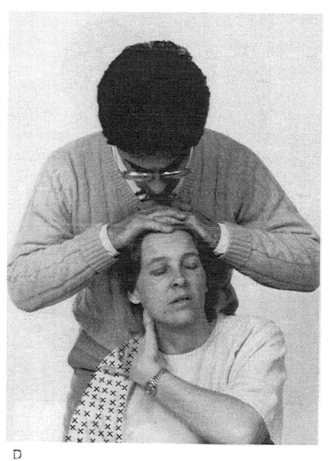

D

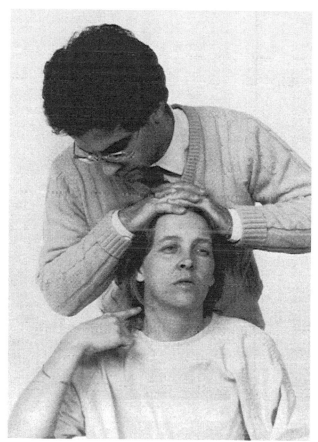

E

8 | *Jackson's Compression Test*

Procedure: The patient is seated. Laterally flex the patient's head to one side and press downward. Repeat this on the opposite side (Figs. A–D).

Rationale: This specifically tests the intervertebral foramina on the side of lateral flexion and thus helps to isolate the complaint. This test is usually performed after a regular compression test. Some apophysitis on the side being tested can be present, as well.

Classical Significance: Radicular symptomatology along a specific dermatome will help to localize the area of the lesion (Fig. E).

Clinical Significance: Ill-defined peripheral symptomatology can indicate scleratogenous pain from the irritated apophyseal joint. Local pain in the cervical spine can be due to stretching of the contralateral cervical muscles (Fig. F).

Follow-up: Perform the distraction test or the extension– and flexion–compression tests.

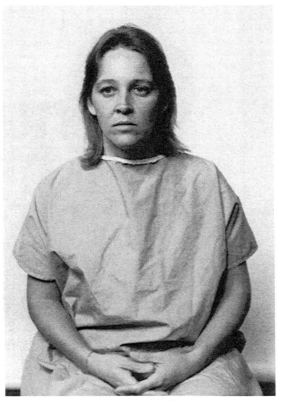

A

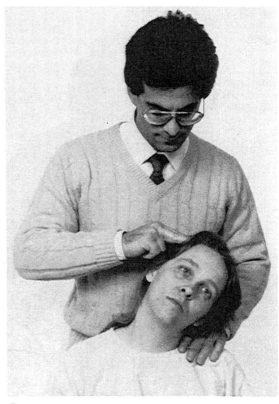

B

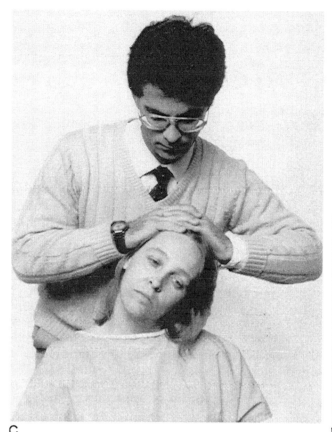

C

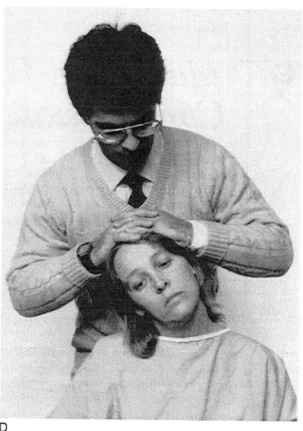

D

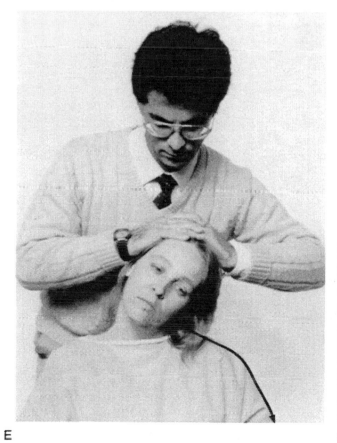

E

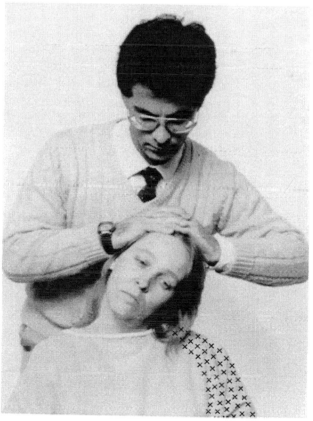

F

9 | *Maximum Foraminal Compression Test*

Procedure: The patient is seated and laterally flexes the head to the shoulder and then brings the chin toward the same shoulder (Figs. A & B). Alternatively, the patient turns the head toward the shoulder and then extends the head (Figs. C & D).

Rationale: The above procedures compress the intervertebral foramina and thus may increase impingement of a nerve root.

Classical Significance: Radicular dermatologic symptomatology is a positive result (Fig. E).

Clinical Significance: Ill-defined scleratogenous pain may indicate a facet involvement on the same side being tested. If pain is felt locally on the opposite side of the neck, consider muscular strain (Fig. F).

Follow-up: Perform the foraminal compression test, Jackson's compression test, the distraction test, or Spurling's test.

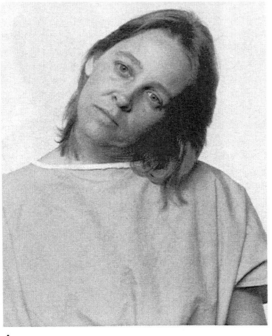

A

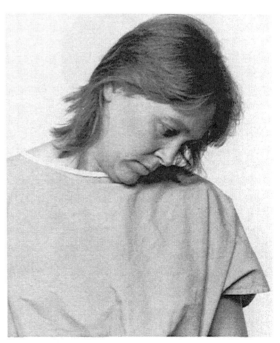

B

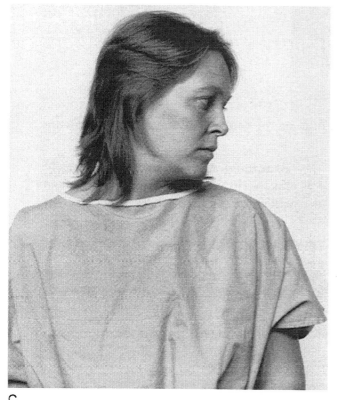

C

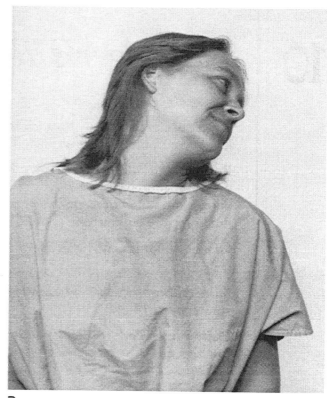

D

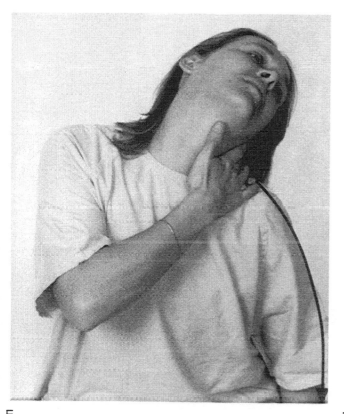

E

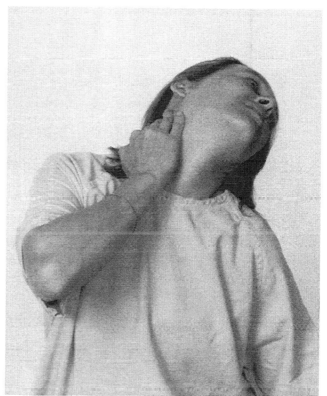

F

10 | *Naffziger's Test*

Procedure: The patient is seated. Stand behind the patient and digitally compress the jugular veins for 30 to 45 seconds (Figs. A–C).

Rationale: This test exacerbates discal lesions throughout the spine. It is generally used in the lumbar spine, but can be just as effective in the cervical and dorsal spine. Spinal cord tumors, especially meningiomas, will increase pain patterns because spinal fluid pressure will increase above the tumor.

Classical Significance: An increase in a dermatologic pain pattern is a positive result (Fig. D).

Clinical Significance: Local nonradicular pain may indicate the site of a strain or sprain injury (Fig. E).

Follow-up: Perform the Valsalva maneuver, distraction test, foraminal compression test, or Jackson's compression test.

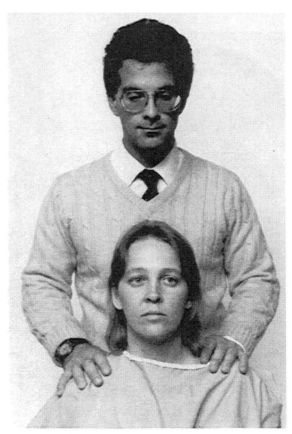

A

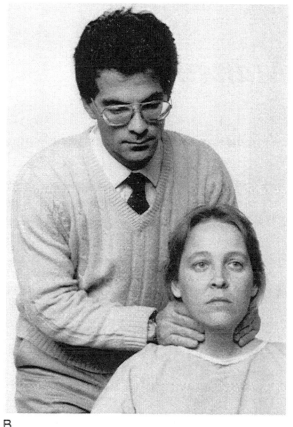

B

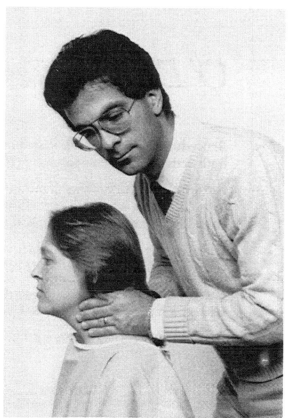

C

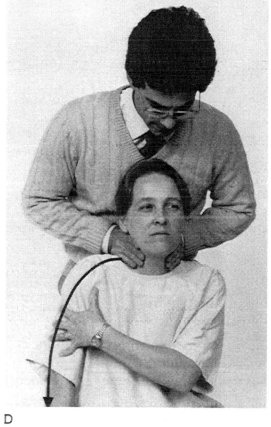

D

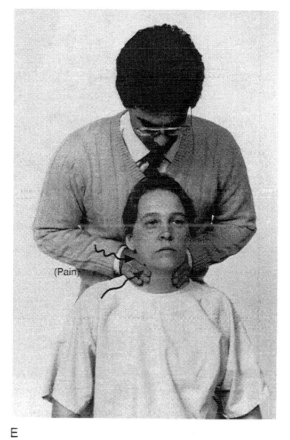

(Pain)

E

11 | *O'Donoghues Maneuver*

Procedure: The patient is seated. Put the cervical spine through its ranges of motion both actively as well as passively (Fig. A).

Rationale: Active ranges of motion will always be less than or equal to passive ranges of motion. This is because, to perform actively, the affected muscles must be used. When passively performed the muscles should not be aggravated.

Classical Significance: If the active ranges of motion are less than the passive ranges, active muscle involvement is the cause of the patient's pain (Figs. B & C).

Clinical Significance: If the active ranges of motion are greater than the passive, suspect a malingerer (Figs. D & E).

Follow-up: Perform Magnuson's test or Mankopf's test (see Ch. 14).

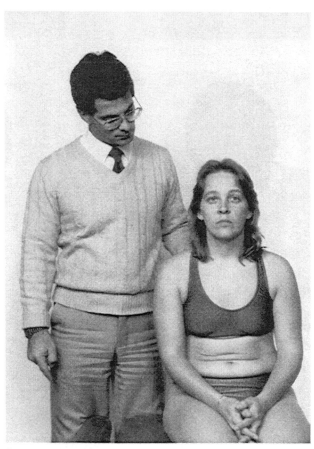

A

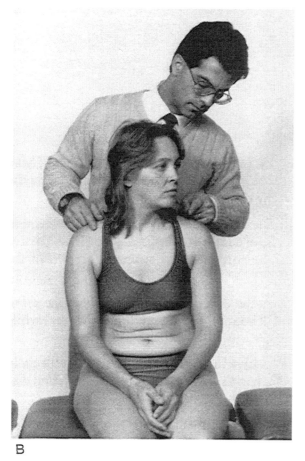

B

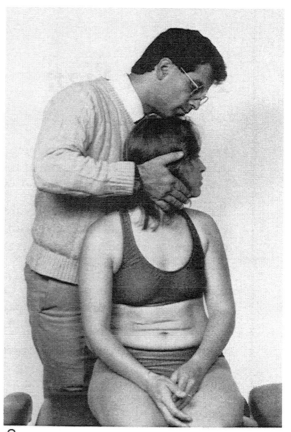

C

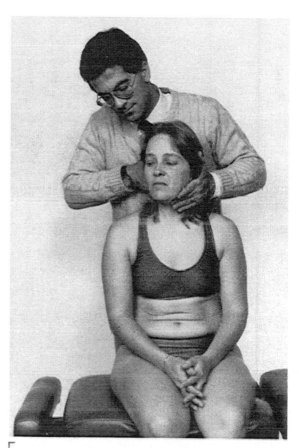

D

E

12 | *Rust's Sign*

Procedure: The patient is supine. Ask the patient to lift the head onto the chest. Alternatively, observe the patient for postural attitude of the head and neck while the patient is seated, lying down, and then rising (Figs. A–D).

Rationale: In acute intervertebral syndrome, the patient will guard every movement of the cervical spine. In strain/sprain, because of damage to the tissue, the active/passive movements will be aggravated because of the normal tensile strength/support of the muscles, tendons, and ligaments.

Classical Significance: Inability to support the weight of the head without the aid of the hands is a positive result. The patient will hold the neck ("cradling" the area) while changing postural positions (Figs. E & F).

Clinical Significance: This test will be positive in severe strain or sprain, especially strain or sprain of the anterior compartment. It is also observed in the intervertebral disc syndrome.

Follow-up: Perform the foraminal compression test or O'Donoghues maneuver, or both.

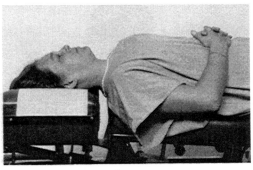

A

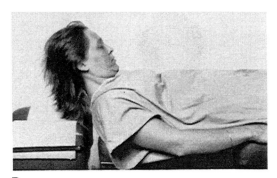

B

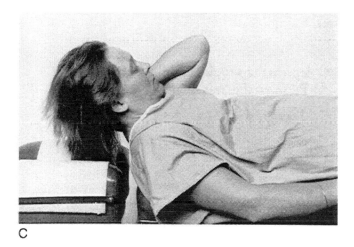

C

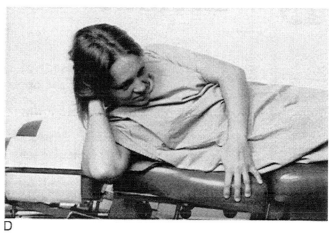

D

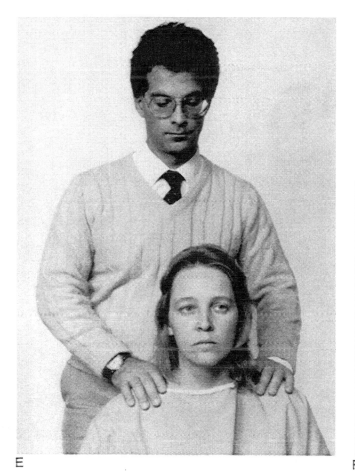

E

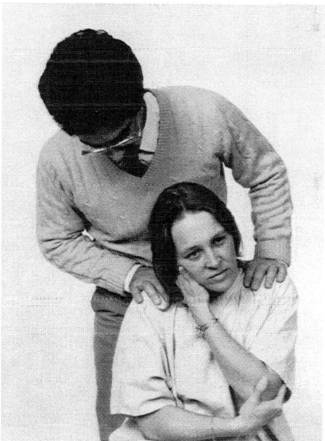

F

13 | *Shoulder Depression Test*

Procedure: The patient is seated. Forcibly depress the shoulder while laterally flexing the patient's head toward the opposite side. Perform this test bilaterally (Figs. A–C).

Rationale: Adhesions of the dural sleeve and nerve root are exaggerated with this test.

Classical Significance: If positive, radicular symptomatology is either produced or already existing and radicular pain is increased (Fig. D).

Clinical Significance: Local muscular pain on the side being stretched may indicate hypertonicity of the sternocleidomastoid or trapezius muscle on that side (Fig. E). A decrease in muscular pain on the side not being tested indicates muscular strain from shortening muscle fibers.

Follow-up: Perform the distraction test or Jackson's compression test.

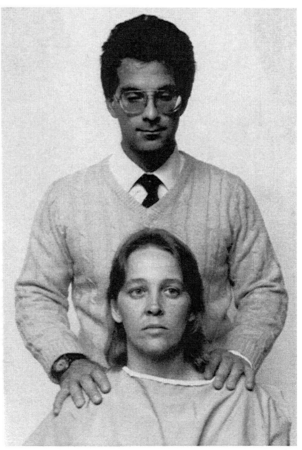

A

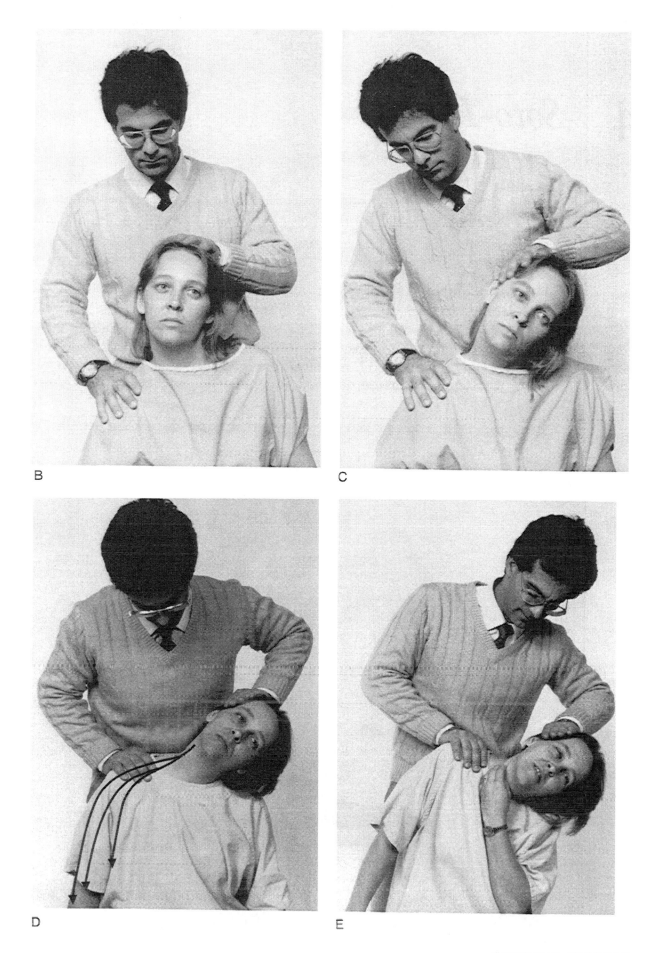

B

C

D

E

14 | *Soto-Hall Test*

Procedure: The patient is supine. Place one hand on the patient's sternum to affix it to the table. Cup your other hand around the patient's head along the occiput and gently flex the chin onto the chest (Figs. A & B).

Rationale: This test places traction along the posterior supraspinous ligaments. When the level of vertebral injury is reached, noticeable local pain occurs.

Classical Significance: If positive, local pain occurs within the cervical and dorsal spinal area but not lower then the T7 level (Fig. C).

Clinical Significance: While not considered truly positive, an increase in pain at the cervicodorsal junction can be due to spasticity of the trapezius muscles. If pain is reported beyond the level of T7, re-evaluate the procedure because the manubrium, which is the fulcrum for this test, does not allow the traction force beyond the T7 level (Figs. D & E).

Follow-up: Perform the spinous percussion test or the tuning fork test (see Ch. 7).

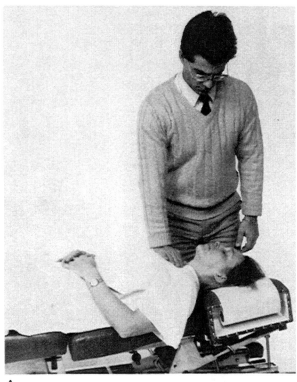

A

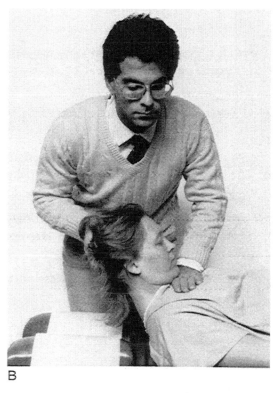

B

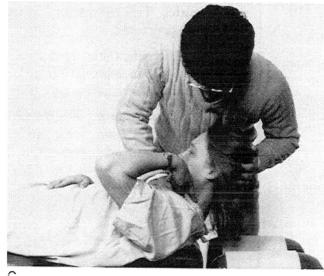

C

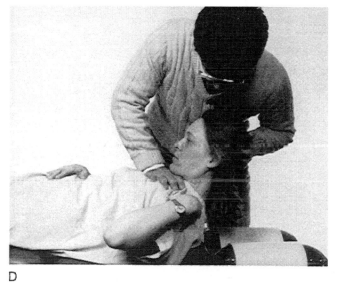

D

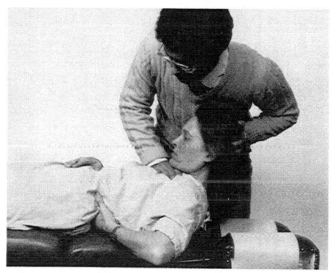

E

15 | *Spinous Percussion Test*

Procedure: The patient is seated with the neck slightly flexed. Using any examining hammer, strike the spinous processes of all exposed vertebrae. Repeat by striking the paraspinal area (Figs. A–C).

Rationale: This test causes irritation to the spinous process and surrounding ligamentous structures.

Classical Significance: Localized pain may indicate a fractured vertebral segment. If radicular pain increases, a disc lesion may be present. Ligamentous sprain will also cause a local nonradiating pain (Fig. D).

Clinical Significance: When striking the paraspinal area, an increase in pain may be due to muscular strain. Some patients may have a low pain tolerance; take care not to cause pain by the percussion alone (Fig. E).

Follow-up: Perform the tuning fork test (see Ch. 7), foraminal compression test, distraction test, or Soto-Hall test.

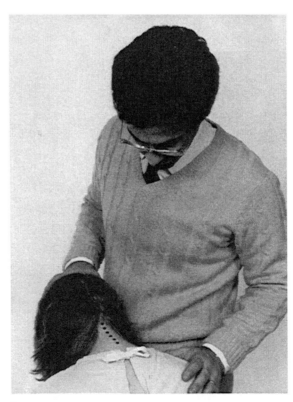

A

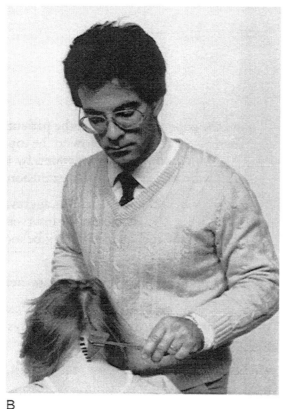

B

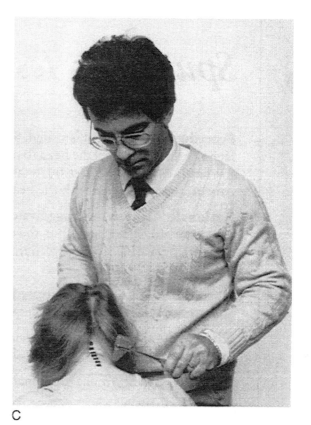

C

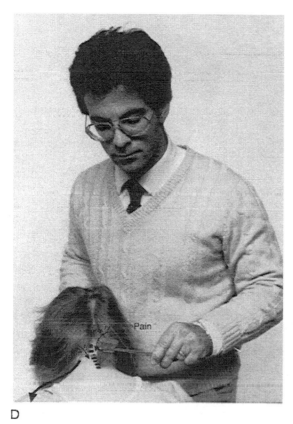

D

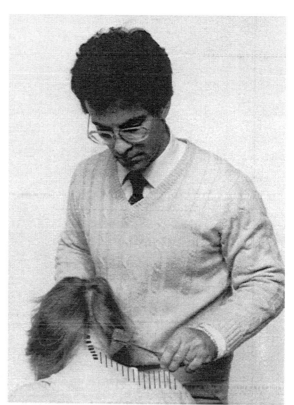

E

16 | *Spurling's Test*

Procedure: The patient is seated. Stand behind the patient and instruct the patient to laterally flex and rotate the head to one side. Then give a downward blow to the top of the head. Perform this test bilaterally (Figs. A–D). When it can be tolerated by the patient, repeat this test with the head in lateral flexion and rotation plus extension.

Rationale: This test will aggravate an irritated apophyseal joint as well as aggravate any nerve root irritation. When the extension is added to the above test the intervertebral foramina are 20 to 30 percent more occluded and the radicular pain may be more acute.

Classical Significance: Increased radicular symptomatology may indicate nerve compression due to cervical spondylosis or disc disease (Fig. E).

Clinical Significance: Scleratogenous pain may indicate irritation to the apophyseal joint on the side being tested (Fig. F).

Follow-up: Perform the foraminal compression test or Jackson's compression test, or both.

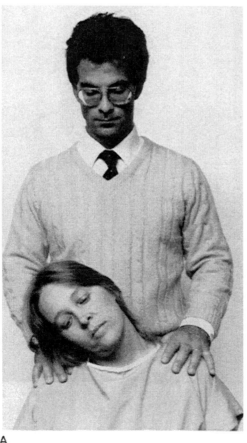

A

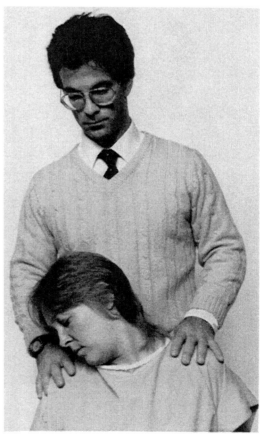

B

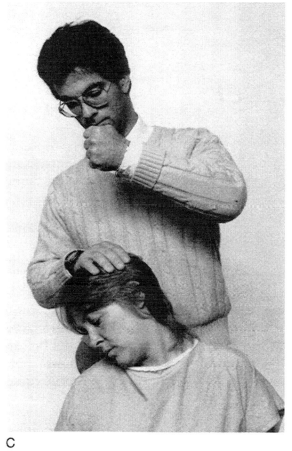

C

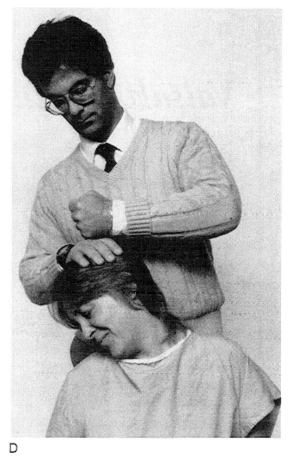

D

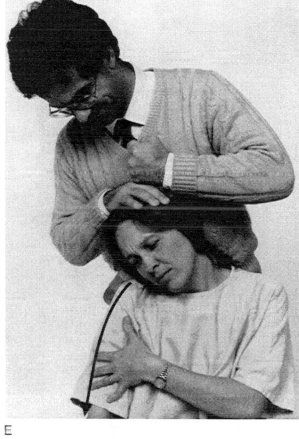

E

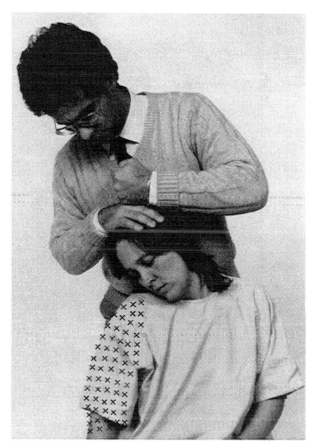

F

17 | *Valsalva Maneuver*

Procedure: The patient is seated. The patient places a thumb within the mouth and then tries to puff the cheeks (increasing the pressure) in an attempt to blow the thumb out of the mouth (Figs. A–C).

Rationale: The increase in pressure will increase the intraspinal pressure if a space-occupying lesion is present.

Classical Significance: An increase in radicular symptomatology along a specific dermatome is a positive result (Fig. D).

Clinical Significance: A space-occupying lesion can indicate disc protrusion, tumor, or foraminal or lateral recess osteophytosis, or both. It is possible to have intervertebral foramen (IVF) encroachment because of soft tissue swelling, even when the IVF are patent as demonstrated on film (Figs. E & F [E: schematic of the oblique cervical spine; F: arrows indicate marked foraminal encroachment]). The resultant edema causes congestion at the nerve root level.

Follow-up: Perform the distraction test and take an oblique cervical radiograph.

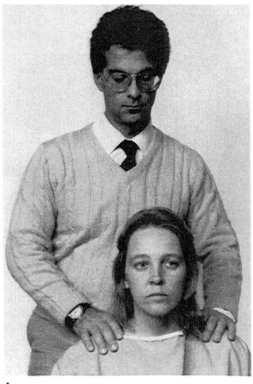

A

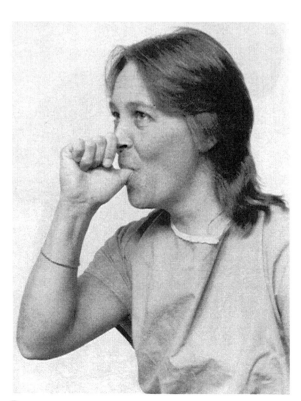

B

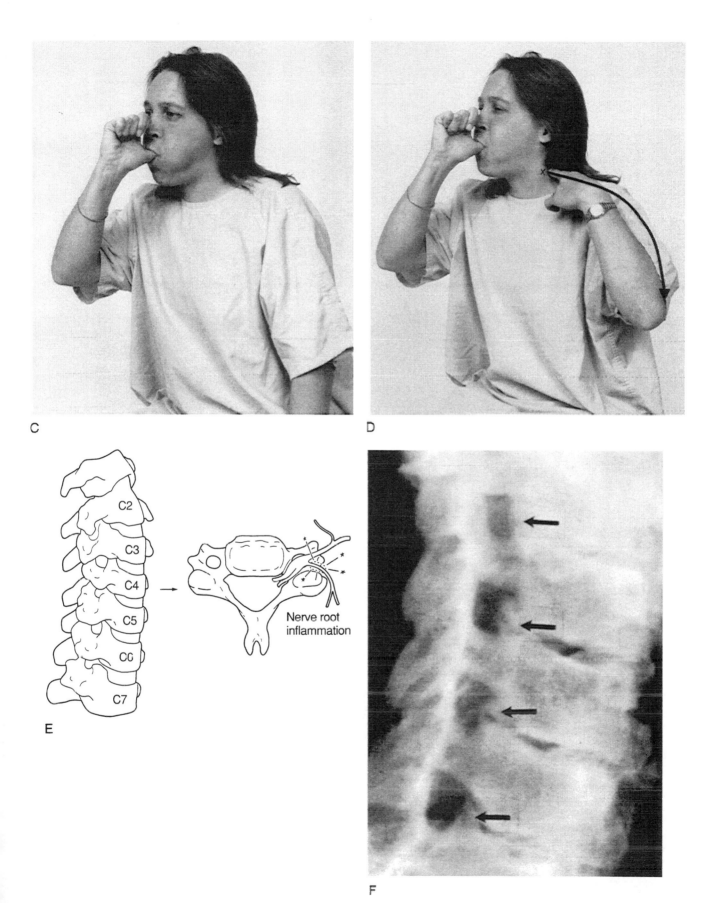

C

D

E

Nerve root
inflammation

C2
C3
C4
C5
C6
C7

F

CHAPTER
3

Thoracic Outlet Syndrome Testing

1. Adson's Test
2. Allen's Maneuver
3. Allen's Test
4. Bikele's Sign
5. Costoclavicular Test
6. Elevated Arm Stress Test
7. Eden's Test
8. Halstead Maneuver
9. Intermittent Claudication Test
10. Pectoralis Stretch Test
11. Traction Test
12. Wright's Test

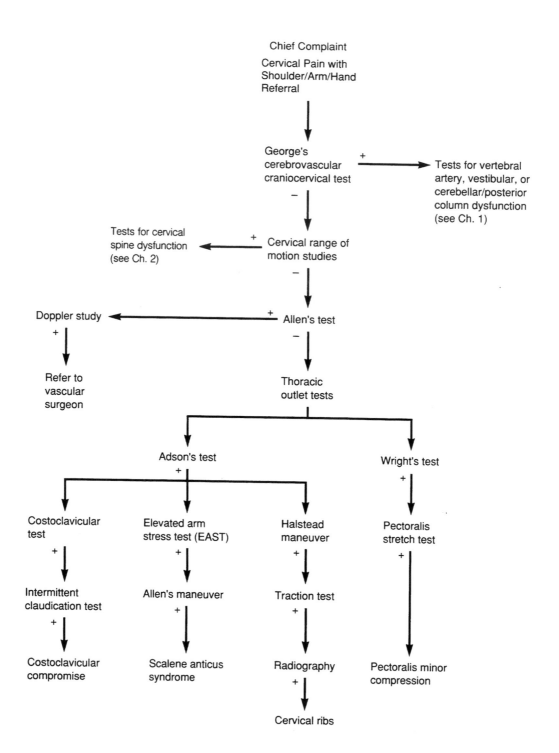

Chief Complaint

Cervical Pain with
Shoulder/Arm/Hand
Referral

George's
cerebrovascular
craniocervical test
→ +
Tests for vertebral
artery, vestibular, or
cerebellar/posterior
column dysfunction
(see Ch. 1)

−

Tests for cervical
spine dysfunction
(see Ch. 2)
← +
Cervical range of
motion studies

−

Doppler study
← +
Allen's test

+

Refer to
vascular
surgeon

−

Thoracic
outlet tests

Adson's test
+

Wright's test
+

Costoclavicular
test
+

Elevated arm
stress test (EAST)
+

Halstead
maneuver
+

Pectoralis
stretch test
+

Intermittent
claudication test
+

Allen's maneuver
+

Traction test
+

Pectoralis minor
compression

Costoclavicular
compromise

Scalene anticus
syndrome

Radiography
+

Cervical ribs

Procedures

1 | *Adson's Test*

Procedure: The patient is seated. Palpate the patient's radial pulse, noting amplitude and frequency. Abduct the arm about 45 degrees while extending it. Have the patient turn the head toward the side being tested, take a deep breath, and hold it for at least 10 seconds while extending the head back. Repeat bilaterally (Figs. A–F). The modified Adson's test is the above procedure with the patient's head turned away from the side being tested.

Rationale: Compression of the neurovascular bundle may be caused by the scalene muscles or by the presence of a cervical rib.

Classical Significance: A dampening of the amplitude or an increase in paresthesia indicates compression of either the neural or vascular component of the neurovascular bundle. A radiograph will rule out a cervical rib.

Clinical Significance: Pressing too hard on the artery can cause neural compression at the wrist and thus a false-positive result.

Follow-up: Perform the costoclavicular test, Wright's test, or Allen's maneuver.

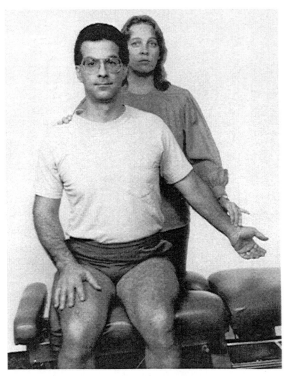

A

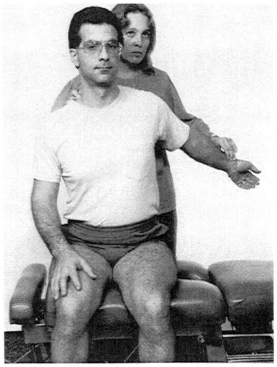

B

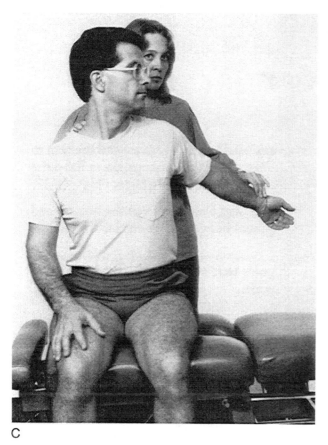

C

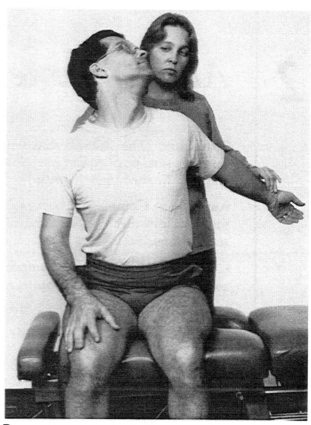

D

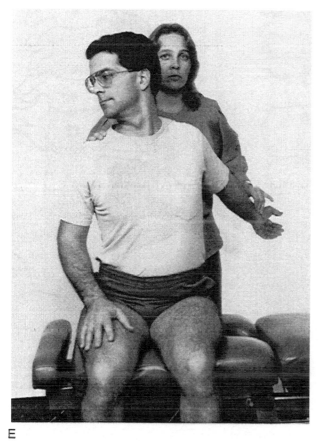

E

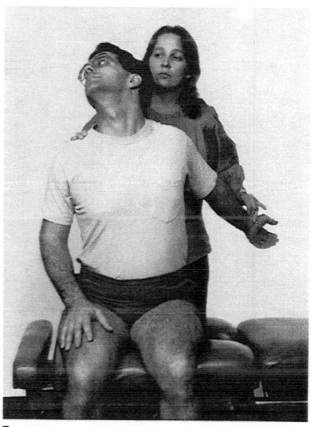

F

2 | *Allen's Maneuver*

Procedure: The patient is seated. Flex the elbow 90 degrees. Then, extend the arm to the horizontal position and externally rotate it. Place digital pressure on the radial pulse and instruct the patient to rotate the head away from the side being tested (Figs. C–F).

Rationale: Compression of the subclavian vessel may occur between the first rib and the clavicle or there may be some scalene entrapment between the anterior and middle scalene muscles (Figs. A & B).

Classical Significance: A dampened radial pulse that occurs as the head is rotated away from the side being tested is a positive result.

Clinical Significance: See Classical Significance.

Follow-up: Perform Adson's test or Allen's test.

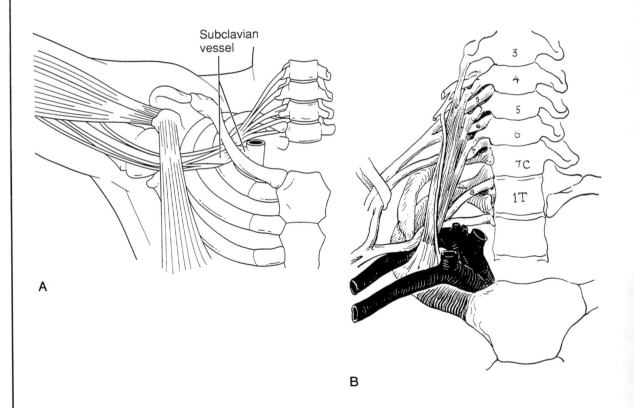

A

B

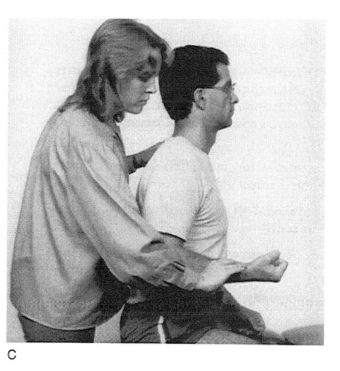

C

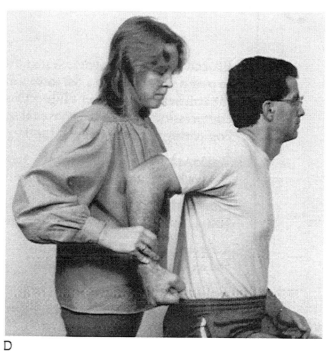

D

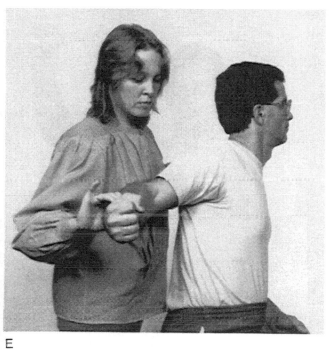

E

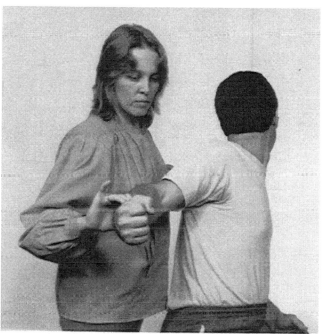

F

3 | *Allen's Test*

Procedure: The patient is seated. Abduct the arm 160 to 180 degrees. Ask the patient to pump the hand into a fist three times and on the third time to sustain the fist. Lower the arm below heart level while occluding the radial and ulnar arteries. Release the ulnar compression. Repeat the above releasing the radial compression. Continue testing by comparing with the opposite arm (Figs. A–F).

Rationale: This is not truly a thoracic outlet syndrome (TOS) test, but it should always be performed first if a TOS condition is suspected.

Classical Significance: Normally the hand should fill with blood within 10 seconds. If not, suspect a thrombus within the vessel tested.

Clinical Significance: Compression may occur anywhere along the distribution of the axillary-brachial-radial-ulnar vessel.

Follow-up: Refer the patient for plethysmography or arteriography.

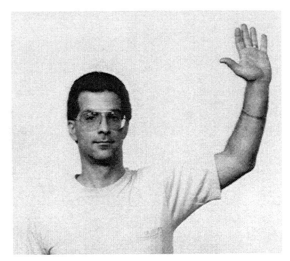

A

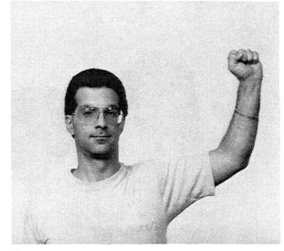

B

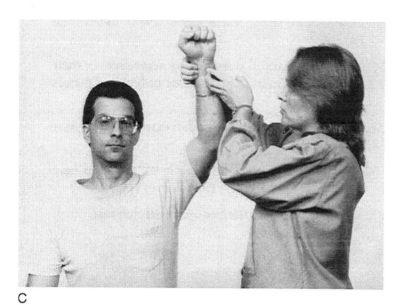

C

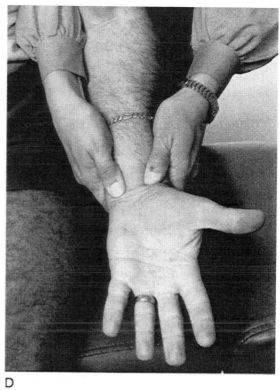

D

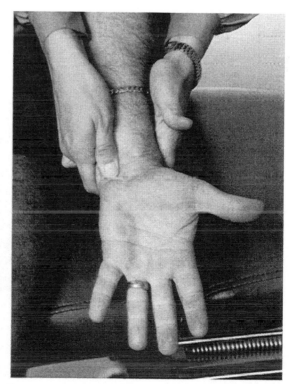

E

F

4 | *Bikele's Sign*

Procedure: The patient is seated. Grasp the patient's arm on the side of the complaint and hold it in abduction at shoulder level with the forearm flexed. Next, extend the forearm (Figs. A–C).

Rationale: Extension of the forearm puts mechanical stress on the nerve roots or their coverings and will exacerbate or re-create the pain in the prescence of brachial plexus neuritis.

Classical Significance: An increase in radicular pain prior to full extension is significant for brachial neuritis (Fig. D).

Clinical Significance: If the patient's arm is above shoulder level, the pain may decrease because of alleviation of tractioning on the dural root sleeves (Fig. E).

Follow-up: Perform Wright's test, Adson's test, or the pectoralis stretch test.

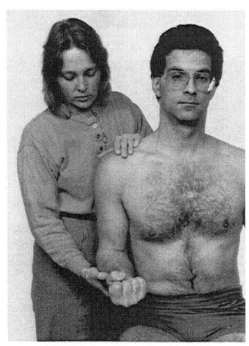

A

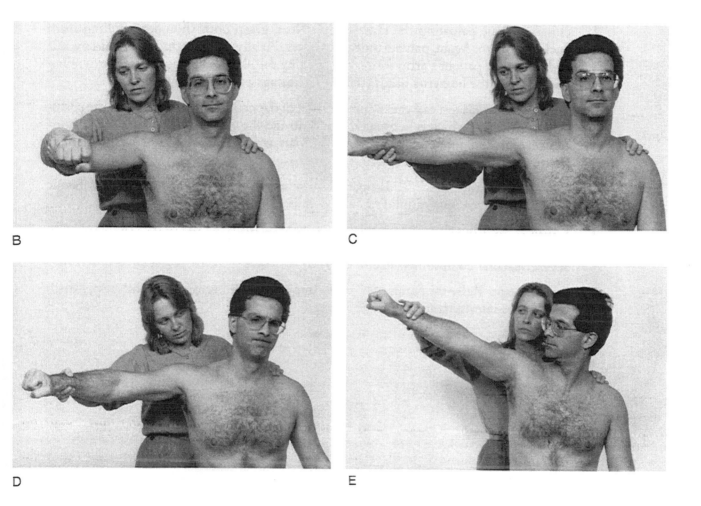

B

C

D

E

5 | *Costoclavicular Test (Hostage Maneuver)*

Procedure: The patient is seated. Palpate the radial pulse, noting amplitude and frequency. Instruct the patient to force the shoulders back and down while flexing the chin; continue palpating the radial pulse. Next, grasp both shoulders, pulling them back and down. Again, palpate the radial pulses. Finally, palpate the radial pulses while abducting the patient's arms 90 degrees, flexing the elbows 90 degrees, and extending and rotating the humerus heads (this is the hostage position) (Figs. A–D).

Rationale: This test can cause compression of the neurovascular bundle at the costo-clavicular space, which is between the first rib and the clavicle. Some medical authorities recommend auscultation of the subclavian and carotid vessels as well, since the above procedure can result in bruits.

Classical Significance: A dampened pulse or an increase in paresthesia, ischemic color changes, or upper limb radicular pain is a positive result.

Clinical Significance: An increase in paresthesia from the site of the compression to the periphery is classical. A marked loss of pallor in the extremity can also be present, if severe vascular compromise occurs (Fig. E).

Follow-up: Refer the patient for plethysmography, or perform Wright's test, Eden's test, or the intermittent claudication test.

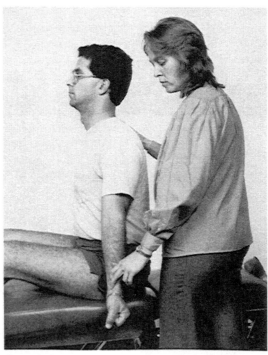

A

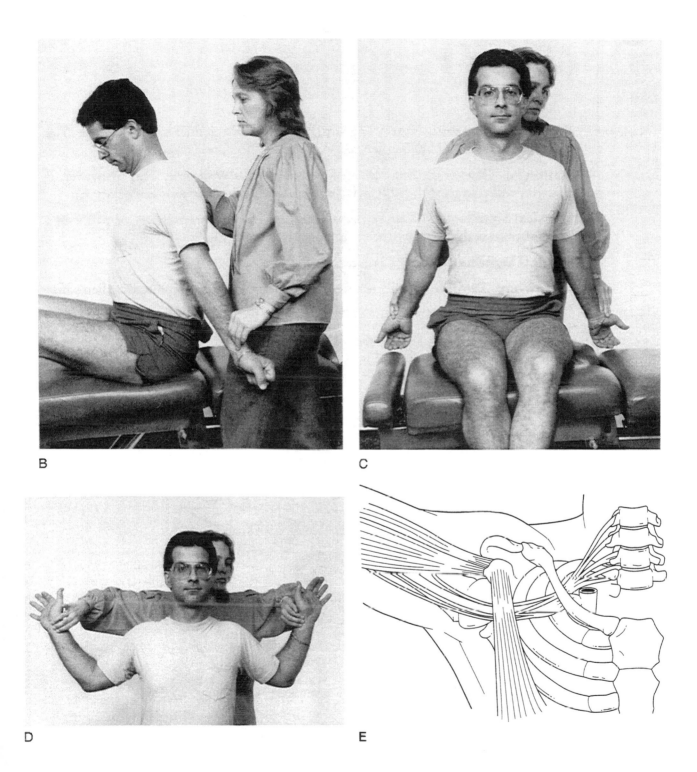

B

C

D

E

6 | *Elevated Arm Stress Test (EAST)*

Procedure: The patient is standing with both arms fully abducted to 90 degrees. The patient then opens and closes the hands for up to 2 minutes (Figs. B–D).

Rationale: This is the best test for scalenus anticus syndrome. This maneuver, if positive, will compress the subclavian or brachial plexus artery, or both (Fig. A).

Classical Significance: Pain or paresthesia distal to the compression, or pallor or a color change in the distal extremity is a positive result (Fig. E).

Clinical Significance: See Classical Significance.

Follow-up: Perform Adson's test, the intermittent claudication test, or Allen's maneuver.

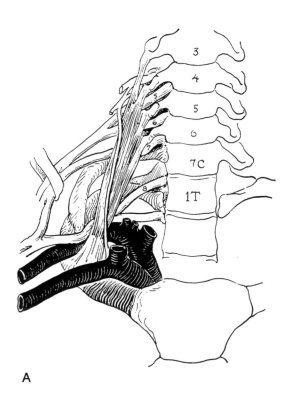

A

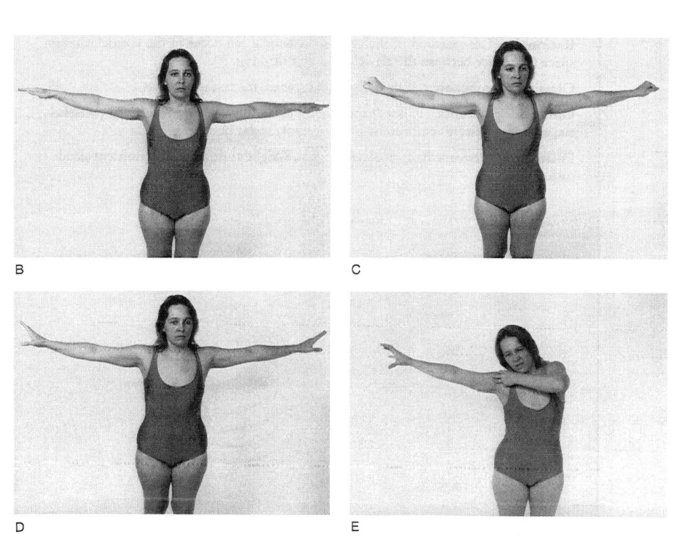

B

C

D

E

7 | *Eden's Test (Soldier's Test)*

Procedure: The patient is standing. Instruct the patient to bring the shoulders back as far as possible while forcing them down. Palpate the radial artery throughout this procedure, noting amplitude and frequency (Figs. B–D).

Rationale: Compression of the neurologic bundle can occur in the costoclavicular space (the space between the clavicle and first rib) (Fig. A).

Classical Significance: If the pulse is dampened, the test is positive.

Clinical Significance: Pallor changes in the extremity or an increase in the paresthesia, or both, indicate compromise of the neurovascular bundle (Fig. E).

Follow-up: Perform the costoclavicular test, Wright's test, or the intermittent claudication test.

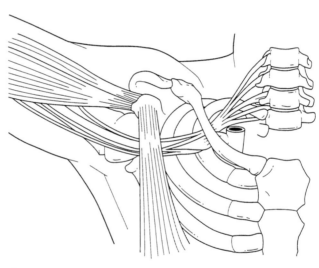

A

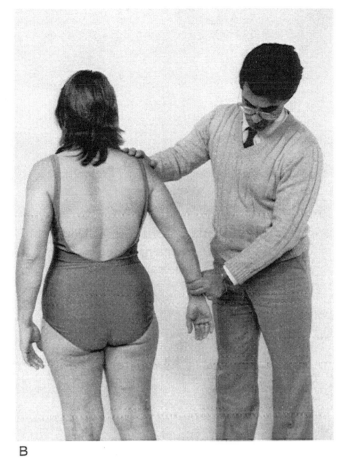

B

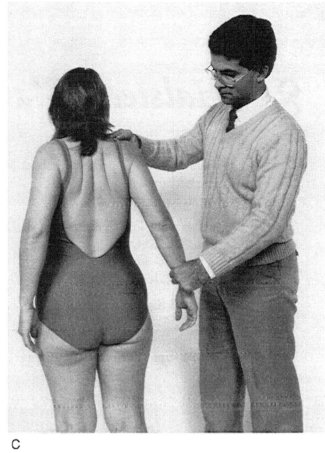

C

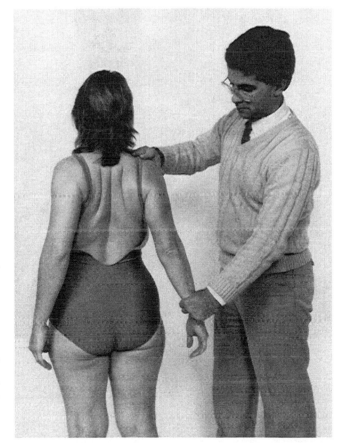

D

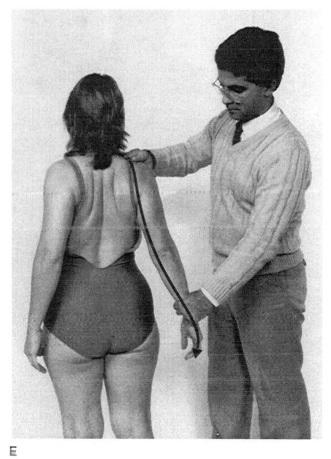

E

8 | *Halstead Maneuver*

Procedure: The patient is seated. Palpate the radial pulse, determining a baseline rate and rhythm. Then apply a downward tractioning on the arm with the patient's head rotated and extended to the side opposite the one being tested (Figs. A–D).

Rationale: Traction on the shoulder causes an approximation of the costoclavicular space. The addition of head rotation and extension tightens the scalene attachment on the first rib and further closes this space (Figs. E & F [Fig. E: left, scalenus anticus; middle, scalenus medius; right, scalenus posticus]).

Classical Significance: If the pulse disappears the test is positive.

Clinical Significance: See Classical Significance.

Follow-up: Perform the traction test, costoclavicular test, or Adson's test.

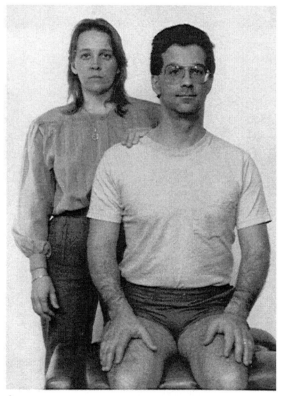

A

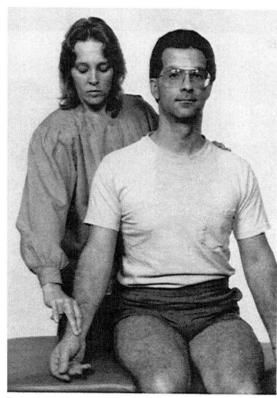

B

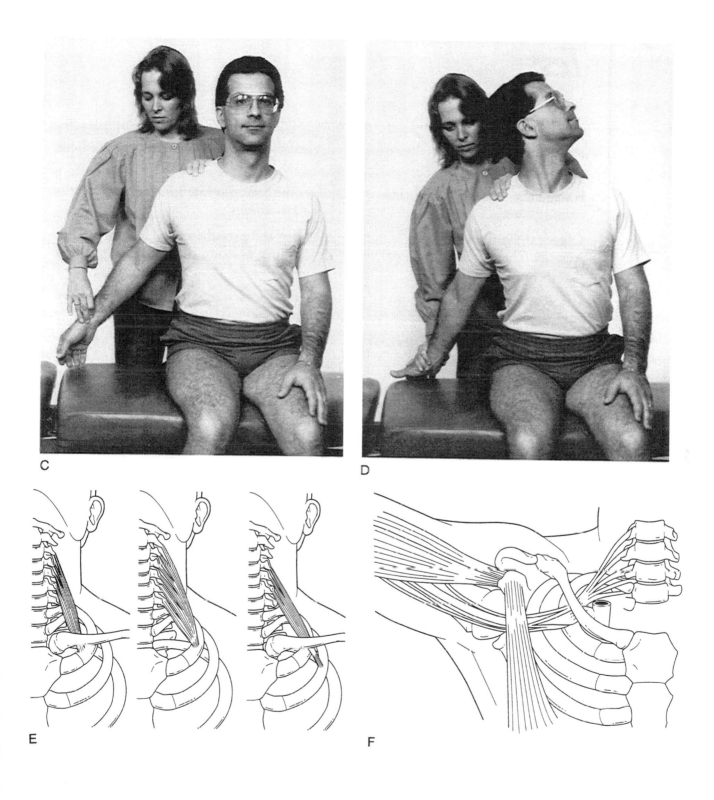

C

D

E

F

9 | *Intermittent Claudication Test*

Procedure: The patient is seated. The arms are elevated, abducted, and externally rotated. The patient flexes the fingers rapidly and should be able to perform this task for 1 minute (Figs. A–D).

Rationale: The above position compromises the costoclavicular interspace. The exercising further taxes the blood supply to the extremities.

Classical Significance: If positive, forearm pain and paresthesia will develop within seconds. The arm may soon collapse with continued testing because of fatigue and discomfort (Figs. E & F).

Clinical Significance: A positive result indicates thoracic outlet syndrome caused by compression of the anterior or middle scalene muscle.

Follow-up: Perform the elevated arm stress test (EAST), Eden's test, or the costoclavicular test.

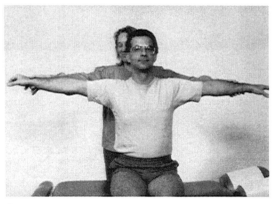

A

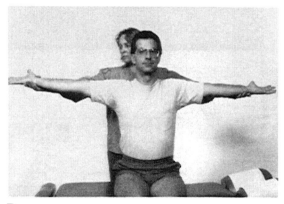

B

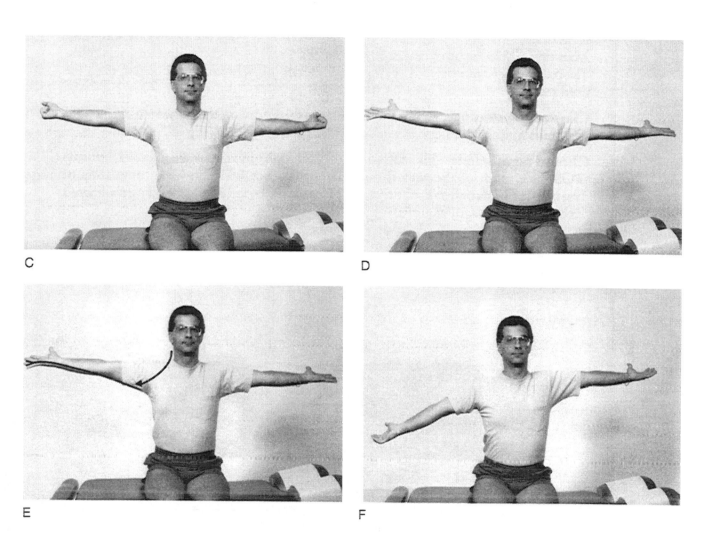

C

D

E

F

10 | *Pectoralis Stretch Test*

Procedure: The patient is supine. Instruct the patient to place the hands behind the head (palms up). Ask the patient to bring the elbows toward one another and then to let the arms relax to the table (Figs. A–D).

Rationale: The pectoralis muscle is primed into action when the elbows are adducted. After the muscle has been used, firing of the fibers will be inhibited and they will relax. The patient with a chronically spasmodic pectoralis muscle will not be able to relax the fired muscle.

Classical Significance: If the test is positive, the elbow on the same side of the tight pectoralis muscle will not relax in a flat fashion on the table (Fig. E).

Clinical Significance: The patient who has complaints of thoracic outlet syndrome (TOS) as a result of the pectoralis minor mechanism will also have complaints of dysesthesia or a dampening of the radial pulse, or both (the classical finding associated with TOS of this nature).

Follow-up: Perform Wright's test.

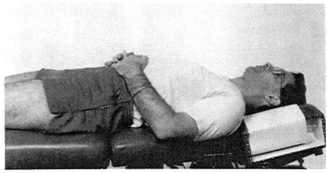

A

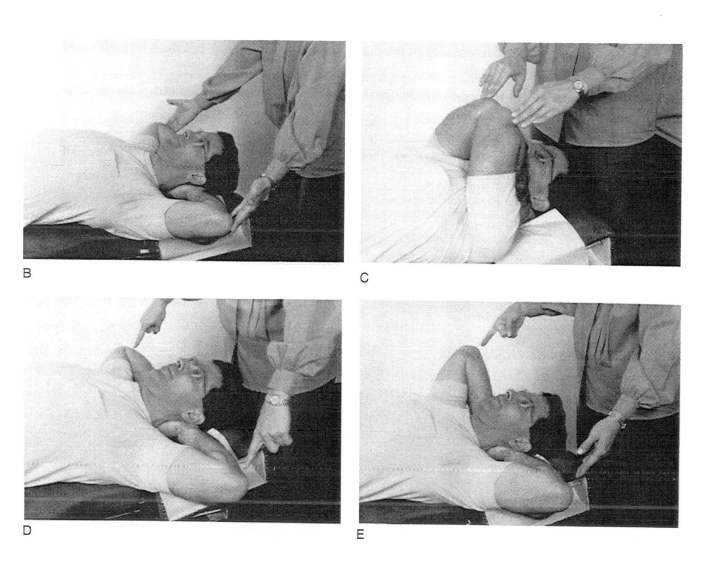

B

C

D

E

11 | *Traction Test*

Procedure: The patient is seated. Palpate the radial pulse, noting amplitude and frequency. Continue palpating the radial pulse and pull the arm anteriorly while stabilizing the torso. Perform this test bilaterally (Figs. A–E).

Rationale: If dampening of the pulse occurs on one side, the test must be performed on the opposite side.

Classical Significance: If dampening occurs on the one side only, suspect a cervical rib on that side.

Clinical Significance: Instances of bilateral cervical rib do occur. If the test is positive bilaterally, refer the patient for radiographic evaluation to rule out the presence of bilateral cervical ribs.

Follow-up: Perform the costoclavicular test, Adson's test, or the Halstead maneuver.

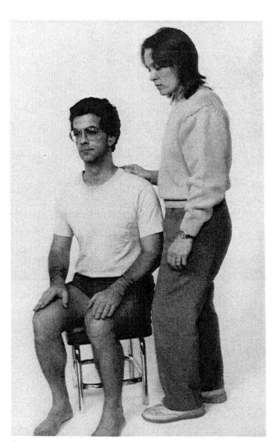

A

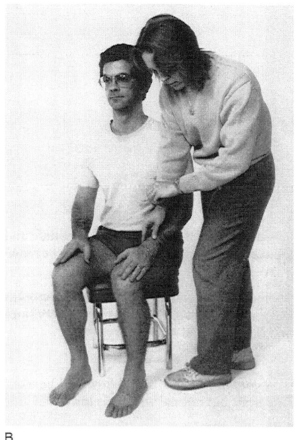

B

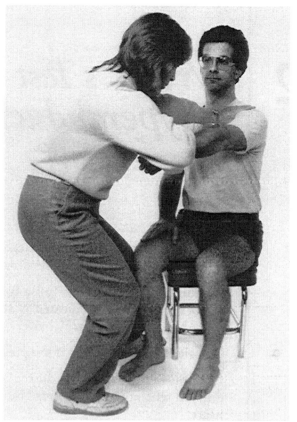

C

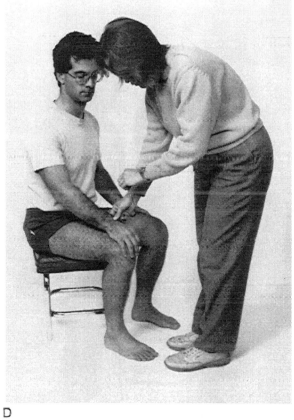

D

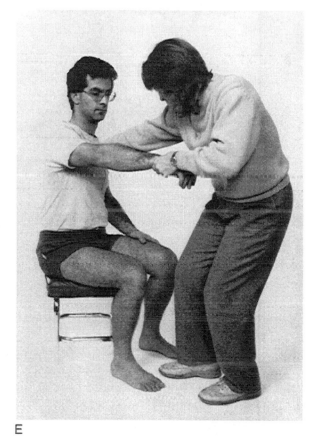

E

12 | *Wright's Test (Hyperabduction Maneuver)*

Procedure: With the patient seated, palpate the radial pulse, noting amplitude and frequency. With the arm fully extended, abduct it 120 degrees while palpating the radial artery. Perform this test bilaterally (Figs. A–F).

Rationale: This test can cause compression of the axillary artery by the pectoralis minor muscle. This is indicated by a dampening or loss of pulse in the radial artery since it is a branch of the brachial artery, which is a branch of the axillary artery.

Classical Significance: If the pulse is dampened the test is positive.

Clinical Significance: If the radial artery contains plaque, blood flow will be more difficult when the arm is elevated above the heart but normal when it is lower than the heart.

Follow-up: Perform the costoclavicular test or the pectoralis stretch test, or refer the patient for plethysmography.

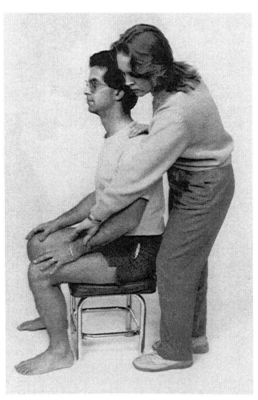

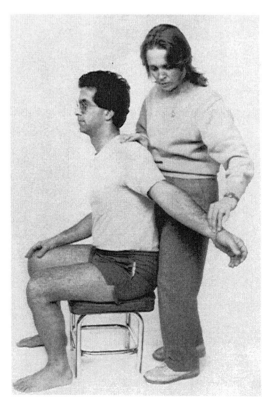

A   B

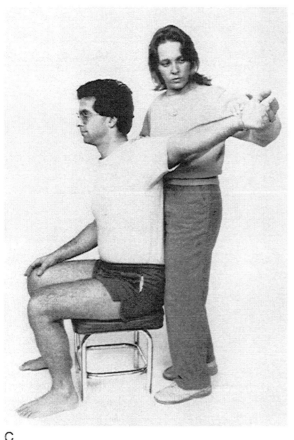

C

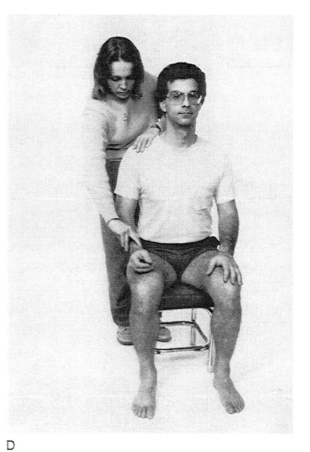

D

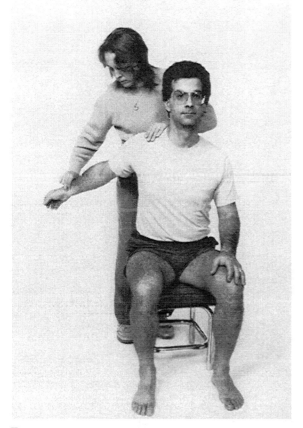

E

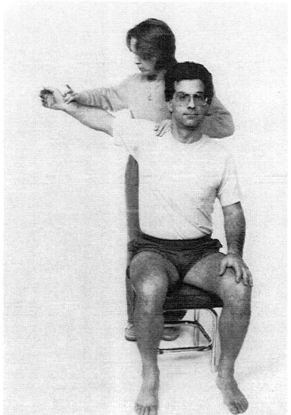

F

Shoulder Testing

1. Range of Motion Studies
2. Abbot-Saunders Test
3. Apley's Scratch Test
4. Apprehension Test
5. Booth-Marvel Transverse Humeral Ligament Test
6. Bryant's Sign
7. Calloway Test
8. Capsular Instability Test
9. Codman's Drop Arm Test
10. Dawbarn's Test
11. Dugas Test
12. Gilcrest Sign
13. Hamilton Ruler Test
14. Hueter's Sign
15. Impingement Sign
16. Lippman Test
17. Locking Position Test
18. Ludington Test
19. Posterior Apprehension Test
20. Quadrant Position Test
21. Scapulothoracic Rhythm
22. Speed's Test
23. Subacromial Push-Button Sign
24. Supraspinatus Arc Test
25. Supraspinatus Test
26. Teres Test
27. Transverse Humeral Ligament Test
28. Yergason's Test

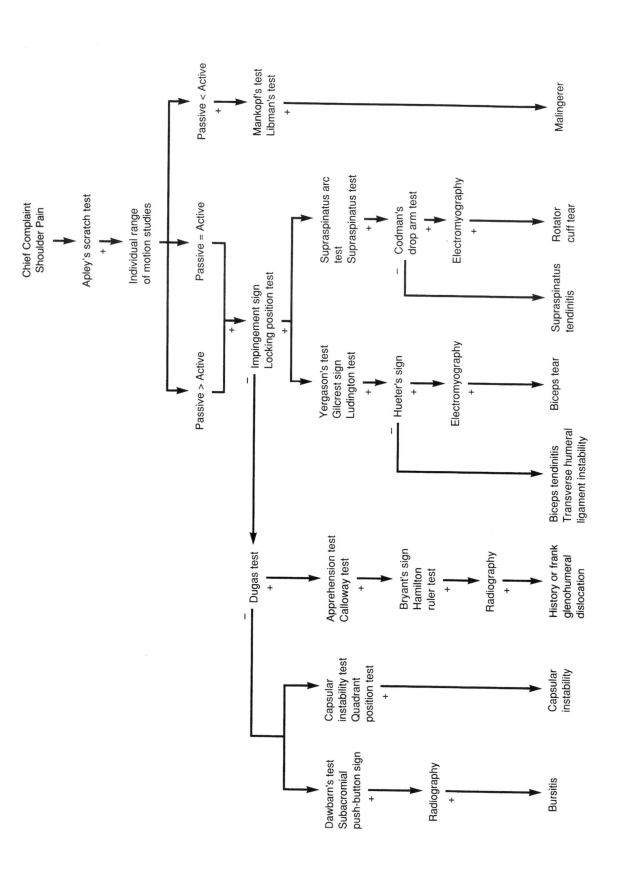

1 | *Range of Motion Studies*

When performing range of motion studies, it is important to use either an arthrodial protractor or an inclinometer. The *American Medical Association Guides for Impairment Ratings* now recommend the use of the inclinometer exclusively. Perform the shoulder ranges of motion bilaterally.

Flexion: The patient is standing. Ask the patient to move the arm, with the palm facing forward, through a forward excursion as far as possible overhead. The patient may complain of pain when flexing the shoulder. This motion is most commonly affected by impingement syndromes and conditions affecting the biceps tendon. Normal flexion is 160 to 180 degrees.

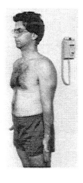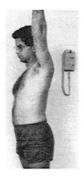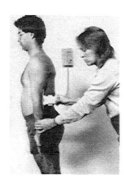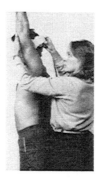

Extension: The patient is standing. Stabilize the shoulder anteriorly so the patient cannot lean forward as the arm is extended. Normal extension is 45 to 60 degrees.

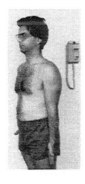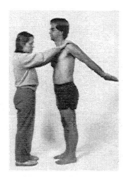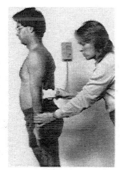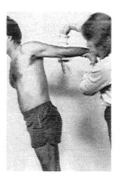

Internal Rotation: The patient is standing. Instruct the patient to stabilize the arm at the elbow against the body while turning the arm inward. Internal rotation is primarily affected by diseases that affect the integrity of the shoulder joint, leaving it vulnerable to dislocation. Expect movement limitations in cases of chronic dislocation. Normal internal rotation is 60 to 90 degrees.

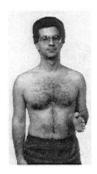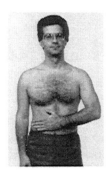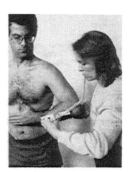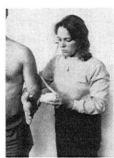

External Rotation: The patient is standing and the arm is stabilized at the elbow against the patient's body. Instruct the patient to rotate the arm laterally away from the body. In the case of subcoracoid bursitis, the external rotators will be limited and painful. Normal external rotation is 80 to 90 degrees.

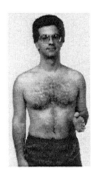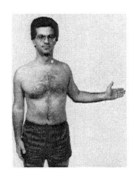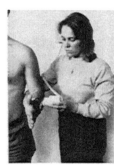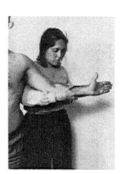

Abduction: The patient is standing. Instruct the patient to raise the arm laterally away from the body. When the arm reaches about 90 degrees, instruct the patient to rotate the palm upward and continue lifting the arm until it is overhead. This is the purest test for abduction as the supination of the palm at 90 degrees allows the greater tuberosity to be moved out and away from the coracoid process. Normal abduction is 170 to 180 degrees.

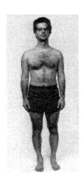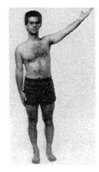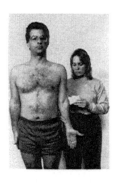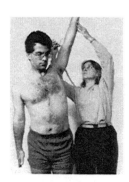

Adduction: The patient is standing. Instruct the patient to cross the extended arm across the midline of the body. If supraspinatus strain or sprain is present, this plane of motion may be limited due to protective guarding of the shoulder joint. Normal adduction is 45 to 75 degrees.

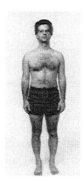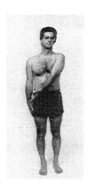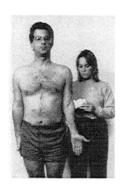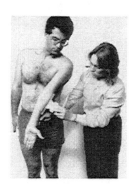

Quick Test: For a quick test of shoulder ranges of motion, ask the patient to reach behind the head and touch the scapula, and then to reach behind the back and touch the inferior part of the opposite scapula. Note any restrictions.

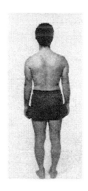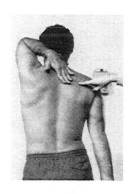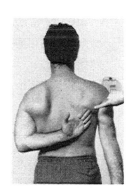

2 | *Abbot-Saunders Test*

Procedure: The patient is standing. Passively raise the arm on the side of the suspected lesion and abduct it 150 degrees. Then externally rotate the arm and lower it to the patient's side (Figs. A–E).

Rationale: Abduction and external rotation of the arm above the horizontal line stresses the biceps tendon at the bicipital groove, making it vulnerable to subluxation.

Classical Significance: Pain in the bicipital groove is considered positive. A palpable or audible click indicates tenosynovitis of the biceps tendon (Fig. F).

Clinical Significance: Carefully screen the patient with a history of shoulder dislocation before performing this test. If pain is elicited, identify the location precisely.

Follow-up: Perform Yergason's test, the Ludington test, or Speed's test.

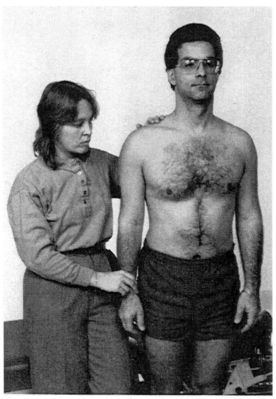

A

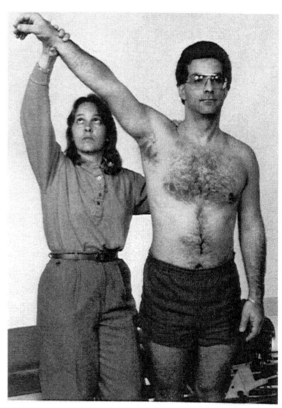

B

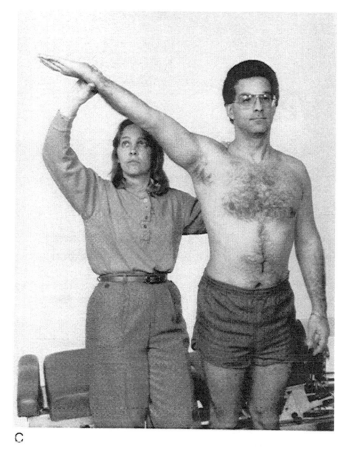

C

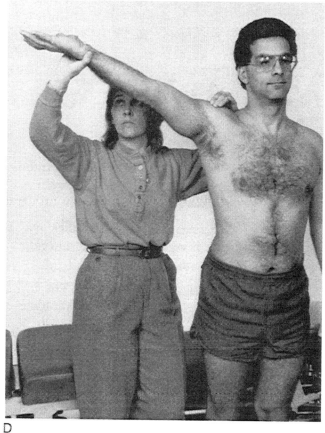

D

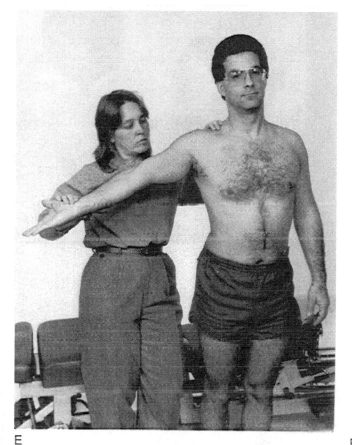

E

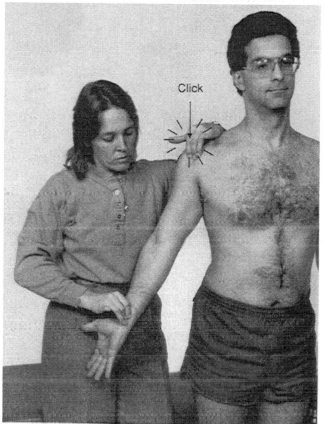

Click

F

3 | *Apley's Scratch Test*

Procedure: The patient is standing. First instruct the patient to reach behind the neck and touch the opposite superior scapula. Then instruct the patient to reach behind the back and touch the inferior border of the opposite scapula (Figs. A–D).

Rationale: This is a quick way to test the shoulder ranges of motion. The first maneuver tests abduction and external rotation; the second tests adduction and internal rotation.

Classical Significance: The inability to perform the above motions indicates the presence of some type of shoulder pathology (Figs. E & F).

Clinical Significance: If a restriction is found, have the patient perform the isolated ranges of motion to narrow down the location of the lesion.

Follow-up: Have the patient perform individual active ranges of motion.

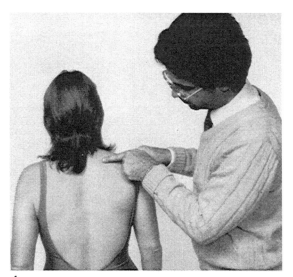

A

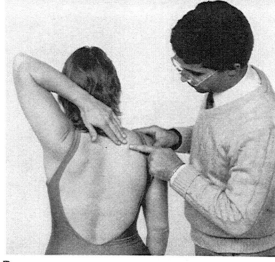

B

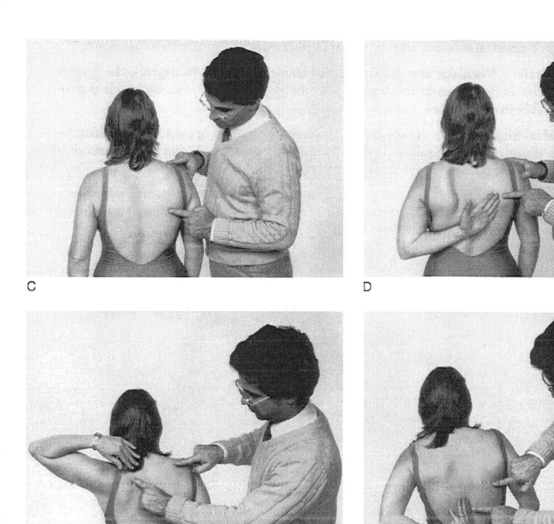

C

D

E

F

4 | *Apprehension Test*

Procedure: The patient is seated. Stand in front of the patient on the side being tested. Bend the forearm 90 degrees and then abduct and externally rotate the arm. Record the patient's physical reaction and response (Figs. A–C).

Rationale: When the arm is externally rotated and flexed 90 degrees, the greater tuberosity is cleared from the acromion of the shoulder. The shoulder joint is then vulnerable to dislocation.

Classical Significance: Reactive guarding from the patient or pain from this maneuver is significant for shoulder dislocation. A facial grimace during this maneuver is significant for possible shoulder dislocation (Fig. D).

Clinical Significance: In patients with thoracic outlet syndrome, pain or paresthesia may be elicited, because this maneuver, in the absence of dislocation, causes tractioning on the neurovascular bundle (Fig. E).

Follow-up: Perform the Dugas test, Calloway test, or Hamilton ruler test.

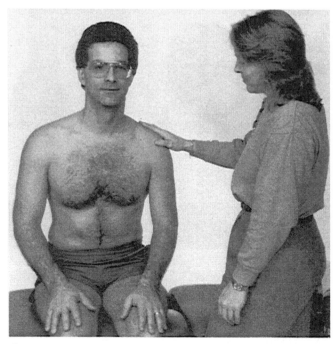

A

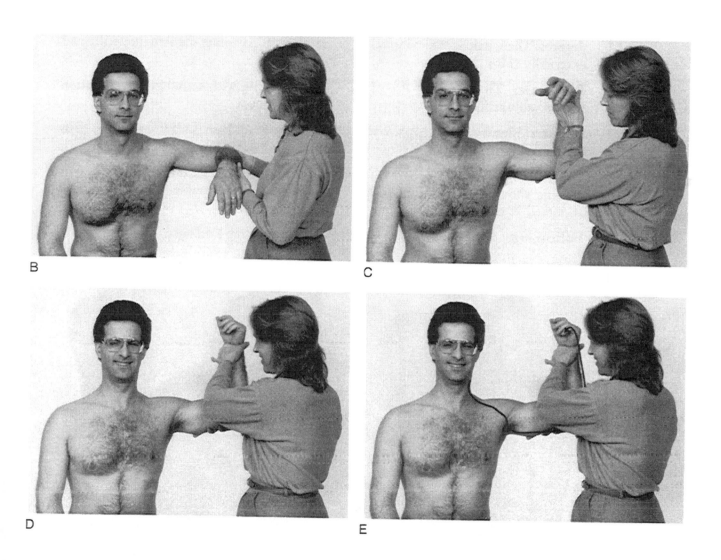

B

C

D

E

5 | *Booth-Marvel Transverse Humeral Ligament Test*

Procedure: The patient is seated. Flex the elbow 90 degrees and abduct the arm 90 degrees. Then, palpate the bicipital groove and passively rotate the arm internally and externally (Figs. A–E).

Rationale: The transverse excursion of the arm along with simultaneous palpation allows subluxation of the biceps tendon from the groove.

Classical Significance: A palpable snap with attendant pain is significant for biceps tendon subluxation due to loss of integrity of the transverse humeral ligament (Fig. F).

Clinical Significance: This test may be detrimental in the patient with a history of chronic shoulder dislocation, because the shoulder is vulnerable when the arm is abducted 90 degrees.

Follow-up: Perform Yergason's test, Speed's test, or the Ludington test.

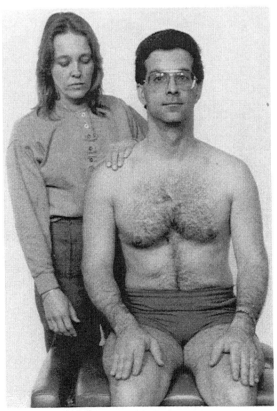

A

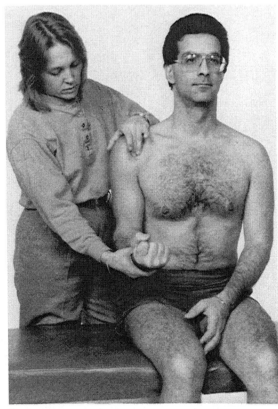

B

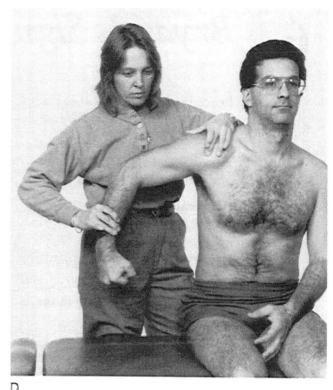

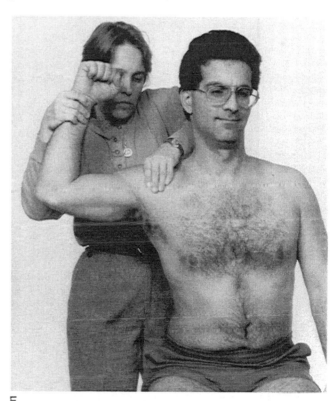

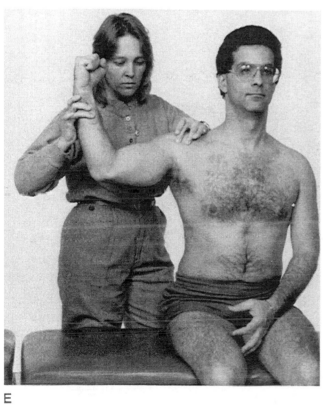

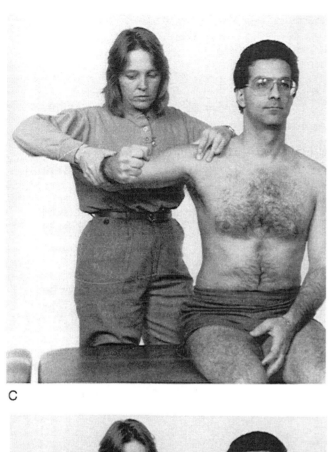

C

D

E

F

6 | *Bryant's Sign*

Procedure: The patient is standing. From either in front of or behind the patient, observe the patient's axillary folds for symmetry and equality in height (Figs. B & C).

Rationale: If the glenohumeral joint is dislocated, the side of the lesion will demonstrate a lower axillary fold, as the slippage of the humerus causes a downward traction of the tissue overlying the joint.

Classical Significance: Lowering of the axillary fold on the side of the lesion indicates a glenohumeral dislocation (Figs. A, D, & E). Changes in contour (the deltoid muscle flattens [Calloway test] and the axillary fold lowers [Fig. A]) are readily noted visually on the side with anterior inferior dislocation (Fig. A inset).

Clinical Significance: Changes in the integrity of the pectoralis muscle should not be confused with a true drop in the axilla. Take care to observe the patient in an upright posture.

Follow-up: Perform the Dugas test, Hamilton ruler test, or Calloway test.

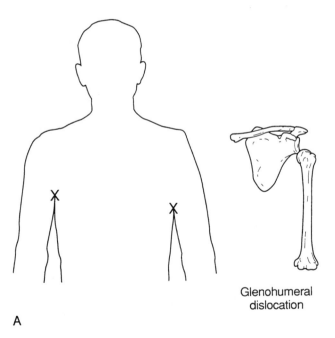

Glenohumeral
dislocation

A

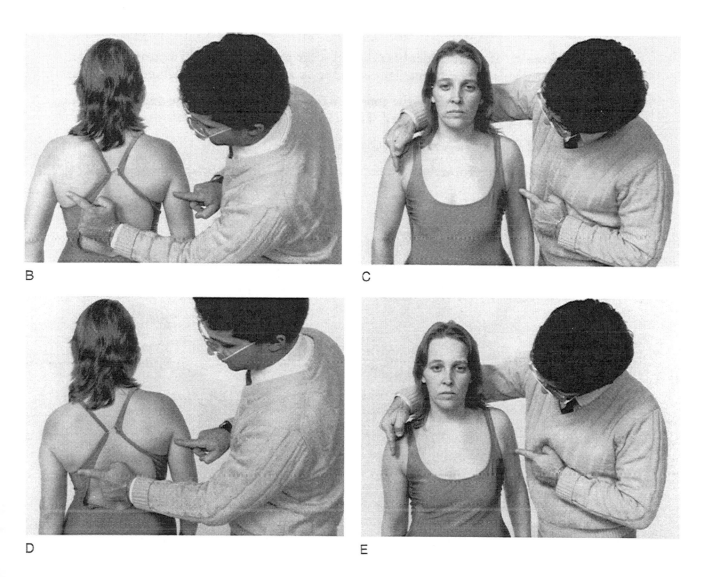

B

C

D

E

7 | *Calloway Test*

Procedure: The patient is seated. Using a tape measure encircle the shoulder under the axilla at the acromion tip. Record the measurement and compare it with the opposite normal shoulder (Figs. A–C).

Rationale: If the shoulder has dislocated, the patient's girth will increase in response to the osseous displacement. This is caused by a flattening of the deltoid musculature.

Classical Significance: If the abnormal shoulder is larger than the opposite shoulder the humeral head has dislocated (Figs. D & E).

Clinical Significance: See Classical Significance.

Follow-up: Perform the Hamilton ruler test, Dugas test, or apprehension test.

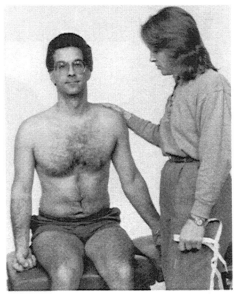

A

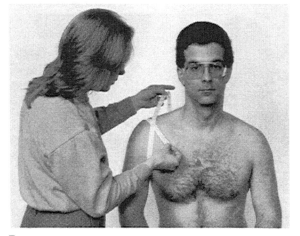

B

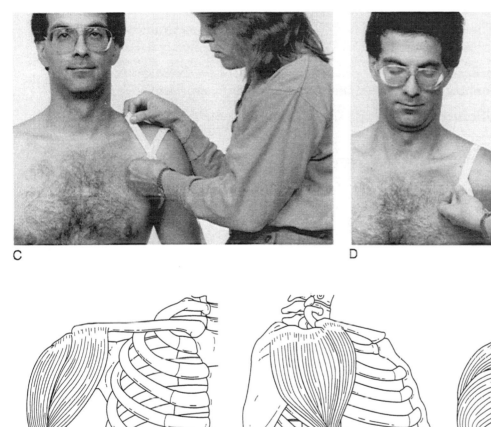

C

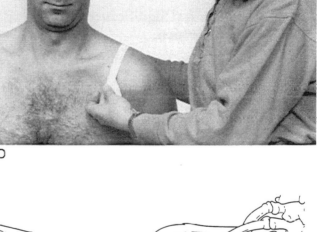

D

E

8 | *Capsular Instability Test*

Procedure: The patient is seated. Flex the elbow 90 degrees and abduct the arm 90 degrees while maximally rotating it. Apply an anterior to posterior force, as well as an inferior to superior and superior to inferior force. Record the patient's response (Figs. A–E).

Rationale: The shoulder is first put into a position of maximal vulnerability. Then forces necessary to stress the capsule in all planes of motion are applied.

Classical Significance: Pain or apprehension, or both, or the dislocation or subluxation of the glenohumeral joint is significant for capsular insufficiency (Fig. F).

Clinical Significance: Do not perform this test on the patient with a history of frank dislocation.

Follow-up: Perform the impingement sign, Dugas test, or apprehension test.

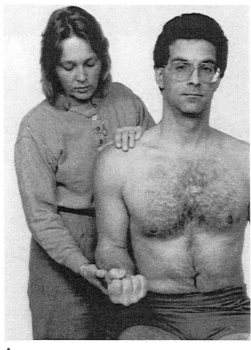

A

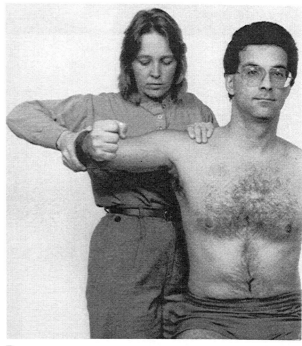

B

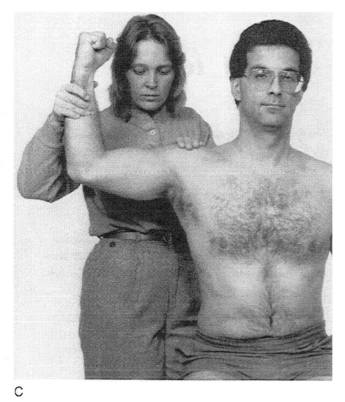

C

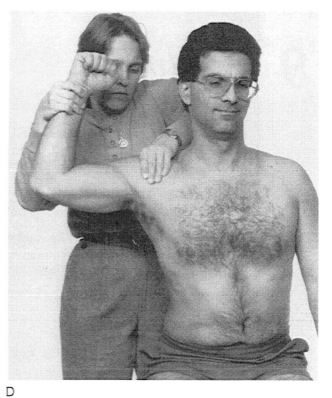

D

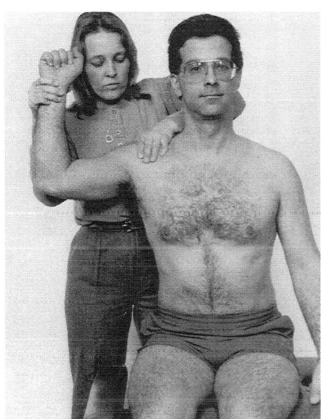

E

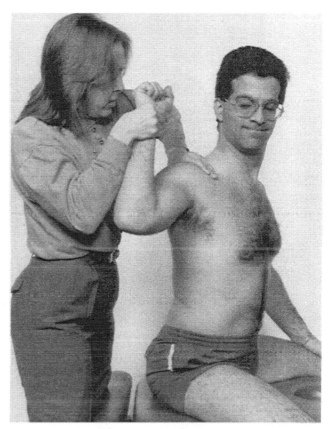

F

9 | *Codman's Drop Arm Test*

Procedure: The patient is standing. Passively abduct the arm 150 degrees. Release the arm and instruct the patient to slowly lower it all the way. Note the patient's ease of motion throughout (Figs. A–D).

Rationale: If integrity of the rotator cuff muscles is lost, the patient will be unable to lower the arm smoothly and rhythmically.

Classical Significance: The sudden contraction of the deltoid muscle with an associated amount of pain or the inability to hold the arm in abduction is significant for rotator cuff lesion. This is especially true if the supraspinatus muscle is the injured muscle (Fig. E).

Clinical Significance: *Do not use this test* if the patient does not have a normally functioning deltoid muscle. If the patient is able to lower the arm alone, then add resistance to the arm lowering. This may bring out a subtle tear (Fig. F).

Follow-up: Perform the supraspinatus arc test or supraspinatus test.

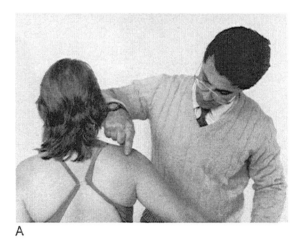

A

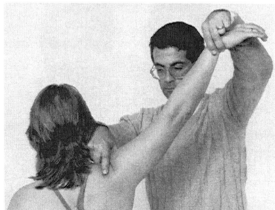

B

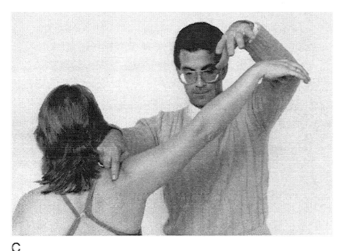

C

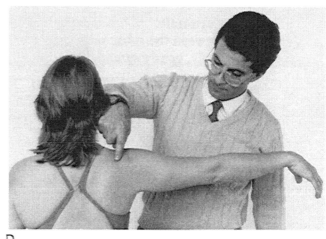

D

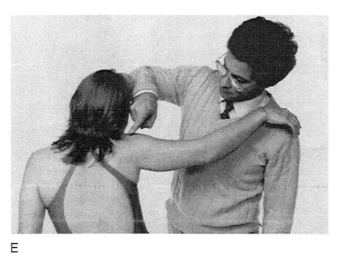

E

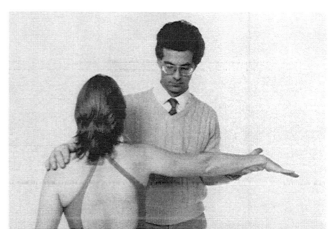

F

10 | *Dawbarn's Test*

Procedure: The patient is seated. Palpate the subacromial bursa for tenderness. If the bursa is tender, abduct the arm 90 degrees. Then ask the patient to describe what is felt as you again palpate the subacromial bursa (Fig. A–D).

Rationale: When the arm is abducted 90 degrees, the deltoid muscle acts as a buffer between the subacromial bursa and the palpating fingers. To palpate the bursa more easily, gently extend the shoulder (move the arm back) while palpating. This further exposes the bursa.

Classical Significance: A decrease in palpable tenderness when the arm is abducted 90 degrees is classical for subacromial bursitis (Fig. E & F).

Clinical Significance: Remember that excessive digital pressure to the bursa will elicit pain in a normal individual.

Follow-up: Perform the subacromial push-button sign.

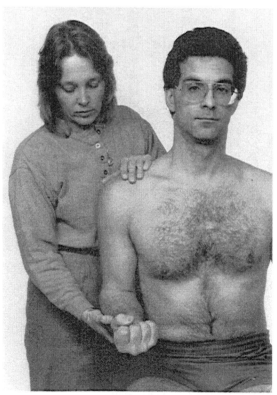

A

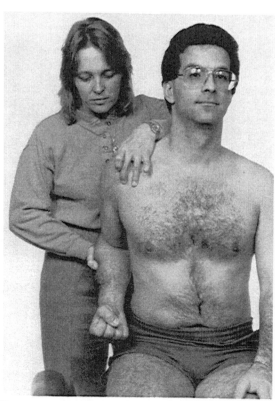

B

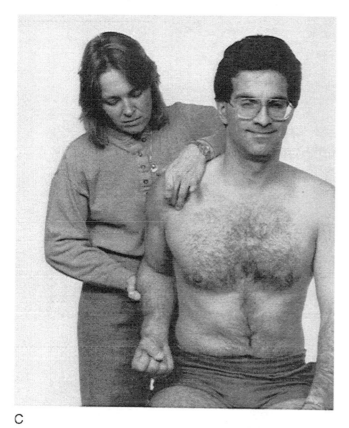

C

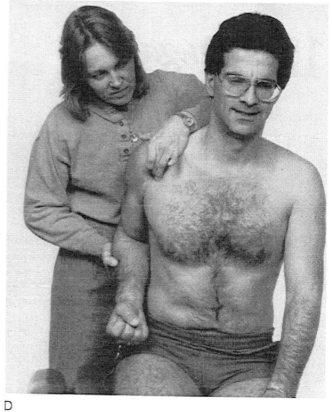

D

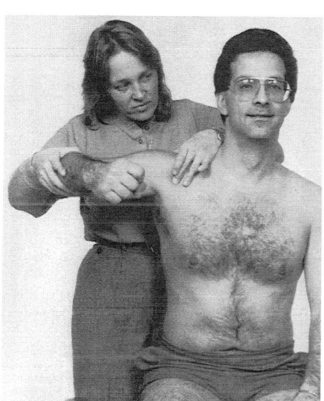

E

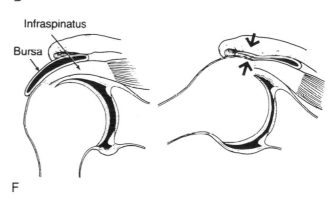

Infraspinatus

Bursa

F

11 | *Dugas Test*

Procedure: The patient is seated. Instruct the patient to touch the opposite shoulder by crossing the arm in front of the body at an angle parallel with the floor. Next, ask the patient to lower the elbow onto the chest (Figs. A–D).

Rationale: In the patient with a shoulder dislocation, internal rotation of the arm is severely limited. The patient with a dislocated shoulder may be able to do the first part of this test, but will not be able to bring the elbow to the chest without severe pain.

Classical Significance: Inability to perform this test is significant for shoulder dislocation (Fig. E).

Clinical Significance: In the case of capsular impingement, the ability to have the arm lie flush with the body may be limited. Pain may be associated with this as well (Fig. F).

Follow-up: Perform the Calloway test, Hamilton ruler test, or impingement sign.

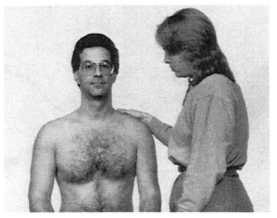

A

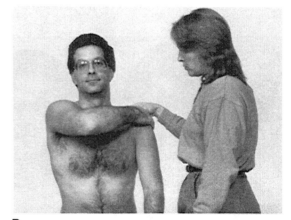

B

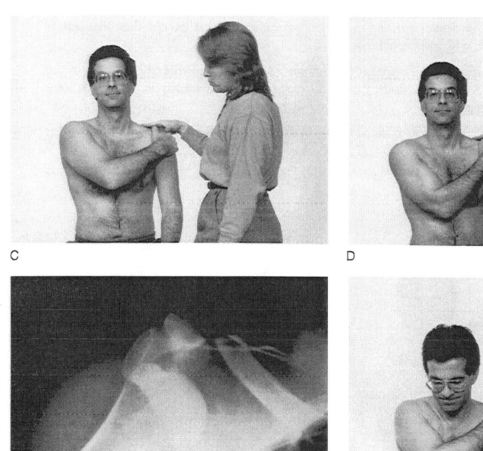

C

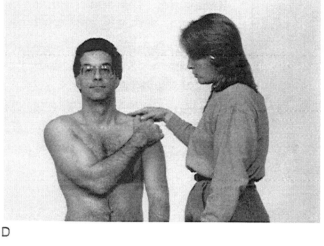

D

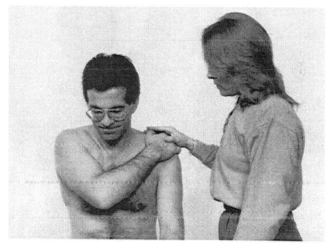

E

F

12 | *Gilcrest Sign*

Procedure: The patient is seated and has a 5-lb weight. Instruct the patient to raise the dumbbell overhead and then to externally rotate the arm. Once this is done, ask the patient to lower the arm to the side (Figs. A–E).

Rationale: This test is similar to the Abbot-Saunders test except that this test is performed with weighted resistance.

Classical Significance: Reproduction of pain in the bicipital area or palpation of the subluxated tendon with an increase in pain is significant for tenosynovitis of the long head of the biceps (Fig. F).

Clinical Significance: As with all testing, establish the integrity of the shoulder joint before performing this test.

Follow-up: Perform Yergason's test, the impingement sign, or the Abbot-Saunders test.

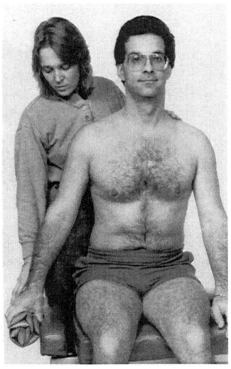

A

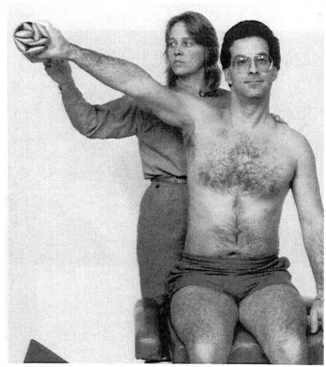

B

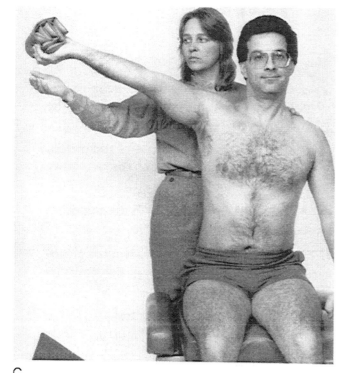

C

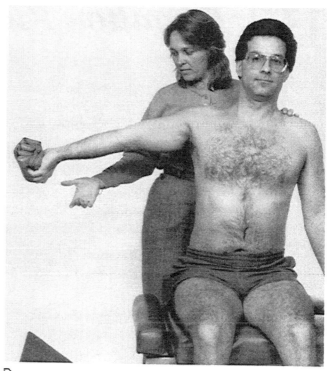

D

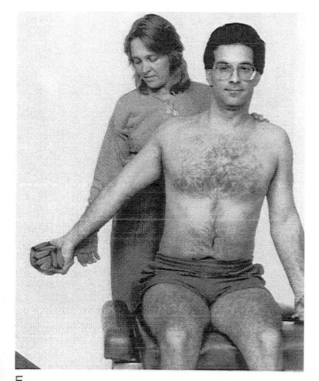

E

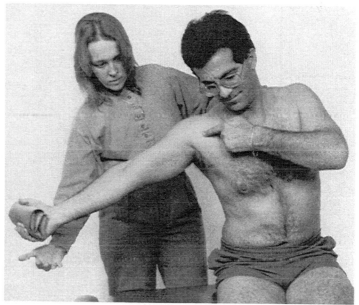

F

13 | *Hamilton Ruler Test*

Procedure: The patient is seated. Place a yardstick along the lateral edge of the epicondyle of the elbow and attempt to align it with the acromion process of the ipsilateral shoulder (Figs. A–D).

Rationale: Shoulder dislocation causes the humeral head to drop inferior and medial to the acromion. This allows the straight edge to form a line between the two bony landmarks.

Classical Significance: The ability to align the lateral epicondyle with the acromion demonstrates loss of integrity of the glenohumeral joint (Figs. E & F).

Clinical Significance: Alignment of this area may be possible even when the glenohumeral joint is secure, if a congenital anomaly that affects the elbow (e.g., deformity) is present.

Follow-up: Perform the Calloway test, Dugas test, or apprehension test.

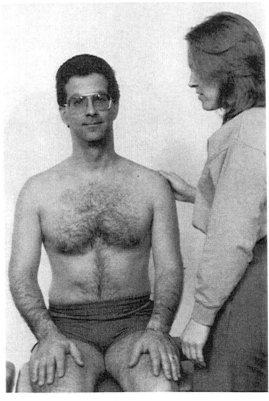

A

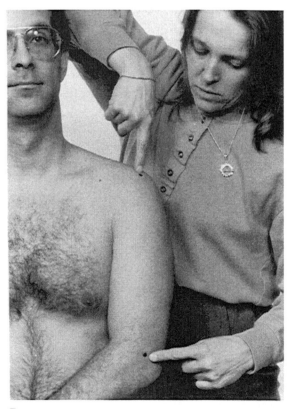

B

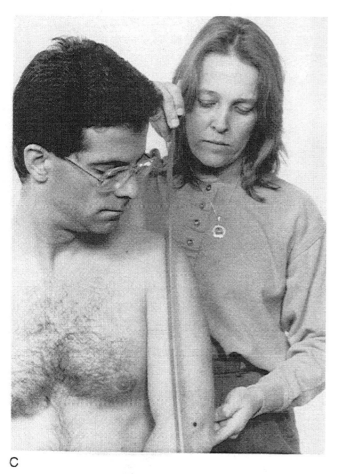

C

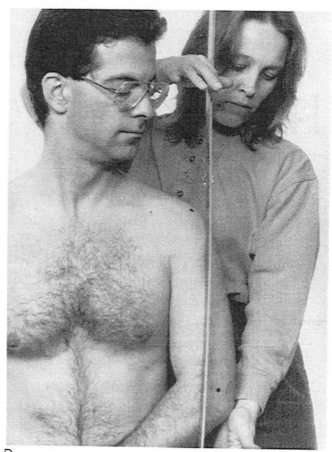

D

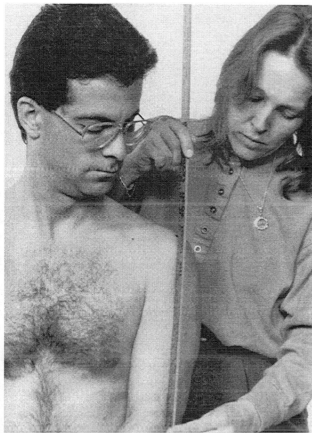

E

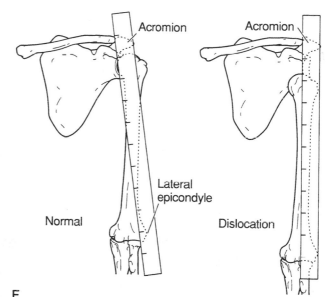

Acromion

Acromion

Lateral
epicondyle

Normal

Dislocation

F

14 | *Hueter's Sign*

Procedure: The patient is seated. Flex the elbow while the patient resists the flexion. Observe the biceps muscle for deformity (Figs. A–D).

Rationale: When the biceps muscle is ruptured, the belly of the muscle is observed to hunch at the lower distal end. On forced resisted flexion, the muscle can be observed as a "ball" just proximal to the elbow joint (Fig. F: biceps tendon tear).

Classical Significance: Pain on resisted flexion is significant for partial rupture (Fig. E).

Clinical Significance: It is our opinion that pain on resisted action is more diagnostic for biceps tendinitis and that an observable hunch of the muscle must be seen to diagnose a ruptured muscle.

Follow-up: Perform Yergason's test or refer the patient for electromyography.

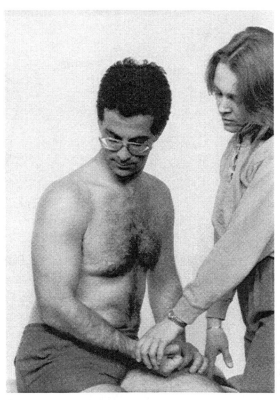

A

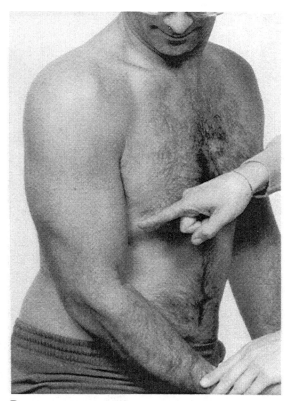

B

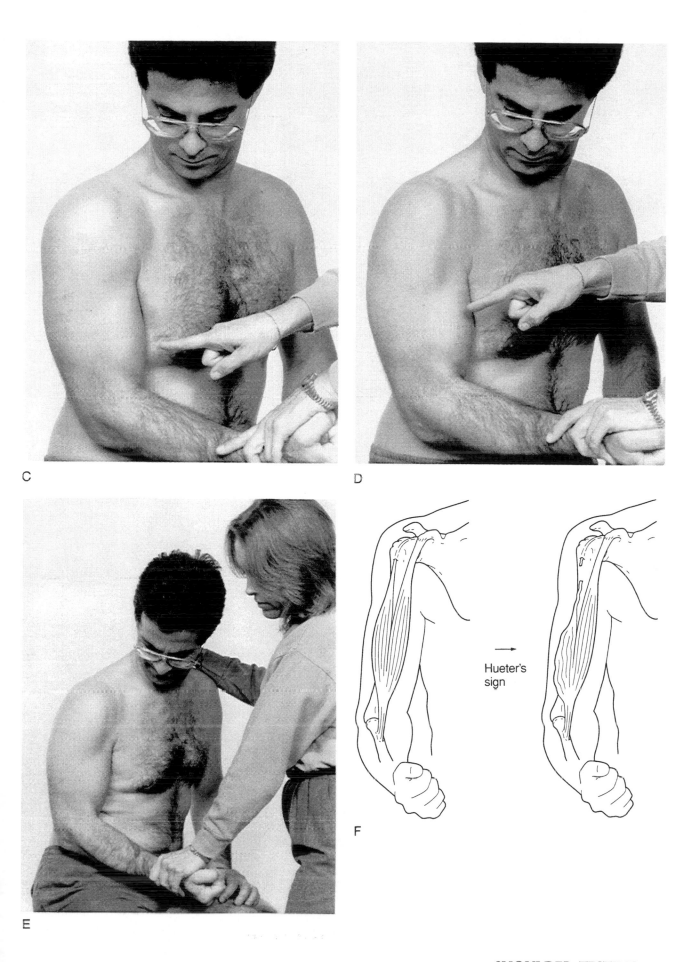

C

D

E

F

Hueter's
sign

15 | *Impingement Sign*

Procedure: The patient is seated. Flex the elbow and pronate the arm. From behind, cup the elbow in your hand and bring the arm through the flexion arc while applying pressure superiorly (Figs. A–E).

Rationale: The flexion and mild abduction of the arm causes a resistance to the biceps and supraspinatus muscles. The upward compression attempts to entrap the tendons where they glide under the acromion.

Classical Significance: Pain on this maneuver is significant for bicipital tendinitis or supraspinatus tendinitis (Fig. F).

Clinical Significance: If the capsule is not stable, pain may be elicited with the upward compression, indicating instability of the glenohumeral joint.

Follow-up: Perform Yergason's test, the supraspinatus test, or the locking position test.

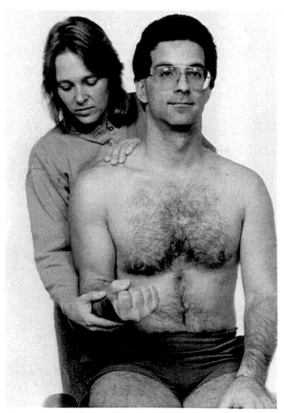

A

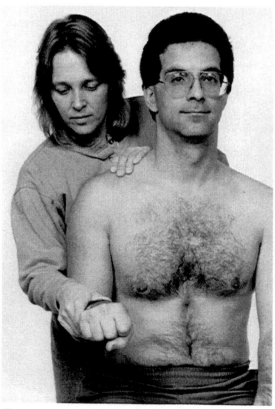

B

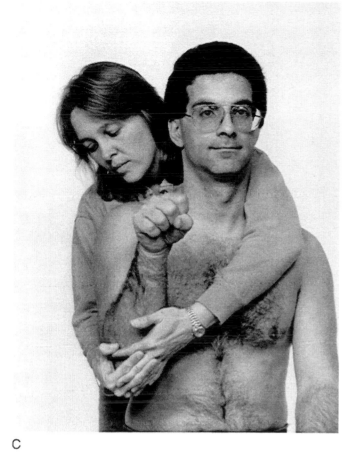

C

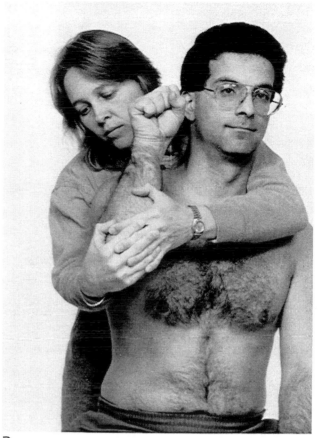

D

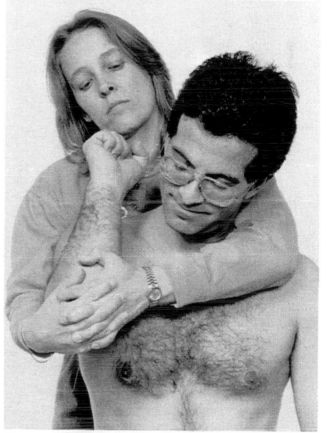

E

F

16 | *Lippman Test*

Procedure: The patient is seated and the elbow flexed 90 degrees. Palpate the biceps tendon approximately 3 inches distal to the glenohumeral joint. Then apply a transverse pressure against the tendon in an attempt to subluxate it from the groove (Figs. A–D).

Rationale: This test is an attempt to dislocate the tendon from the bicipital groove by direct manual pressure.

Classical Significance: The ability to palpate the tendon slipping from the groove or the reproduction of pain at the groove is significant for instability of the transverse ligament (Fig. E: left, tendon dislocation [transverse ligament rupture]; right, tendon rupture).

Clinical Significance: If pain is reproduced without subluxation of the transverse ligament, consider biceps tendinitis (Fig. F).

Follow-up: Perform Yergason's test, the Ludington test, or the Gilcrest sign.

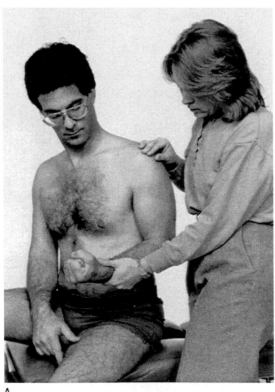

A

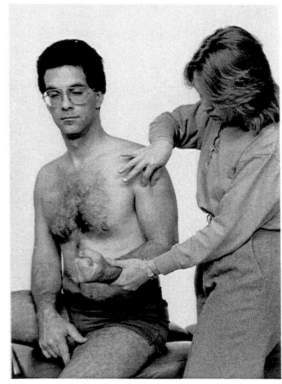

B

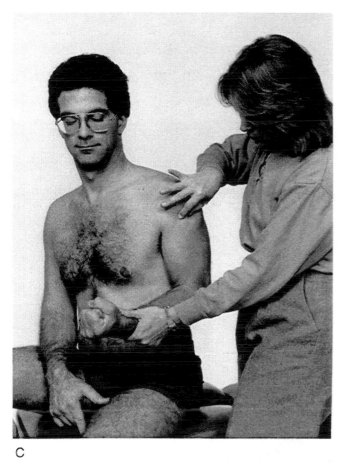

C

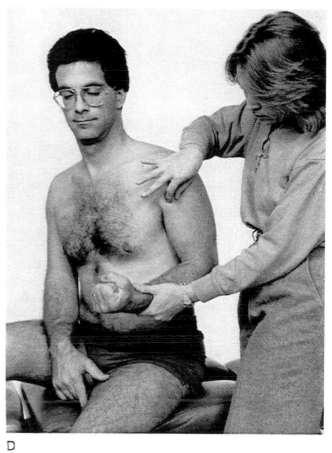

D

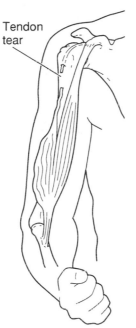

Ligament
tear

Tendon
tear

E

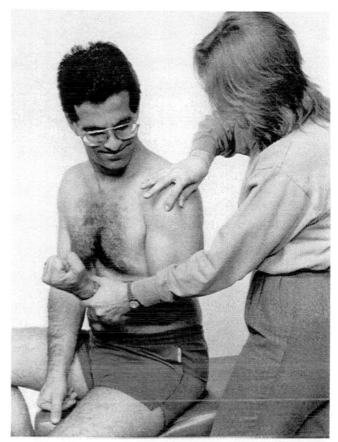

F

17 | *Locking Position Test*

Procedure: The patient is supine. Allow the patient's arm on the side being tested to drop into extension while internally rotating the arm (Figs. A–D).

Rationale: Extension coupled with internal rotation places maximum stress on the biceps and supraspinatus tendons as they cross under the acromial ledge.

Classical Significance: Reproduction of pain in the above position is significant for an impingement syndrome (Fig. E).

Clinical Significance: Capsular instability may also cause a painful response because the joint is stressed from posterior to anterior in this position.

Follow-up: Perform the impingement sign or the capsular instability test, or both.

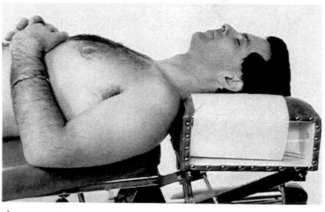

A

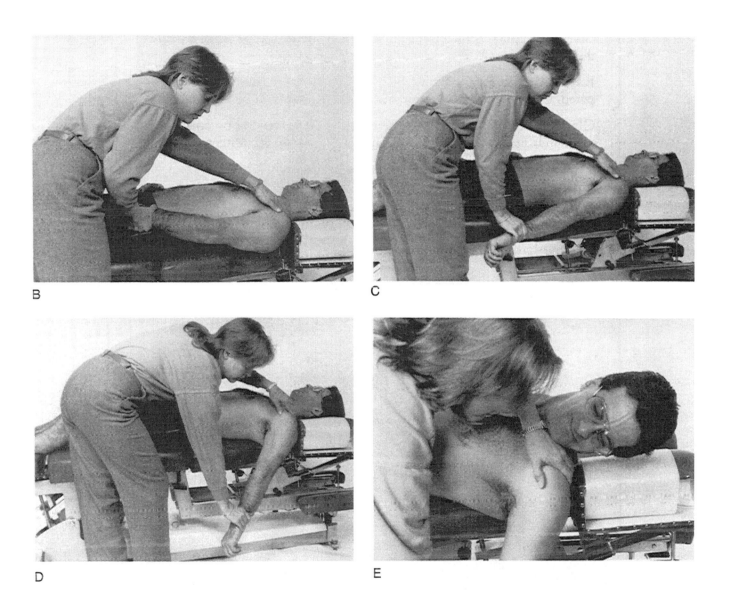

B

C

D

E

18 | *Ludington Test*

Procedure: The patient is seated. Ask the patient to clasp both hands behind the head and to support the weight of the upper limbs in this position. Next, ask the patient to alternately contract the biceps muscles. Palpate the biceps tendon while the patient is doing this (Figs. A–E).

Rationale: In this position, the biceps tendons are readily observed and easily palpated. On the side of the lesion, the biceps tendon will be absent.

Classical Significance: The absence of the biceps tendon on one side and not on the other indicates biceps tendon rupture on the side of the absent tendon.

Clinical Significance: See Classical Significance.

Follow-up: Perform Hueter's sign.

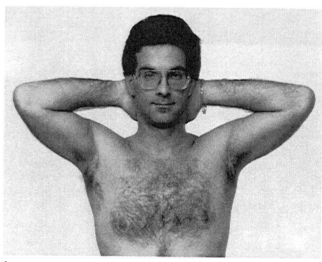

A

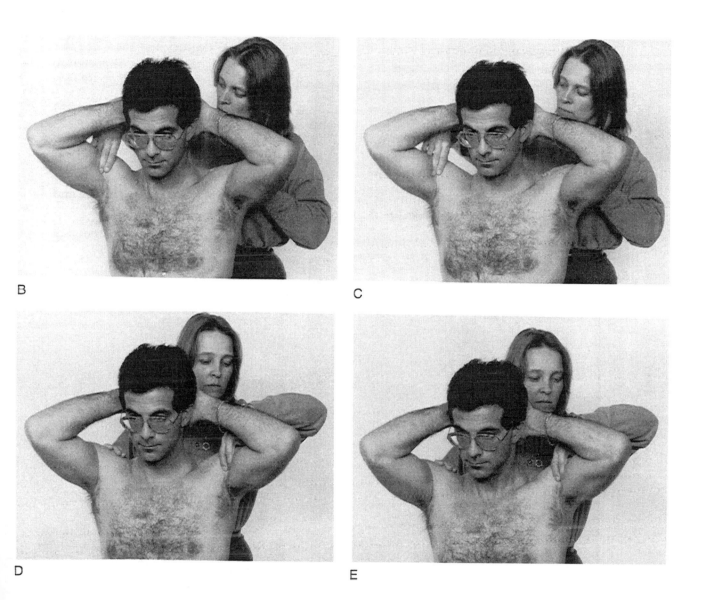

B

C

D

E

19 Posterior Apprehension Test

Procedure: The patient is supine. First raise the arm 90 degrees and then flex the elbow. Next, adduct the elbow across the chest. Finally, apply an anterior to posterior pressure while noting the resistance and facial expression of the patient (Figs. A–E).

Rationale: This test will cause apprehension in the patient, if the glenohumeral joint is dislocated.

Classical Significance: Reproduction of pain or the resistance to further motion is significant for shoulder dislocation (Fig. F).

Clinical Significance: Impingement syndromes also will result in apprehension and pain produced by compression of the joint.

Follow-up: Perform the impingement sign, locking position test, or apprehension test.

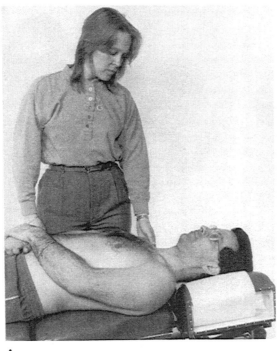

A

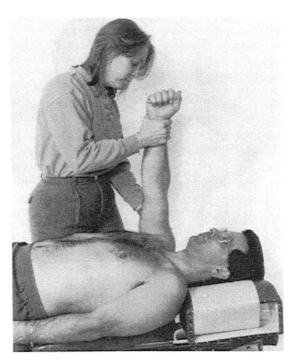

B

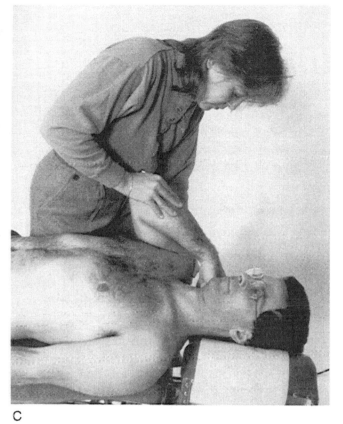

C

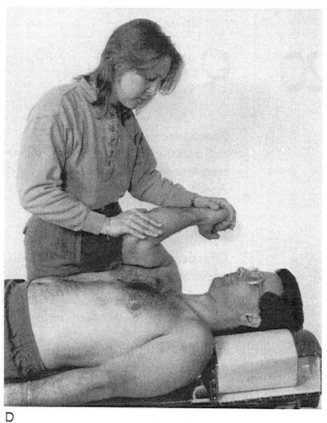

D

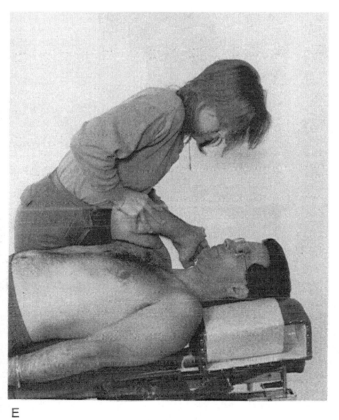

E

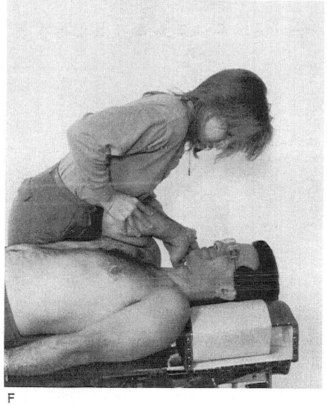

F

20 | *Quadrant Position Test*

Procedure: The patient is supine. Externally rotate the arm and flex it fully over the patient's head. Apply pressure to the arm, moving it backward. Record the patient's response to this maneuver as well as the amount of excursion of the humeral head (Figs. A–E).

Rationale: The pressure applied to the joint stresses the joint capsule and compresses the acromioclavicular joint.

Classical Significance: Pronounced forward motion of the humeral head by the addition of pressure is significant for laxity of the anterior capsule (Fig. F).

Clinical Significance: Pain produced by this maneuver may be due to an acromioclavicular joint lesion or an impingement syndrome.

Follow-up: Perform the posterior apprehension test or locking position test.

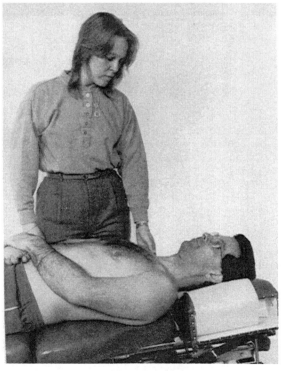

A

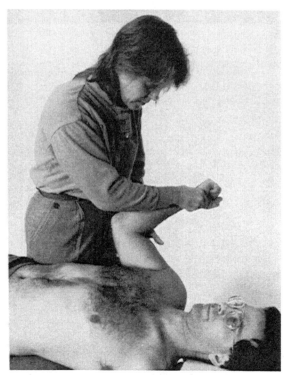

B

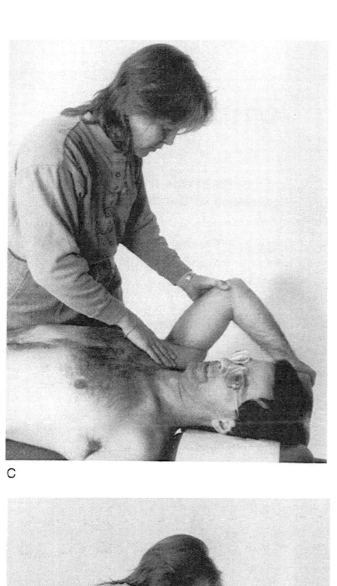

C

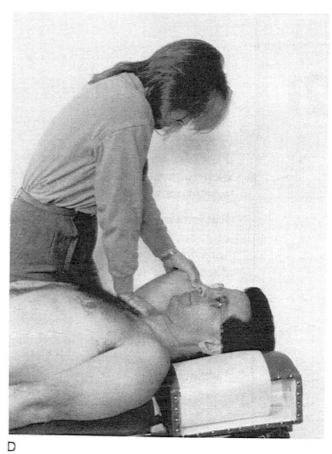

D

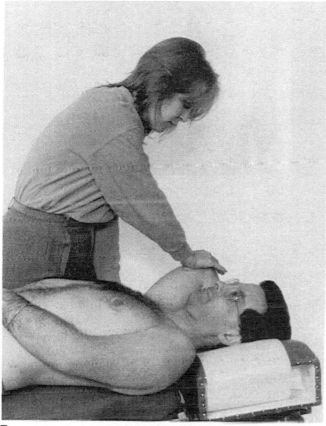

E

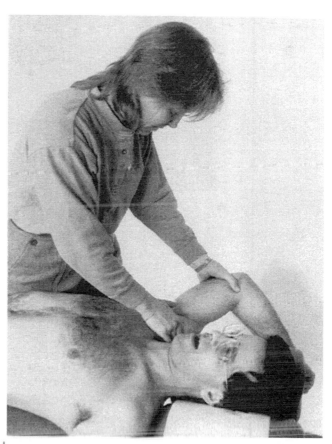

F

21 | *Scapulothoracic Rhythm*

Procedure: Observe the ratio of the amount of movement that occurs between the glenohumeral joint and the scapulothoracic articulation of the shoulder when the patient actively abducts the arm (Figs. A–C).

Rationale: The normal scapulothoracic rhythm is 2:1. Therefore, for every 3 degrees of abduction, 2 degrees occurs at the glenohumeral joint and 1 degree occurs at the scapulothoracic articulation. This is often observed when, at about 30 degrees of abduction, the medial border of the scapula moves laterally.

Classical Significance: A scapulothoracic rhythm of 2:1 indicates normal shoulder motion (Figs. D–F).

Clinical Significance: In frozen shoulder syndrome, only early glenohumeral motion is present. Acromioclavicular dysfunction can cause interruption of the normal rhythm.

Follow-up: Perform active range of motion studies or Apley's scratch test.

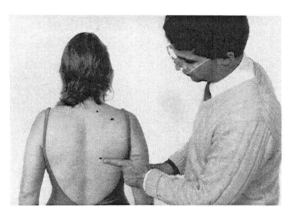

A

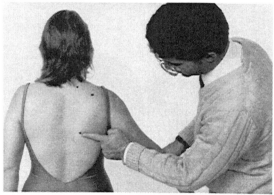

B

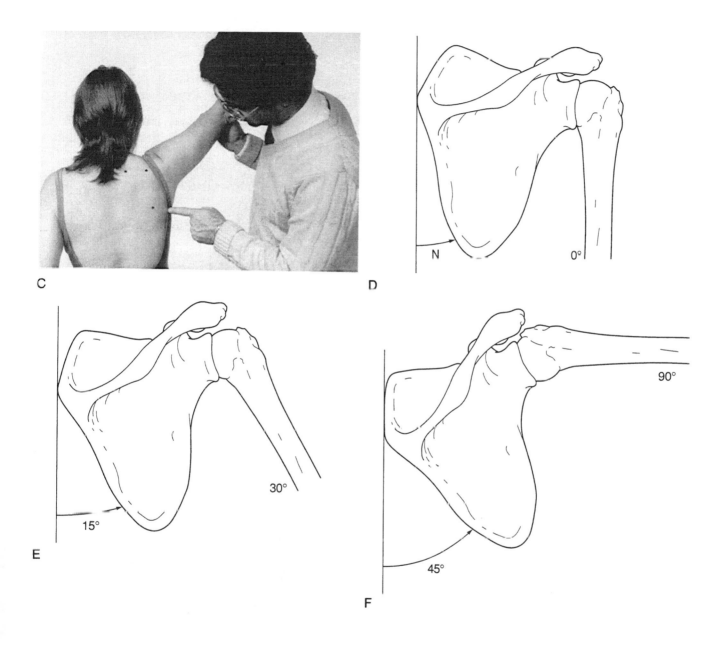

Speed's Test (Biceps Test)

Procedure: The patient is seated. Stand on the side being tested and supinate the hand while maintaining full extension of the elbow. Then ask the patient to flex the limb at the shoulder while you resist this move. Record the response (Figs. A–D).

Rationale: Resisted limb flexion with the elbow extended allows movement of the humerus anteriorly, which forces the biceps tendon from the bicipital groove floor.

Classical Significance: Tenderness elicited from the bicipital area indicates biceps tendinitis (Fig. E).

Clinical Significance: If there is an insufficiency of the transverse humeral ligament, a subluxation of the tendon may also occur associated with a palpable and/or audible click (Fig. F).

Follow-up: Perform the transverse humeral ligament test or the Abbot-Saunders test.

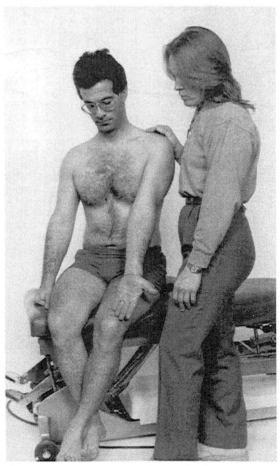

A

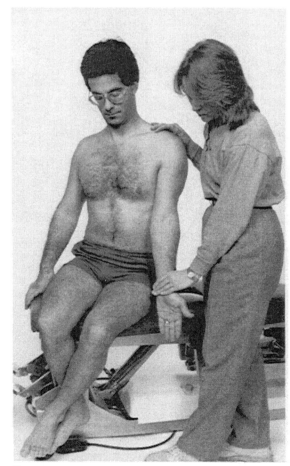

B

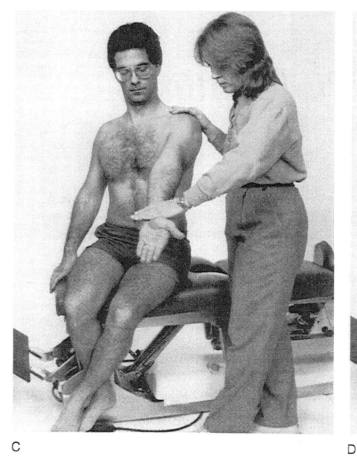

C

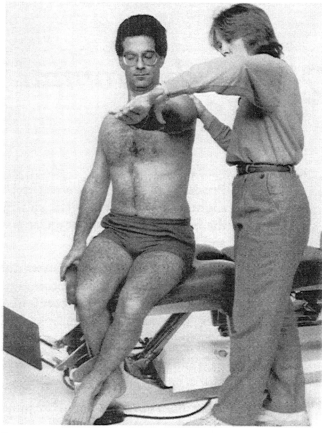

D

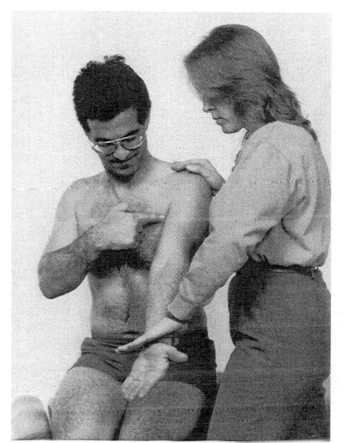

E

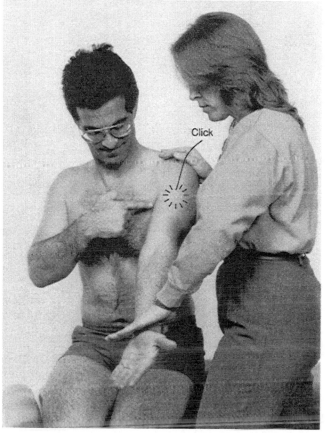

Click

F

23 | *Subacromial Push-Button Sign*

Procedure: The patient is seated. Stand behind the patient on the side being tested and slightly extend the arm while palpating the area of the bursa. Apply digital pressure to the bursa and then allow the arm to fall back into the neutral position (Figs. A–C and E).

Rationale: With the arm extended, the subacromial bursa moves from its location under the acromion and becomes palpable. Digital pressure causes tenderness to the inflamed bursa at the site of the lesion. When the arm is returned to the neutral position, there is a translocation of the pain back to the acromion.

Classical Significance: Exquisite tenderness on palpation and the translocation of pain is a positive sign for subacromial bursitis (Fig. D).

Clinical Significance: In the normal individual, the use of excessive pressure will cause pain on palpation. This must be gauged accordingly and compared with the uninvolved extremity (Fig. E).

Follow-up: Perform Dawbarn's test.

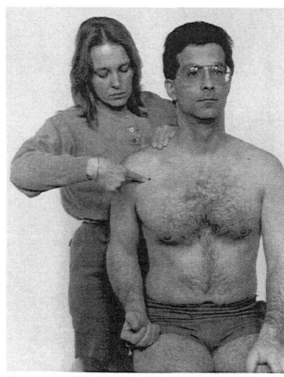

A

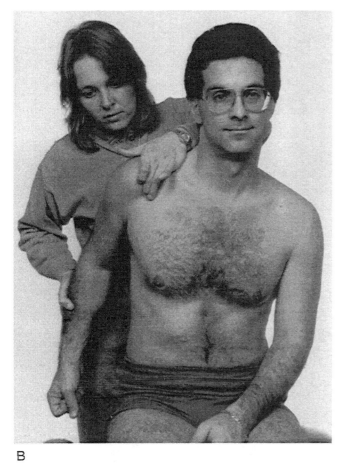

B

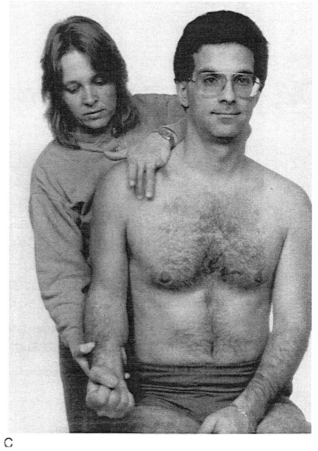

C

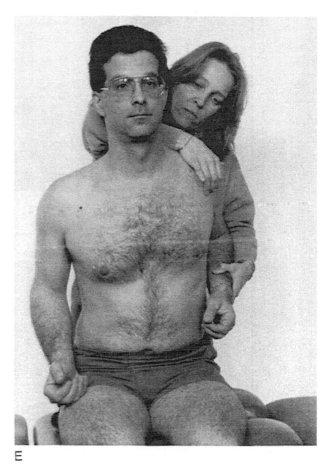

D

E

24 | *Supraspinatus Arc Test*

Procedure: The patient is standing with the arm flush against the side. Apply resistance while the patient abducts the arm through the normal abduction arc (Figs. A–E).

Rationale: In a positive test, pain will occur at 10 to 20 degrees, go away at 20 to 90 degrees, and return at 90 to 110 degrees. This is because at 20 to 90 degrees most of the motion in abduction is from the lateral deltoid muscle and not the supraspinatus muscle.

Classical Significance: Pain at 10 to 20 degrees that goes away at 20 to 90 degrees and returns at 90 to 110 degrees is significant for supraspinatus tendinitis.

Clinical Significance: Patients with frozen shoulder syndrome will be unable to perform this test since the shoulder cannot be put through its normal arc (Fig. F).

Follow-up: Perform the supraspinatus test.

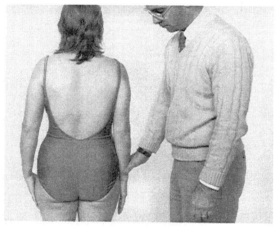

A

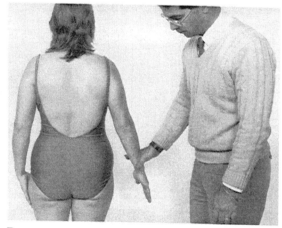

B

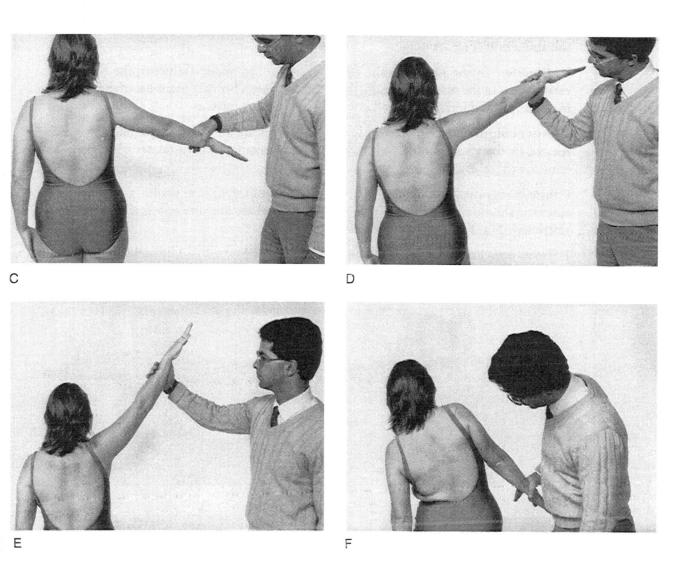

C

D

E

F

25 | *Supraspinatus Test*

Procedure: The patient is seated and the arms are abducted 90 degrees with no rotation. Apply resistance to the abduction. Grade the response and then angle the shoulders forward 30 degrees and internally rotate them while applying resistance to the abduction (Figs. A–D).

Rationale: In the first position, the integrity of the major abductor, the deltoid, is established. In the second position, the deltoid action is limited and most of the stress of maintaining abduction is placed on the supraspinatus muscle.

Classical Significance: Weakness when the arms are angled forward and internally rotated or the elicitation of pain when tested in this position indicates supraspinatus tendinitis (Fig. E).

Clinical Significance: Patients with frozen shoulder will be unable to do this test since the shoulder cannot be put through its normal arc and abduction will be severely restricted (Fig. F).

Follow-up: Perform the supraspinatus arc test.

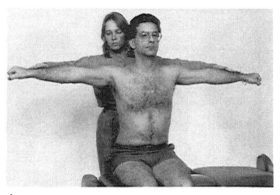

A

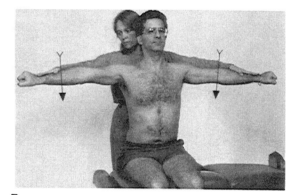

B

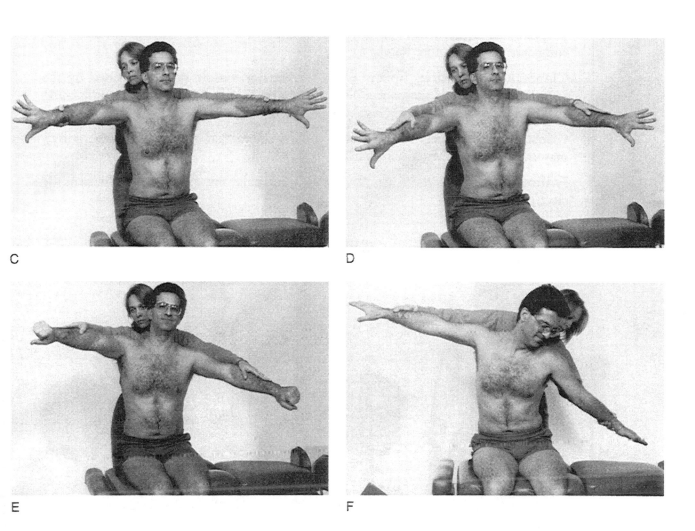

C

D

E

F

26 | *Teres Test*

Procedure: The patient is standing. Ask the patient to assume a relaxed posture and observe the position of the hands (Figs. A & B).

Rationale: The teres major muscle causes internal rotation of the arm. If the muscle is in spasm, the affected arm will internally rotate and the hand will face posteriorly as compared with the other hand.

Classical Significance: Spasm of the teres major muscle is demonstrated by the asymmetric facing of the palms. The affected palm will face posteriorly, indicating spasm of teres major muscle (Figs. C–F).

Clinical Significance: Rotator cuff weakness or brachial plexus palsy (Erb's palsy), may cause an asymmetric hand position as well.

Follow-up: Perform muscle testing of the teres major muscle or refer the patient for electromyography.

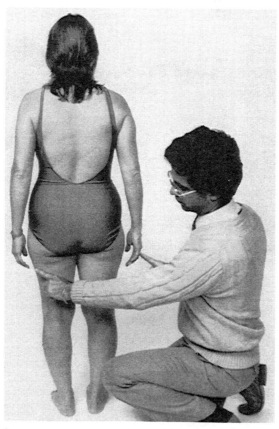

A

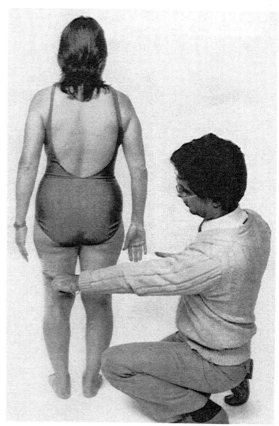

B

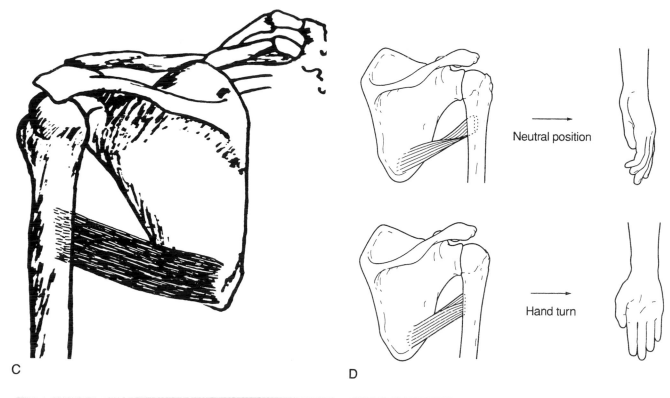

C

D

Neutral position

Hand turn

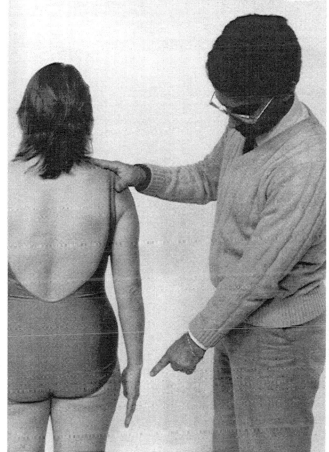

E

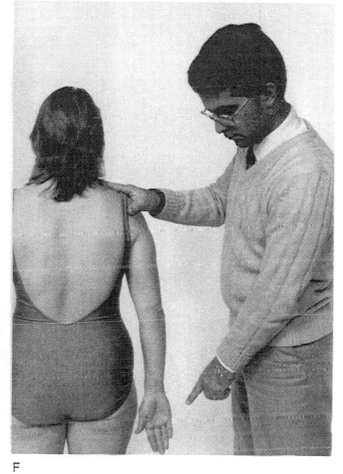

F

27 | Transverse Humeral Ligament Test

Procedure: The patient is seated. Extend the elbow and abduct and internally rotate the arm. Palpate the bicipital groove while externally rotating the arm to check whether the biceps tendon pops or snaps (Figs. A–C).

Rationale: If the transverse humeral ligament is insufficient, this motion will cause a spontaneous dislocation of the biceps tendon from the bicipital groove.

Classical Significance: Popping associated with a palpable dislocation of the tendon is significant for transverse humeral ligament laxity (Fig. D).

Clinical Significance: Pain from the area of palpation without the accompanying pop may indicate tendinitis (Fig. E).

Follow-up: Perform the Gilcrest sign or Yergason's test.

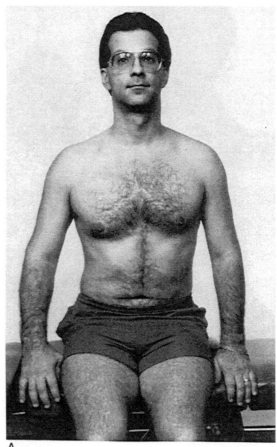

A

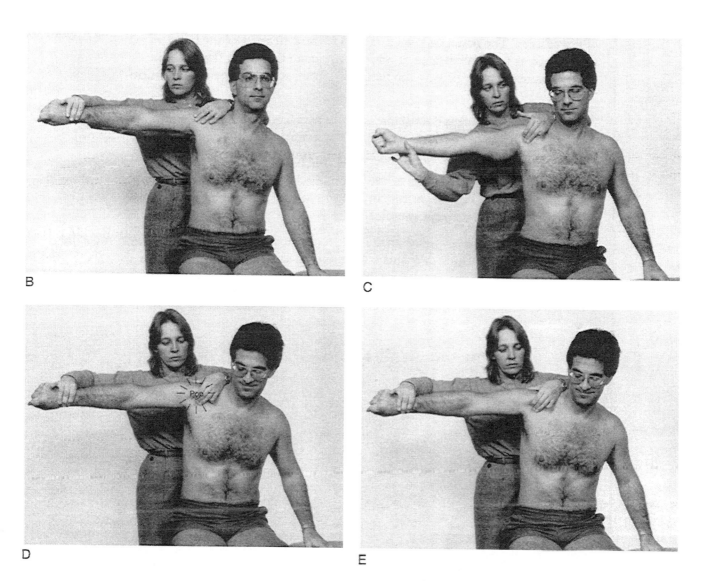

B

C

D

E

28 | *Yergason's Test (Biceps Tendon Stability Test)*

Procedure: The patient is seated with the elbow flexed and the hand pronated. Apply resistance as the patient tries to actively supinate the hand, flex the elbow, and externally rotate the arm. Palpate the bicipital groove while the patient attempts this (Figs. A–D).

Rationale: The biceps is a supinator of the forearm as well as a flexor. The addition of external rotation makes the bicipital groove more vulnerable or accessible to palpation. Resistance against these motions places maximum stress on the tendon.

Classical Significance: Pain at the bicipital groove or the reproduction of a palpable or audible click is significant for subluxation of the biceps tendon or tenosynovitis of the long head of the biceps muscle (Fig. E).

Clinical Significance: This maneuver may cause pain at the elbow and must be further differentiated from tennis elbow (lateral epicondylitis) (Fig. F).

Follow-up: Perform the Ludington test, Speed's test, or the Gilcrest sign.

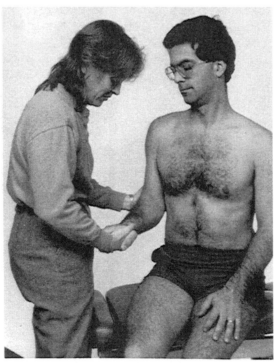

A

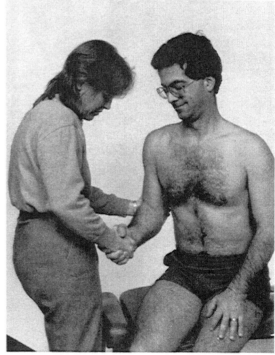

B

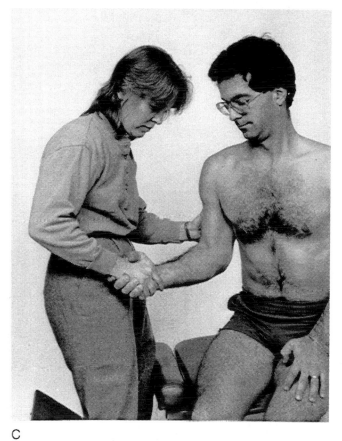

C

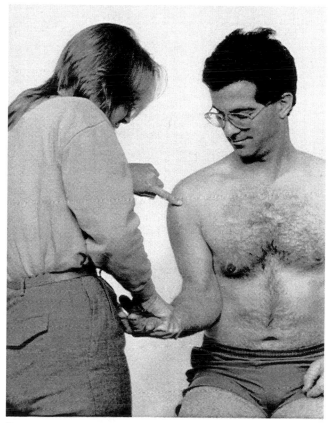

D

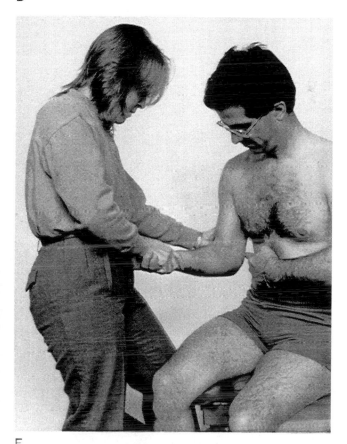

E

F

Elbow Testing

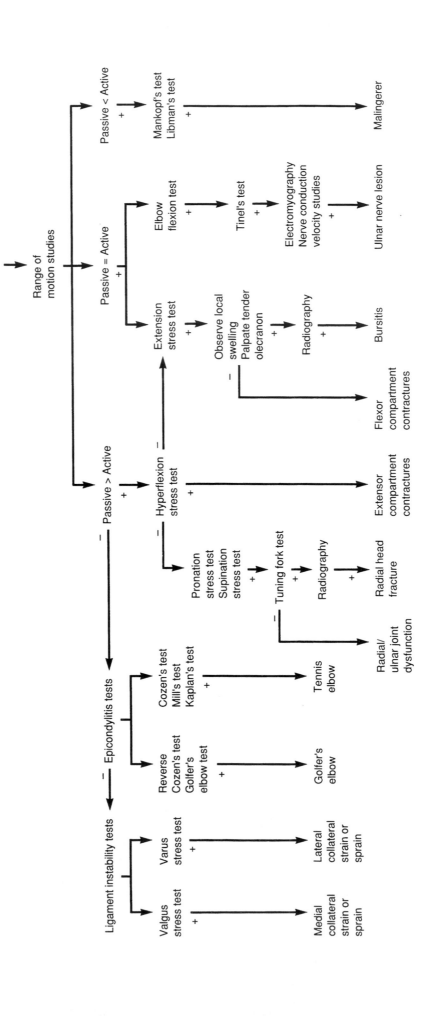

Range of Motion Studies

1

When performing range of motion studies, it is important to use either an arthrodial protractor or an inclinometer. The *American Medical Association Guides for Impairment Ratings* now recommend the use of the inclinometer exclusively. It is our opinion that for elbow mensuration, a good goniometer be used because measuring supination and pronation is difficult with the inclinometer.

Flexion: The patient is standing with the arm next to the body in anatomic position. Ask the patient to bend the elbow and try to touch the ipsilateral shoulder with the fingertips. Normal flexion is 135 to 150 degrees.

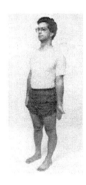 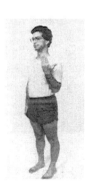 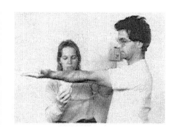 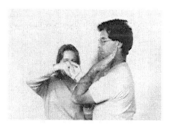

Extension: The patient is standing with the arm next to the body in anatomic position. Ask the patient to straighten the arm out to the maximum that the joint will allow. In females, extra play at the elbow joint may be possible, allowing up to 10 degrees of hyperextension. Most males can extend the elbow to the zero-degree mark. In males with very muscular arms, the biceps tendon does not allow the arm to reach zero degrees. Normal extension is 0 to minus 10 degrees.

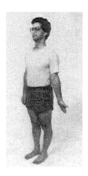 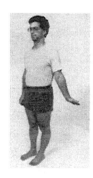 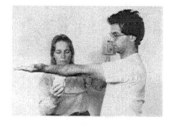

Supination: The patient is seated with the elbow bent about 90 degrees. Ask the patient to rotate the forearm so that the palm faces upward. Normal supination is 90 degrees.

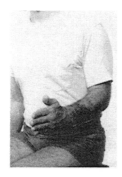 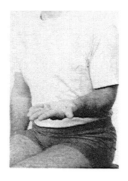 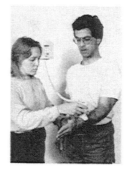 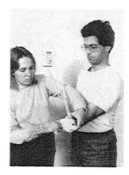

Pronation: The patient is seated with the elbow bent about 90 degrees. Ask the patient to rotate the forearm so that the palm faces downward. Normal pronation is 90 degrees.

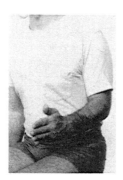 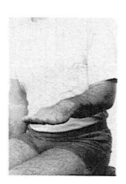 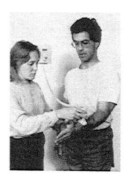 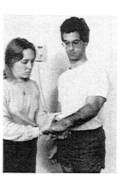

Note: If possible, both elbows should be tested simultaneously for flexion and extension. However, supination and pronation should be tested together in one elbow before testing the opposite since they basically describe one arc of motion.

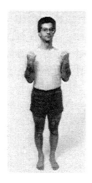 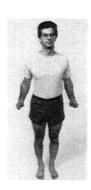 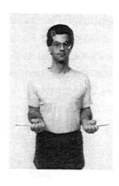 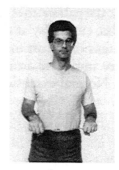

Procedures

2 | *Cozen's Test*

Procedure: The patient is seated with the elbow flexed 90 degrees. Palpate the lateral epicondyle while the patient extends the wrist against your resistance (Figs. A–D).

Rationale: The extensors of the wrist originate at the lateral epicondyle. The resisted action causes stress at the origin of this muscle group.

Classical Significance: Reproduction of pain that is acute and lancinating from the lateral epicondyle indicates lateral epicondylitis (tennis elbow) (Fig. E).

Clinical Significance: Take care to have the hand and elbow stabilized. Pronation of the forearm may cause pain from median nerve entrapment at the elbow. The pain would follow a distinct nerve pathway. The differential diagnosis would be median nerve entrapment (Fig. F).

Follow-up: Perform Mill's test or Kaplan's test or both.

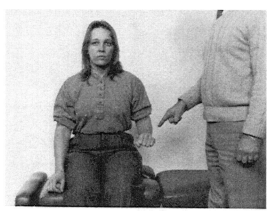

A

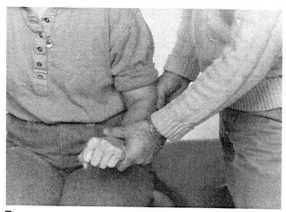

B

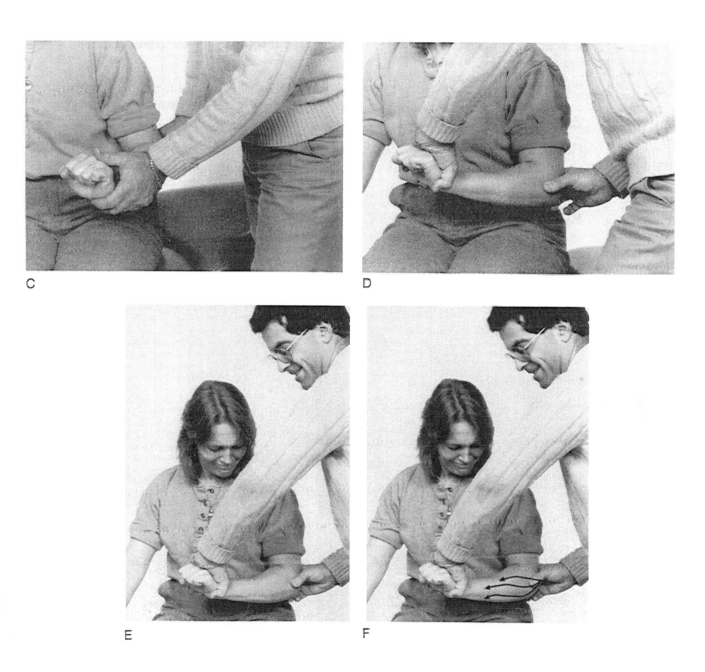

3 | *Elbow Flexion Test*

Procedure: The patient is seated. Ask the patient to fully flex the elbow and mildly flex the wrist and to stay in this position for 5 minutes (Figs. A–C).

Rationale: The ulnar nerve passes through the cubital tunnel formed by the ulnar collateral ligaments and the flexor carpi ulnaris muscle. In full flexion of the elbow along with slight wrist flexion, the ulnar nerve is in full traction.

Classical Significance: Reproduction of an ulnar nerve palsy or dysesthesia along the course of the ulnar nerve is significant for ulnar nerve entrapment (Fig. D).

Clinical Significance: See Classical Significance.

Follow-up: Refer the patient for electromyography of the wrist flexors or perform nerve conduction velocity studies.

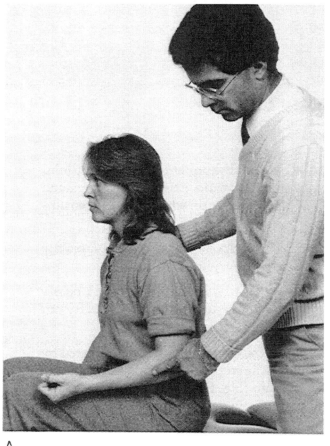

A

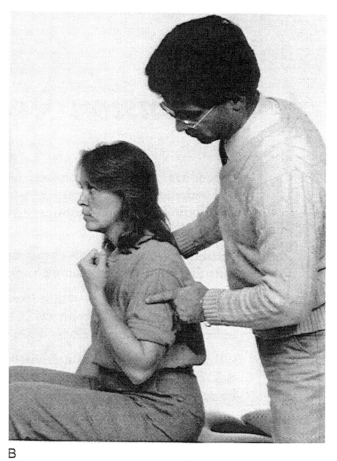

B

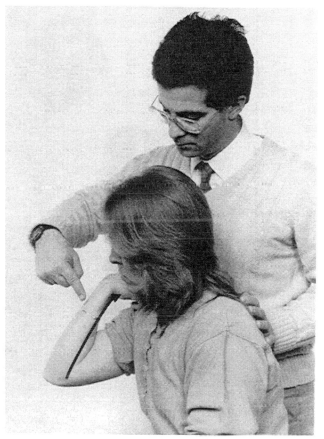

C

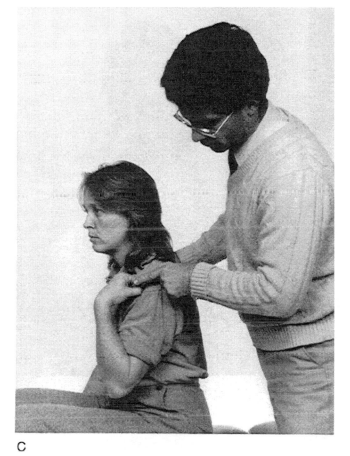

D

4 | *Extension Stress Test*

Procedure: The patient is seated. Grasp the elbow at the posterior aspect of the joint and with the other hand grasp the wrist of the supinated hand. Attempt to hyperextend the elbow by applying pressure from posterior to anterior while the arm remains extended (Figs. A–C).

Rationale: This test stresses many structures in the elbow joint. However, it mainly tests the integrity of the annular ligaments of the elbow joint.

Classical Significance: A decrease or increase in joint motion associated with pain is definitely cause for further investigation. Joint pathology and ligament instability can indicate a tendency for elbow dislocation or tendinitis (Fig. D).

Clinical Significance: Bursal problems within the elbow joint can be provoked by this test. Look for swelling and tenderness around the area of the bursa. Palpation of the bursa without forced extension will also elicit pain (Fig. E).

Follow-up: Perform the valgus and varus stress tests.

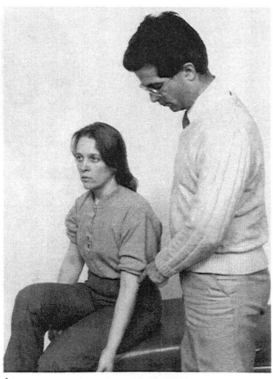

A

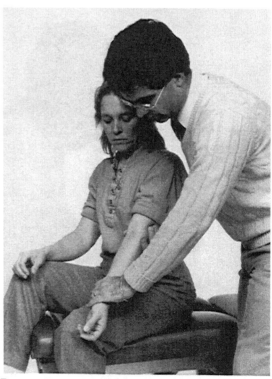

B

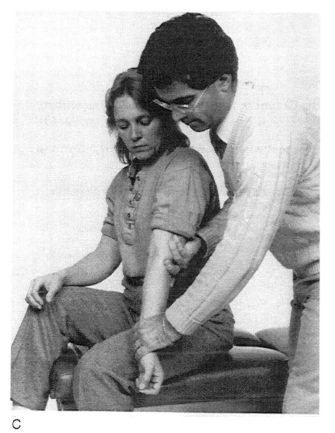

C

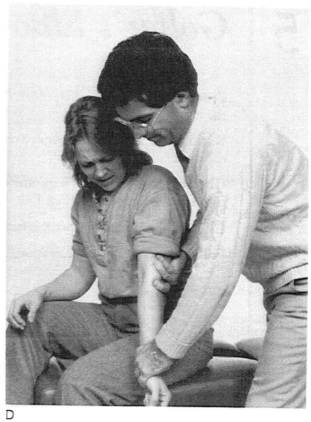

D

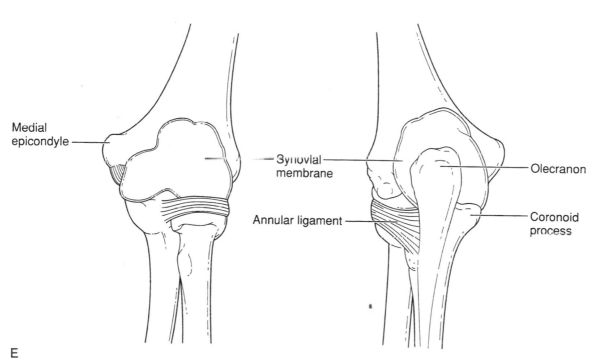

Medial
epicondyle

Synovial
membrane

Annular ligament

Olecranon

Coronoid
process

E

5 | *Golfer's Elbow Test*

Procedure: The patient is seated. Ask the patient to flex the elbow and then supinate the hand. Then apply resistance to the forearm as the patient extends it (Figs. A–D).

Rationale: This test is designed to stress the medial epicondyle, thereby re-creating the pain.

Classical Significance: Reproduction of pain at the medial epicondyle is significant for medial epicondylitis (Fig. E).

Clinical Significance: See Classical Significance.

Follow-up: Perform the reverse Cozen's test.

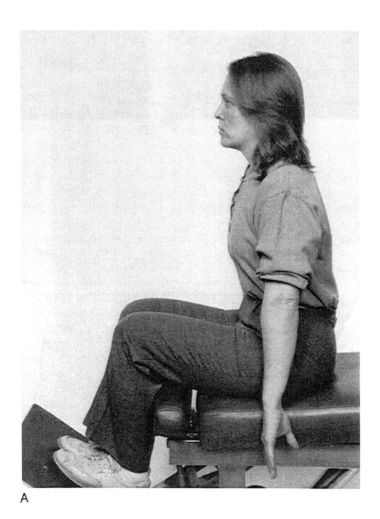

A

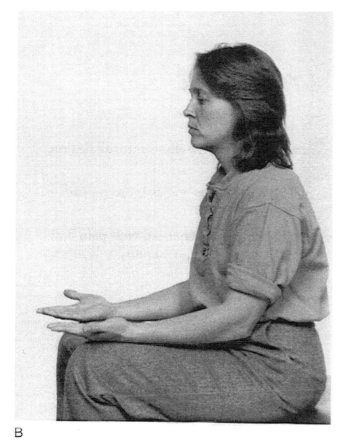

B

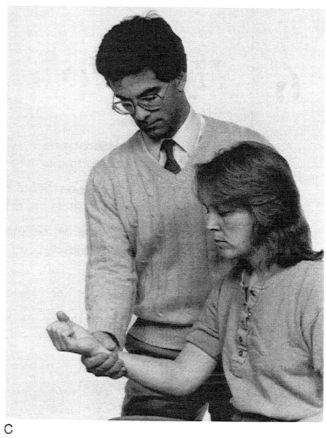

C

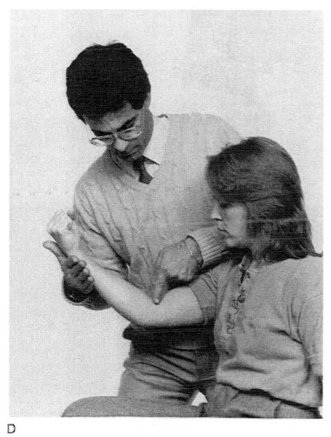

D

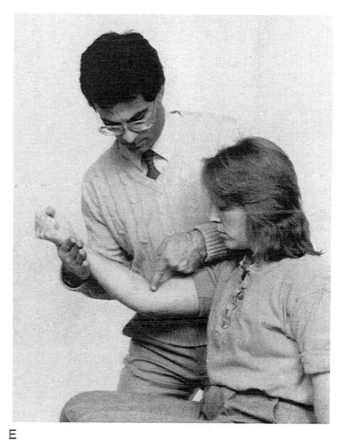

E

6 | *Hyperflexion Stress Test*

Procedure: The patient is seated. Grasp the wrist and force the elbow into full flexion, noting any restrictions in this motion (Figs. A–D).

Rationale: This position causes stress on many structures and is more limited in capsular patterns of dysfunction than any other motion.

Classical Significance: A decrease or increase of motion associated with pain indicates joint pathology, muscle contracture of the posterior arm, tendinitis, or ligament strain (Fig. E).

Clinical Significance: See Classical Significance.

Follow-up: Perform the valgus and varus stress tests or the extension stress test.

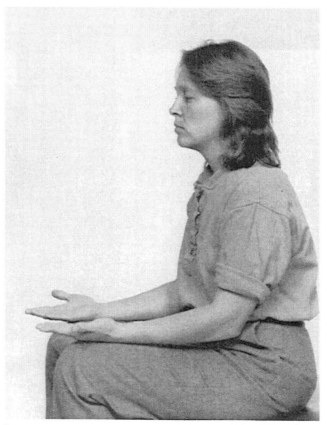

A

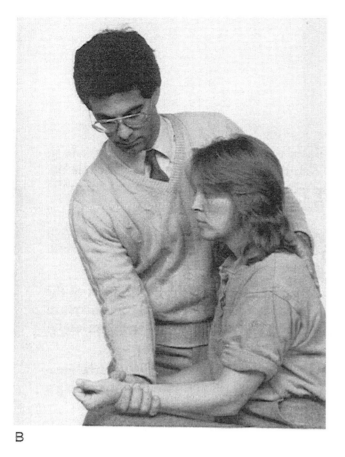

B

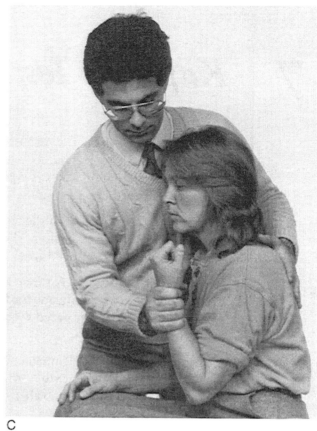

C

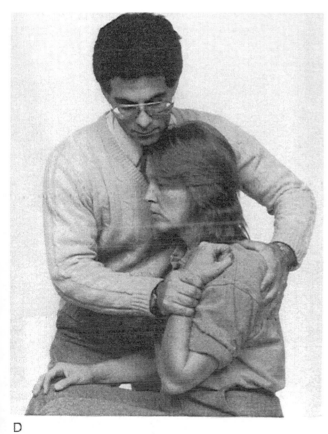

D

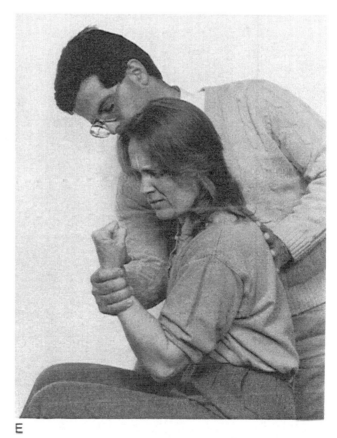

E

7 | *Kaplan's Test*

Procedure: The patient is seated with the arm fully extended and the wrist held in mild extension. Use a dynamometer to record the grip strength. Next, encircle the forearm approximately 2 inches below the elbow joint and have the patient repeat the maneuver. Record this grip strength (Figs. A–D).

Rationale: The first part of the test measures the baseline strength of the wrist when stressed in maximum extension. The second part of the test measures the grip strength when the tension is removed from the lateral epicondyle.

Classical Significance: An increase in dynamometer strength with support of the extensor tendons is significant for lateral epicondylitis. A decrease in the amount of pain with support as compared with no support is also significant for lateral epicondylitis (Fig. E).

Clinical Significance: If median nerve entrapment at the elbow is present, the pressure used to support the extensor tendons may aggravate this entrapment, causing a decrease in grip strength as well as paresthesia (Fig. F).

Follow-up: Perform Cozen's test or Mill's test.

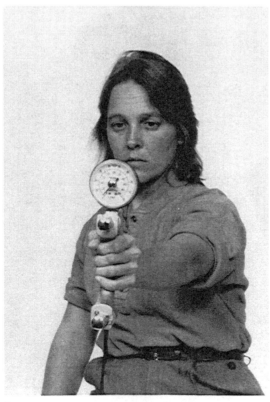

A

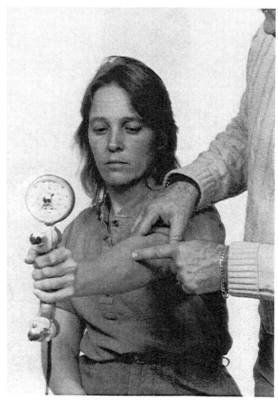

B

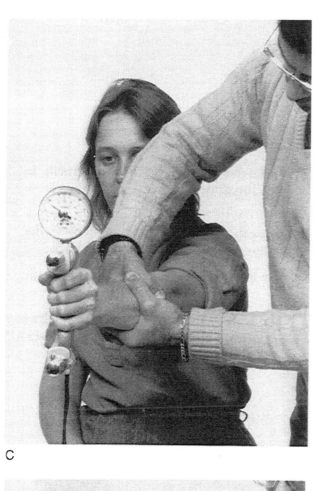

C

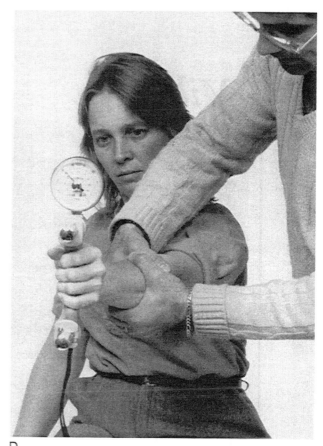

D

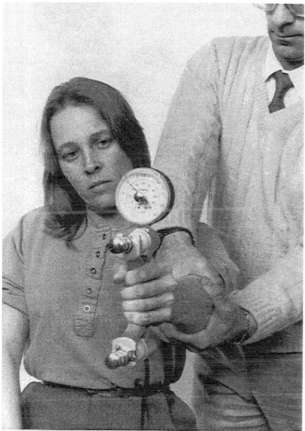

E

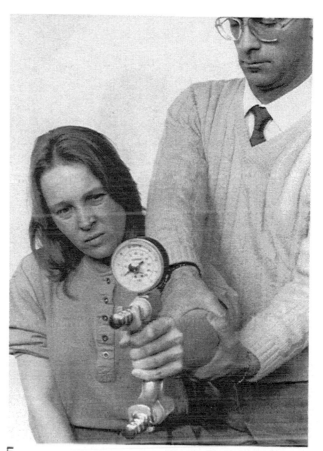

F

8 | *Mill's Test*

Procedure: The patient is seated. Palpate the lateral epicondyle while the patient, in one fluid motion, flexes the wrist, pronates the forearm, and then extends the elbow (Figs. A–E).

Rationale: Pronation and wrist flexion causes the greatest amount of stress at the lateral epicondyle.

Classical Significance: Reproduction of pain at the lateral epicondyle is significant for lateral epicondylitis (Fig. F).

Clinical Significance: This position may also create pain and paresthesia as a result of median nerve entrapment from the pronator muscles, which contract in this maneuver.

Follow-up: Perform Cozen's test or Kaplan's test.

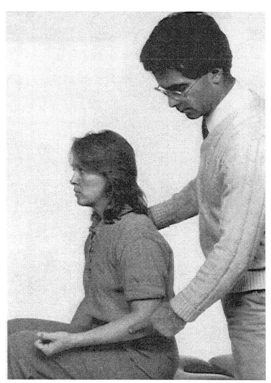

A

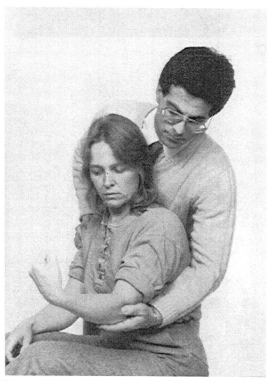

B

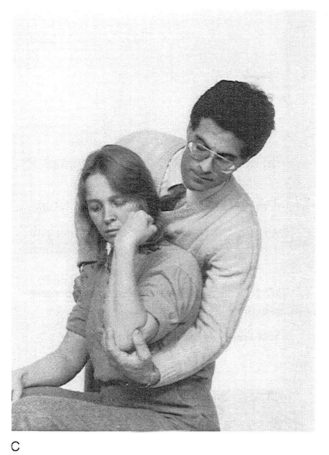

C

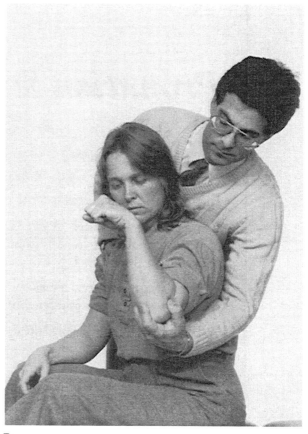

D

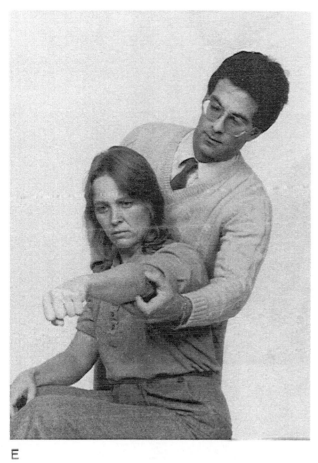

E

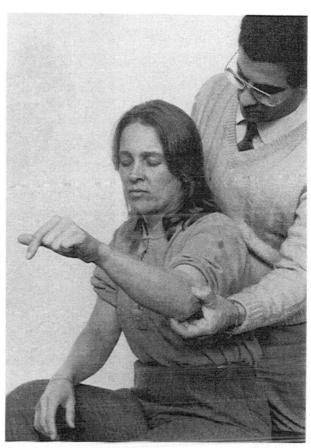

F

9 | *Pronation Stress Test*

Procedure: The patient is seated. Grasp the forearm at the wrist and attempt to pronate it excessively (Figs. A–D).

Rationale: This test stresses the integrity of the osseous and ligamentous structures.

Classical Significance: A decrease or increase in the motion associated with pain indicates radial/ulnar joint dysfunction, because this maneuver requires the radial head to rotate on the ulnar (Fig. E).

Clinical Significance: Pronator teres/quadratus entrapment of the median interosseous nerve may be simulated by this maneuver.

Follow-up: Perform Tinel's test, Phalen's test (see Ch. 6), or Kaplan's test.

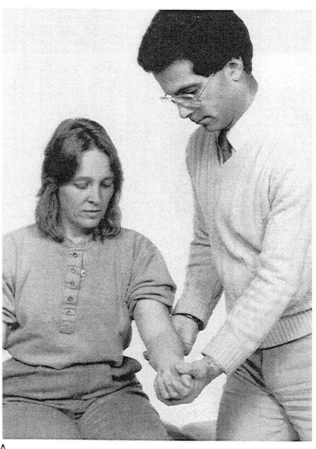

A

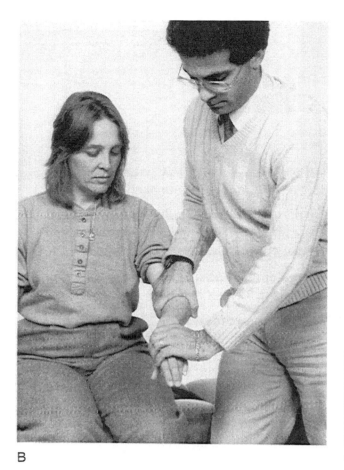

B

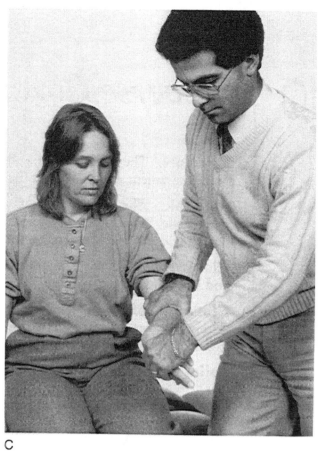

C

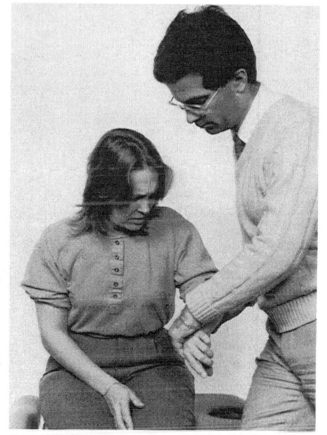

D

E

10 | *Reverse Cozen's Test*

Procedure: The patient is seated. Palpate the medial epicondyle. Continue palpating while the patient attempts to flex the wrist against resistance of your hand (Figs. A – C).

Rationale: The wrist flexors as well as the pronators originate from the medial epicondyle. Resisted action of either of these muscle groups puts stress at the medial epicondyle and will create or aggravate medial epicondylitis and cause pain.

Classical Significance: Reproduction of pain at the medial epicondyle that is acute and lancinating indicates medial epicondylitis (Fig. D).

Clinical Significance: As with other testing, take care to stabilize the elbow. Otherwise, excessive pronation may aggravate entrapment syndromes related to the pronator group at the elbow.

Follow-up: Perform the golfer's elbow test.

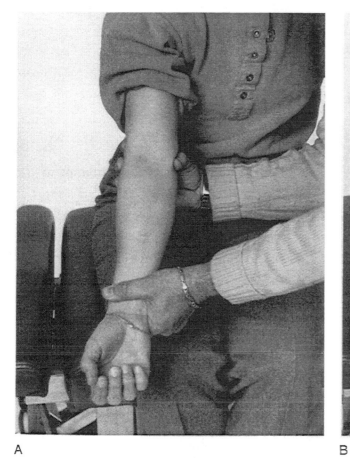

A

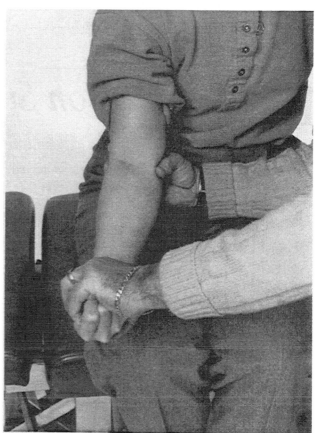

B

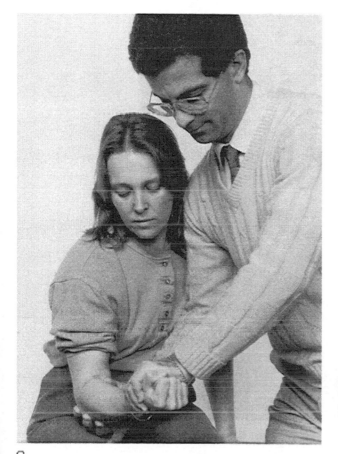

C

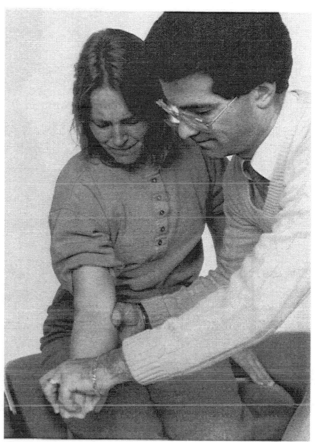

D

11 | *Supination Stress Test*

Procedure: The patient is seated. Grasp the forearm at the wrist and attempt to forcefully supinate it (Figs. A–C).

Rationale: This test stresses the integrity of the elbow joint inclusive of the osseous and ligamentous structures.

Classical Significance: Limitation and pain on this motion indicates a joint dysfunction, which should be further investigated (Fig. D).

Clinical Significance: In the case of radial head fracture (Little Leaguer's elbow), this maneuver will exacerbate pain (Fig. E: multiple fractures; 1, neck of radius; 2, head of radius).

Follow-up: Perform the tuning fork test or radiography.

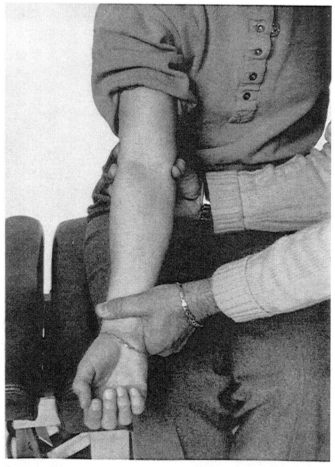

A

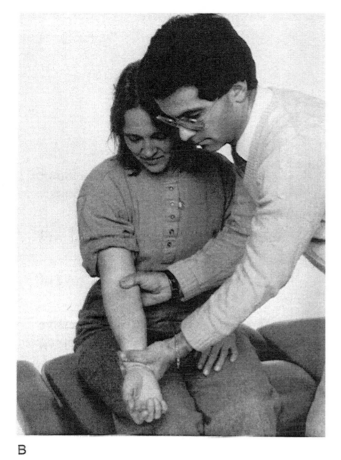

B

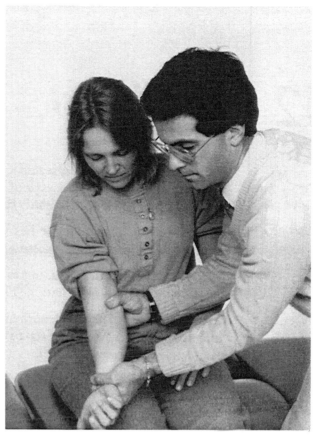

C

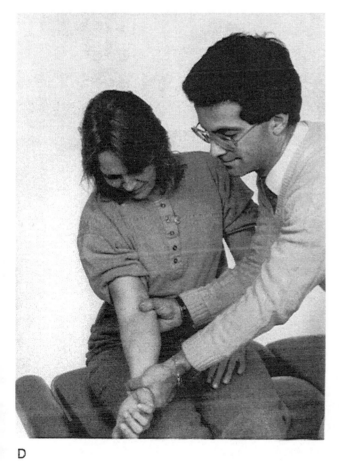

D

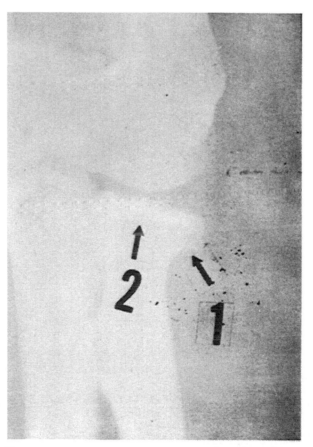

E

12 | *Tinel's Test*

Procedure: The patient is seated. Grasp the patient's arm and strike the groove found between the olecranon process and the medial epicondyle with a neurologic hammer. Be careful not to strike too hard (Figs. A–C).

Rationale: The ulnar nerve lies very superficial at this point and if irritated will produce a tingling along its distribution.

Classical Significance: An increase in tingling distal to the tapping is indicative of ulnar nerve neuritis or irritation (Figs. D & E).

Clinical Significance: In normal individuals, tapping at this level with excessive force may result in tingling distal to the nerve along its pathway. Also, repeated tapping can damage the nerve (Fig. F).

Follow-up: Perform the palm sweeping test, Froment's cone test, or the needle threading pinch test (see Ch. 6 for all three).

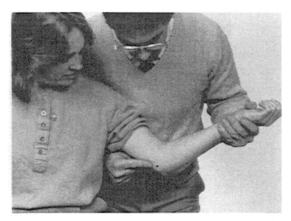

A

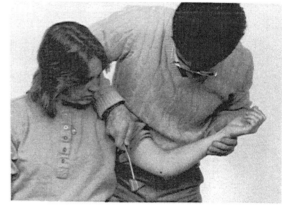

B

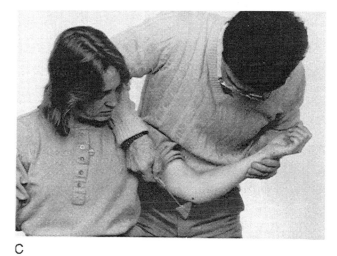

C

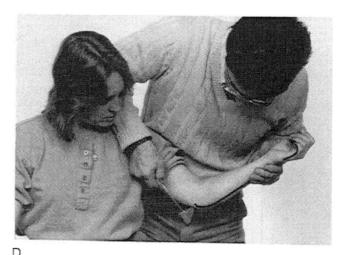

D

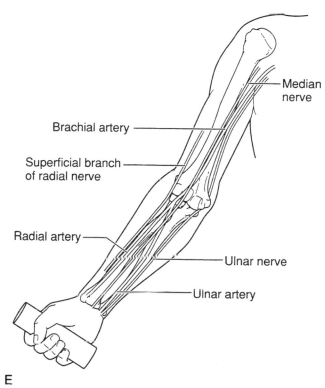

E

Median
nerve

Brachial artery

Superficial branch
of radial nerve

Radial artery

Ulnar nerve

Ulnar artery

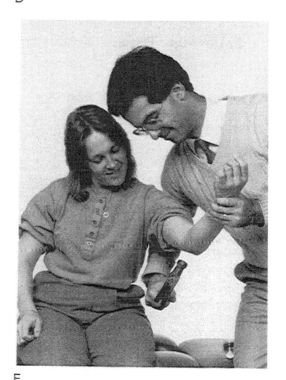

F

13 | *Valgus Stress Test (Abduction Stress Test)*

Procedure: The patient is seated with the arm out in front of the body. Stabilize the upper arm while grasping the forearm and pulling away from the body. This places a valgus stress at the elbow (Figs. A–C).

Rationale: This tests for stability of the medial collateral ligament of the elbow joint. Note any excessive play and compare with the other elbow.

Classical Significance: Medial collateral ligament laxity is a positive result. An increase in pain at the elbow should be compared with the other side as a lesion may be present within the elbow itself (Fig. D).

Clinical Significance: An increase in pain on the lateral side of the elbow may be due to compression of the radial head into the capitellum or to irritation of the lateral epicondyle (Fig. E).

Follow-up: Perform the varus stress test, Cozen's test, or Mill's test.

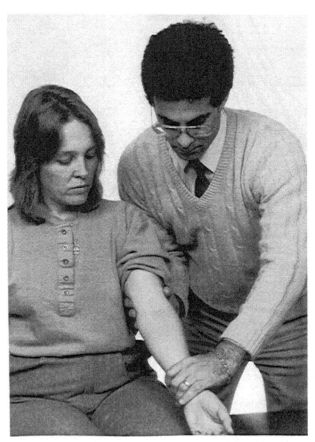

A

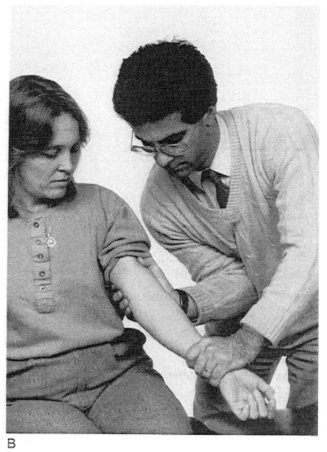

B

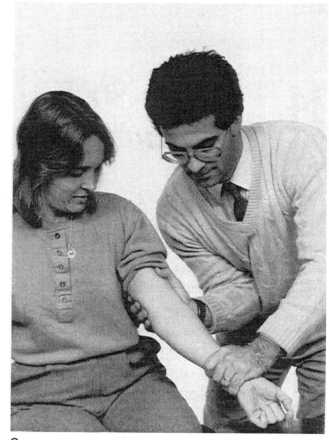

C

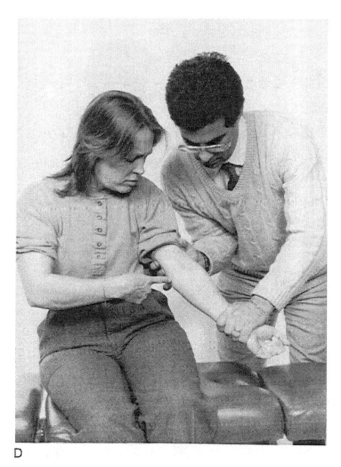

D

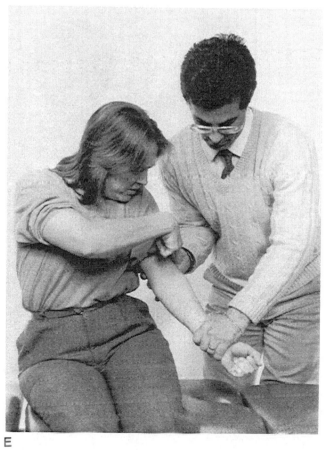

E

14 | *Varus Stress Test (Adduction Stress Test)*

Procedure: The patient is seated with the arm out in front of the body. Stabilize the upper arm while grasping the forearm and pushing into the body. This places a varus stress at the elbow (Figs. A–D).

Rationale: This tests for stability of the lateral collateral ligament of the elbow joint. Note any excessive play and compare with the other elbow.

Classical Significance: Lateral collateral ligament laxity is a positive result. An increase in pain at the elbow should be compared with the other side as a lesion may be within the elbow itself (Fig. E).

Clinical Significance: An increase in pain on the medial side of the elbow may be due to inflammation within the olecranon fossa (Fig. F).

Follow-up: Perform the valgus stress test, Cozen's test, or Mill's test.

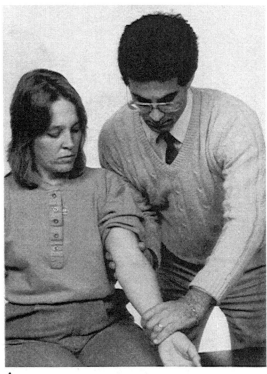

A

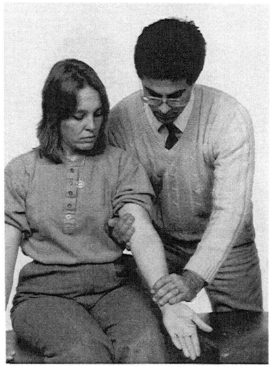

B

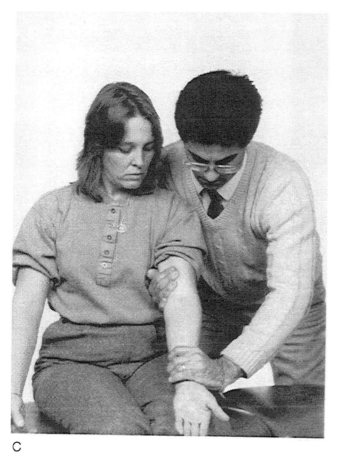

C

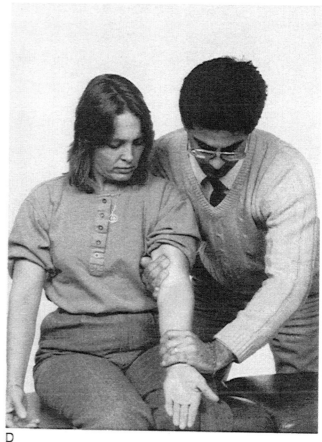

D

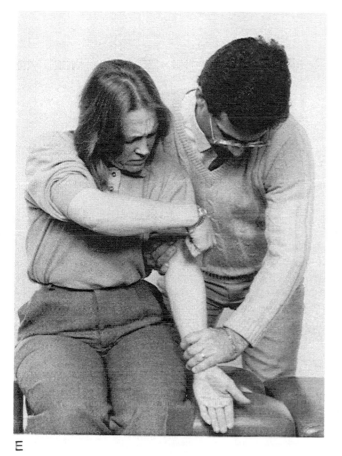

E

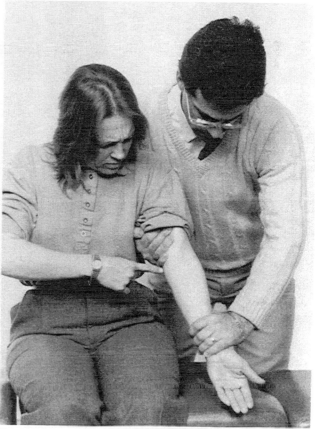

F

Wrist and Hand Testing

1. Wrist Range of Motion Studies
2. Hand Range of Motion Studies
3. Allen's Test
4. Bracelet Test
5. Bunnel-Littler Test
6. Dellon's Two Point Discrimination Test
7. Desk Scratching Test
8. Extension Stress Test
9. Finkelstein's Test
10. Finsterer's Test
11. Fist Making Test
12. Flexion Stress Test
13. Froment's Cone Test
14. Froment's Sign
15. Index Extension Test
16. Maisonneuve's Test
17. Needle Threading Pinch Test
18. Oschner's Test
19. Palm Sweeping Test
20. Phalen's Test
21. Pinch Grip Test
22. Pronation Test
23. Radial Stress Test
24. Resisted Passive Supination Test
25. Supination Test
26. Thumb and Index Circle Test
27. Thumb Joint Extension Test
28. Thumb Tip to Fingertips Test
29. Tinel's Test
30. Ulnar Stress Test
31. Wartenburg's Oriental Prayer Sign
32. Weber Two Point Discrimination Test
33. Wrinkle Shrivel Test
34. Wrist Drop Test
35. Wrist Extension Test
36. Wrist Flexion Test

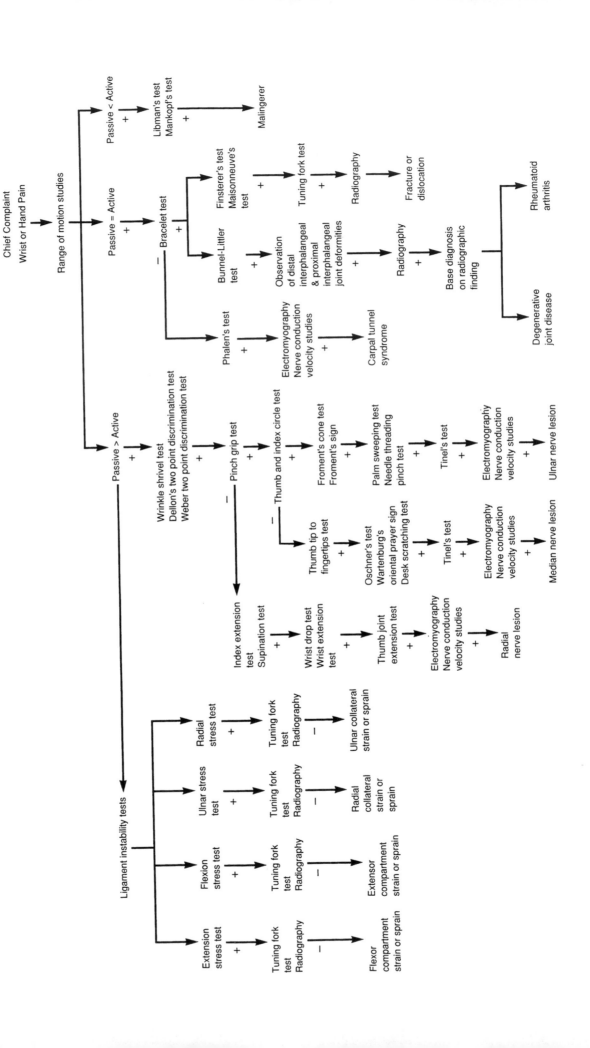

1 | *Wrist Range of Motion Studies*

When performing range of motion studies, it is important to use either an arthrodial protractor or an inclinometer. The *American Medical Association Guides for Impairment Ratings* now recommend the use of the inclinometer exclusively. The patient is seated throughout this examination, the elbow is flexed 90 degrees and held into the waist, and the hand is supinated when testing radial and ulnar deviation. Test the most painful ranges of motion last.

Pronation and Supination: Ask the patient to make a closed fist around a pencil with the pencil pointing up. Then ask the patient to pronate the wrist as far as possible and then to supinate it as far as possible. Use the pencil as the reference point as if it is going around an arc. These two motions should be performed as one test because they are one arc of motion. Normal pronation and supination are each 85 to 90 degrees; the combined total is normally 170 to 180 degrees.

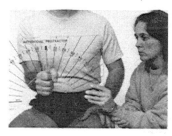 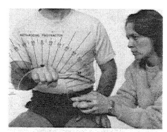 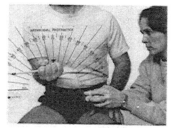

Flexion and Extension: Ask the patient to hold the hand out palm down and to flex the wrist as far as possible. Then ask the patient to extend the wrist as far as possible. Normal flexion is 80 to 90 degrees; normal extension is 70 to 90 degrees.

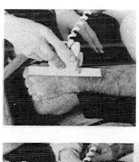 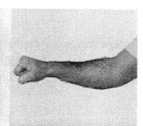 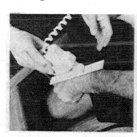 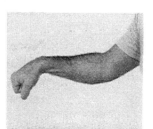

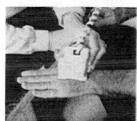 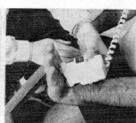 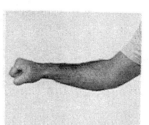 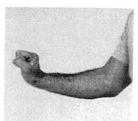

Radial Deviation: Ask the patient to hold the hand in supination (palm upward) and to force the wrist in the direction of the thumb. Normal radial deviation is 15 to 20 degrees.

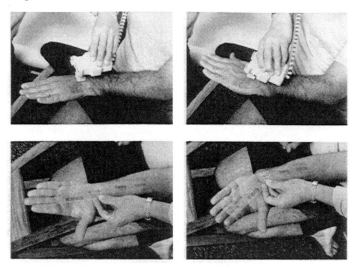

Ulnar Deviation: Ask the patient to hold the hand in supination (palm upward) and to force the wrist in the direction of the fifth digit. Normal ulnar deviation is 30 to 45 degrees.

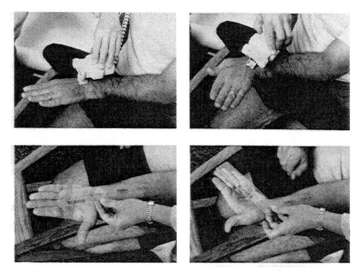

Note: Active ranges of motion of the wrist can be affected by neurologic problems, as well as by contractile ones, such as median nerve entrapment, tenosynovitis, ganglionic cyst, and collagen disease. Therefore, a comparison with the opposite side is very important.

2 | Hand Range of Motion Studies

When performing range of motion studies, it is important to use either an arthrodial protractor or an inclinometer. The *American Medical Association Guides for Impairment Ratings* now recommend the use of the inclinometer exclusively. It is our opinion that a good goniometer be used for hand mensuration, because it is difficult to use an inclinometer when testing the small joints of the hand. The hand ranges of motion are divided into three compartments: (1) the metacarpophalangeal (MCP) joint, (2) the proximal interphalangeal (PIP) joint, and (3) the distal interphalangeal (DIP) joint. The thumb is tested separately.

Metacarpophalangeal Joint

Flexion: Stabilize the patient's hand at the carpal joint and MCP joint so the patient cannot recruit the wrist. Ask the patient to bend the fingers at the MCP joint down while keeping the rest of the fingers straight. Normal flexion is 75 to 90 degrees.

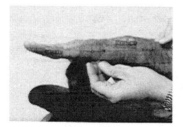 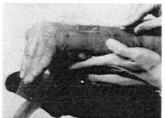

Extension: Stabilize the patient's hand at the carpal joint and MCP joint so the patient cannot recruit the wrist. Ask the patient to bend the fingers at the MCP joint backward as far as possible while keeping the rest of the fingers straight. Normal extension is 20 to 30 degrees.

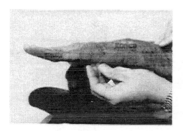 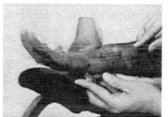

Abduction: Ask the patient to place the hand out in front of the body and to spread the fingers as wide as possible. Observe the spacing between each finger; it should be fairly equal, as measured from the third digit. Normal abduction is 20 degrees.

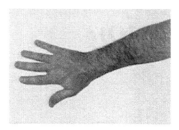 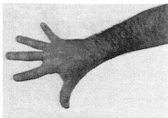

Adduction: Ask the patient to place the hand out in front of the body and to approximate the fingers so they all touch side to side. Normal adduction is 0 degrees.

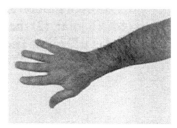 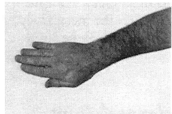

Proximal Interphalangeal Joint

Flexion: Ask the patient to place the hand out in front of the body. Stabilize one MCP joint and ask the patient to flex that finger as far as possible. Test each finger separately. Normal flexion is 90 to 100 degrees.

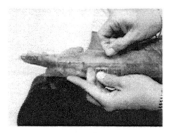 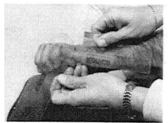

Extension: Ask the patient to place the hand out in front of the body. Stabilize one MCP joint. Ask the patient to extend that finger as far back as possible. Test each finger separately. Normal extension is 0 to 5 degrees.

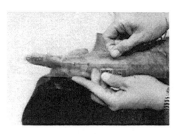 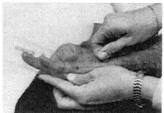

Distal Interphalangeal Joint

Flexion: Ask the patient to place the hand out in front of the body. Stabilize each PIP joint. Ask the patient to flex the most distal joint in each finger. Normal flexion is 60 to 70 degrees.

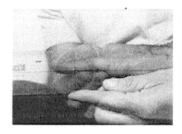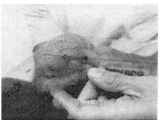

Extension: Ask the patient to place the hand out in front of the body. Stabilize each PIP joint. Ask the patient to extend as far as possible the most distal joint in each finger. Normal extension is 0 to 5 degrees.

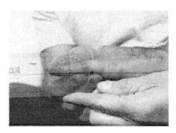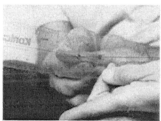

Thumb Metacarpophalangeal Joint

Flexion: This is also known as transpalmar abduction. Ask the patient to bring the thumb tip toward the base of the fifth MCP joint. Normal flexion is 40 to 50 degrees.

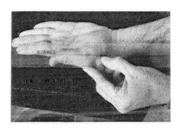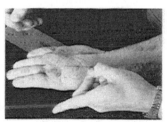

Extension: This is also known as radial abduction. Ask the patient to bring the thumb out as far as possible in the horizontal plane. Normal extension is 80 to 90 degrees.

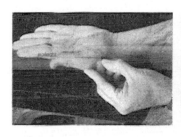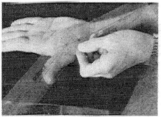

Thumb Interphalangeal Joint

Flexion: Stabilize the MCP joint while the patient fully flexes the remaining part of the digit. Normal flexion is 80 to 90 degrees.

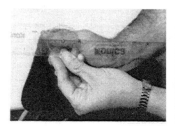 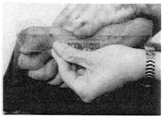

Extension: Stabilize the MCP joint while the patient fully extends the remaining part of the digit. Normal extension is 10 to 20 degrees.

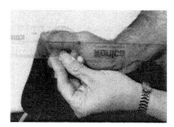 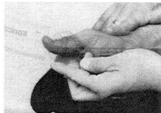

Palmar Abduction

Ask the patient to move the thumb as a unit vertically away from the palm as far as possible. Normal palmar abduction is 70 degrees.

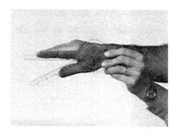 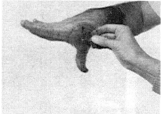

Palmar Adduction

Ask the patient to move the thumb as a unit back to the palm of the hand. Normal palmar adduction is 0 degrees.

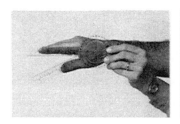 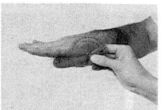

Finger Opposition

Ask the patient to touch the tip of the thumb to the tip of each of the other fingers. No measurement is taken. Observe the relative ease with which the patient is able to perform this test.

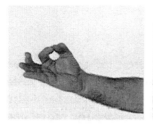 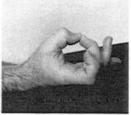 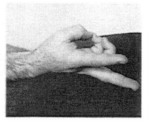 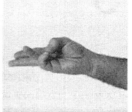

3 | *Allen's Test*

Procedure: The patient is seated with the arm abducted 160 to 180 degrees. Ask the patient to pump the hand into a fist three times and on the third time to sustain the fist. Lower the patient's arm below heart level while occluding the radial and ulnar arteries. Release the ulnar compression. Repeat the above and release the radial compression. Continue testing by comparing with the opposite arm (Figs. A–F).

Rationale: Always perform this test when the patient has a history of pain or dysesthesia within the wrist. Not all dysesthesia is due to nerve compression; the patient's complaint may have a vascular component.

Classical Significance: Normally the hand should fill with blood within 10 seconds. If not, suspect a thrombus within the vessel tested.

Clinical Significance: Compression may be present anywhere along the distribution of the axillary-brachial-radial-ulnar vessel.

Follow-up: Refer the patient for plethysmography or arteriography.

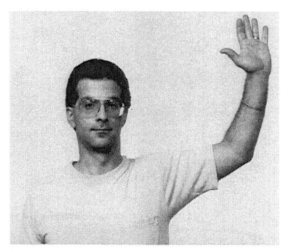

A

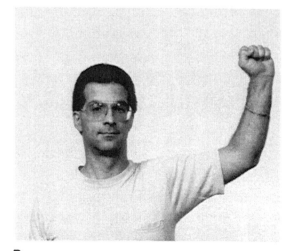

B

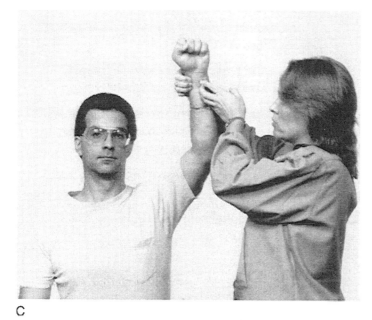

C

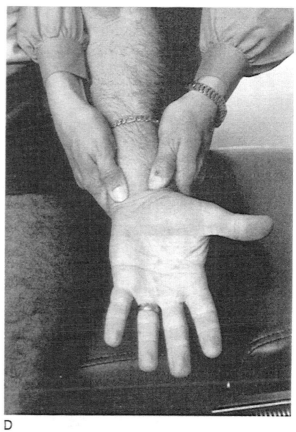

D

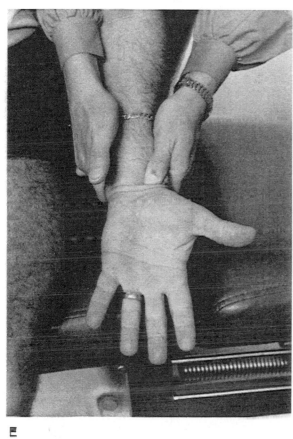

E

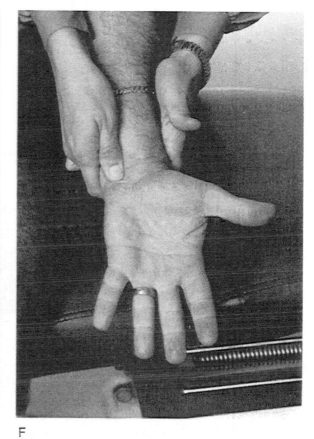

F

4 | *Bracelet Test*

Procedure: The patient is seated with the hand supinated. Grasp the most distal end of the radius and ulnar bones and compress them (Figs. A–C).

Rationale: This test produces direct pressure at the wrist and forearm. If the patient has acute arthritis, pain associated with the inflammation will be produced.

Classical Significance: Reproduction of pain in the forearm, wrist, and hand is significant for rheumatoid arthritis (Figs. D & E [E: advanced rheumatoid arthritis; 1, gross loss of interarticular spaces with subluxations; 2, advanced osteoporosis]).

Clinical Significance: Also, pain will occur with this compressive maneuver, if the patient has a carpal tunnel or ganglionic cyst (Fig. F).

Follow-up: Perform Phalen's test, Tinel's test, or Finkelstein's test.

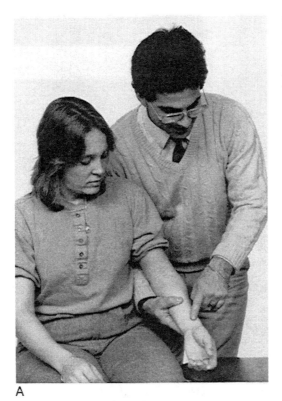

A

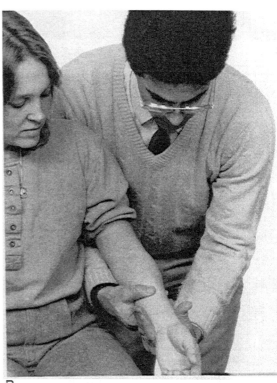

B

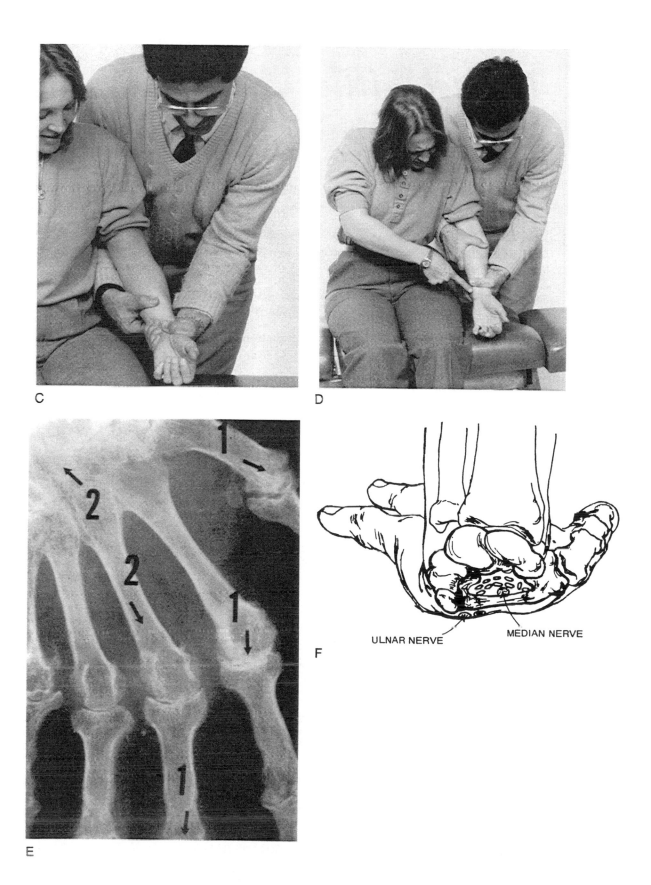

C

D

E

ULNAR NERVE   MEDIAN NERVE

F

5 | *Bunnel-Littler Test*

Procedure: The patient is seated. Perform the following two-stage procedure: (1) slightly extend the patient's metacarpophalangeal (MCP) joint, and then attempt to flex the proximal interphalangeal (PIP) joint. (2) Flex the MCP joint and attempt to fully flex the PIP joint. Record the patient's responses (Figs. A–E).

Rationale: If, with the MCP joint extended, the patient is unable to fully flex the joint, the intrinsic muscles or the joint capsule is tight. If, with the MCP joint flexed the PIP joint can be flexed to a fuller degree, the intrinsic muscles are tight.

Classical Significance: If the same amount of restriction is met when performing both aspects of this test then a joint capsule is tight.

Clinical Significance: Comparative restriction with and without extension and flexion indicates a tight capsule. The intrinsics are at fault if the degree of flexion at the PIP joint changes.

Follow-up: Perform individual muscle tests for the C8 and T1 nerve roots.

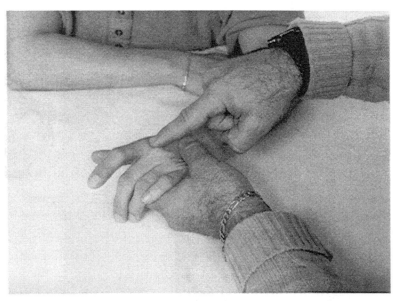

A

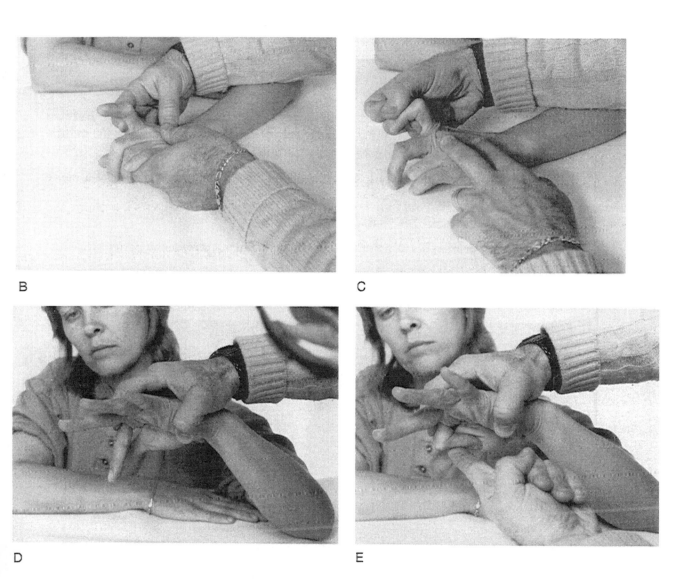

B

C

D

E

6 | *Dellon's Two Point Discrimination Test*

Procedure: The patient is seated with the palm supinated. Using two blunt points, touch the patient's palm or digits from the proximal to the distal axis. Randomly touch the patient with either one or two points. Decrease the distance between the points until the patient distinguishes only one point when two are used (Figs. A–F).

Rationale: If sensation in the extremity is normal, distinction between one and two points will be possible. The normal distance for the distal digit is 4 mm; for the middle digit, 6 mm; and for the palm, 5 to 8 mm (± 2 mm).

Classical Significance: Early loss of two point discrimination is a sign of a nerve lesion.

Clinical Significance: See Classical Significance.

Follow-up: Perform nerve conduction velocity studies, or refer the patient for electromyography.

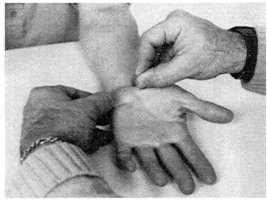

A

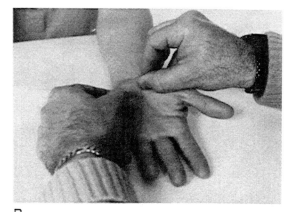

B

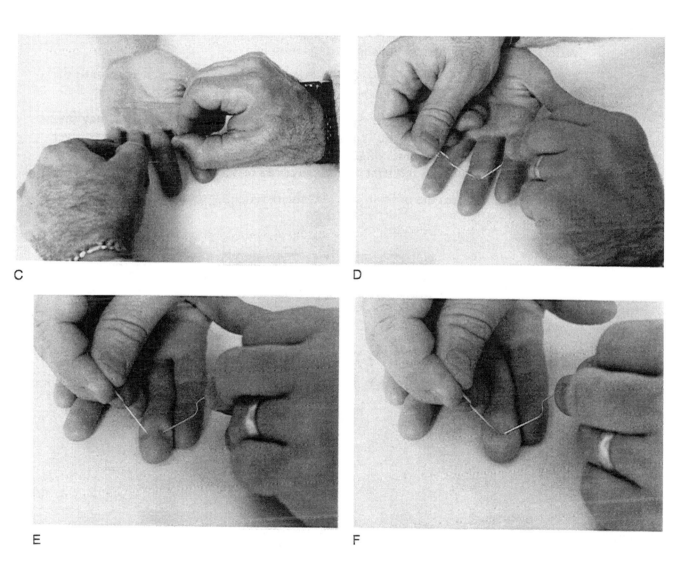

C

D

E

F

7 | *Desk Scratching Test*

Procedure: The patient is seated with the forearm pronated and lying on a flat surface. Ask the patient to scratch the surface with the index finger (Figs. A–C).

Rationale: This test requires normal functioning of the median nerve with its innervation into the flexor digitorum superficialis muscle.

Classical Significance: Inability to perform this maneuver indicates a lesion to the median nerve. The lesion is probably at the elbow (Fig. D).

Clinical Significance: Patients with rheumatoid arthritis or osteoarthritis may find this test painful or difficult to do. However, they will be able to attempt this maneuver since the median nerve is intact (Fig. E: advanced rheumatoid arthritis; 1, gross loss of interarticular spaces with subluxations; 2, advanced osteoporosis).

Follow-up: Perform the pronation test or the fist making test.

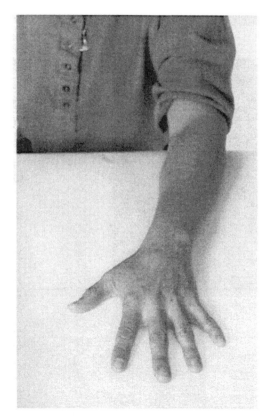

A

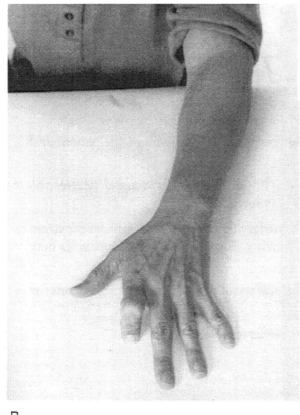

B

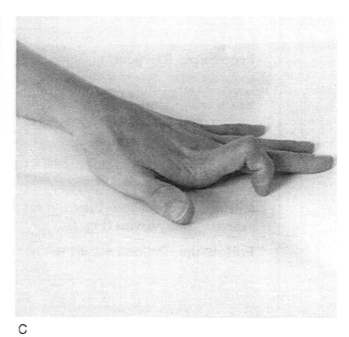

C

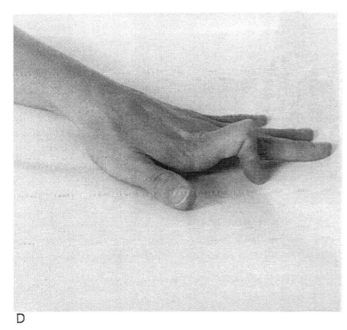

D

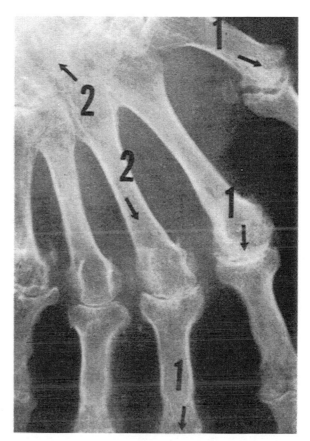

E

8 | *Extension Stress Test*

Procedure: The patient is seated. Oppose your palm to the palm of the patient and force the wrist into extension (Figs. A & B).

Rationale: This test compresses the wrist joint at its dorsal aspect and stresses the flexor compartment and ligaments of the volar surface.

Classical Significance: Pain over the volar surface of the wrist is significant for strain of the wrist flexors or sprain of the wrist ligaments (Fig. C). Pain with dysesthesia may represent carpal tunnel syndrome (Fig. D).

Clinical Significance: Pain over the dorsal surface of the joint may be significant for extensor tenosynovitis (Fig. E).

Follow-up: Perform muscle testing or Kaplan's test (see Ch. 5).

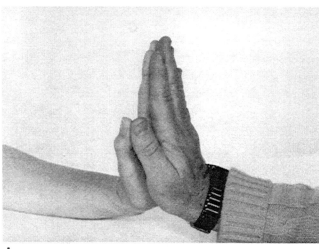

A

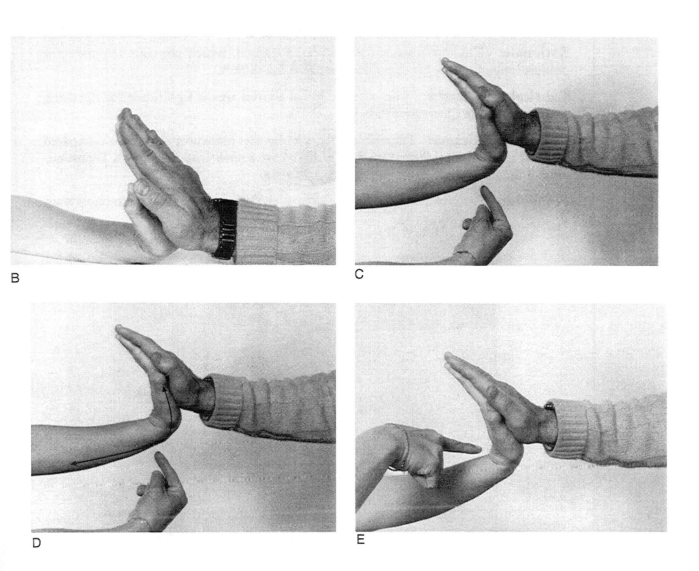

B

C

D

E

9 | *Finkelstein's Test*

Procedure: The patient is seated with the hand pronated. Instruct the patient to make a fist with the thumb tucked inside the other fingers. Then stabilize the forearm and gently force the wrist into ulnar deviation (Figs. A–D).

Rationale: This test stresses the first carpal tunnel, which contains the abductor pollicis longus and extensor pollicis brevis of the thumb.

Classical Significance: Pain over the radial styloid area is significant for stenosing tenosynovitis (de Quervain's disease) (Fig. E).

Clinical Significance: The pain reproduced by this maneuver should be compared with the uninvolved side because some people have a sensitivity to this test. Tenosynovitis of the thumb is known as Hoffman's disease.

Follow-up: Perform Tinel's test or the extension, flexion, radial, and ulnar stress tests.

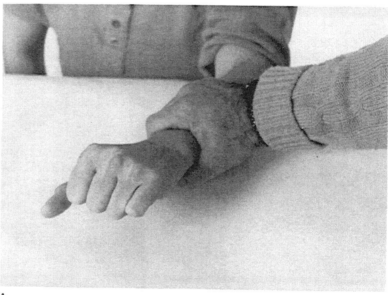

A

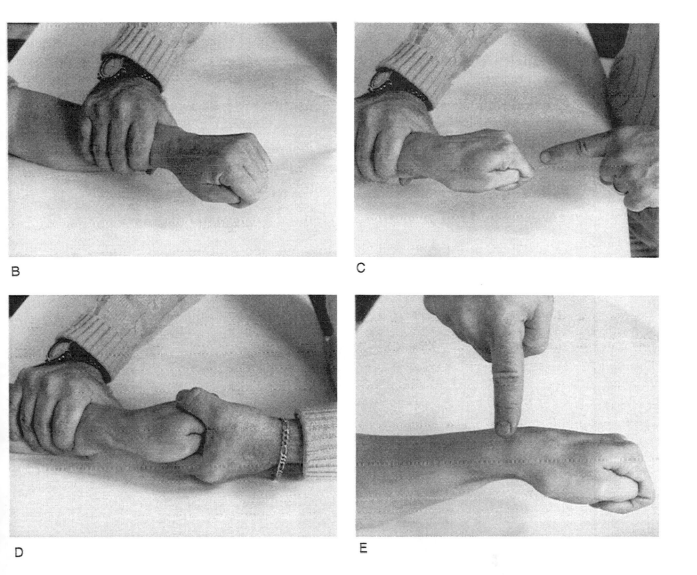

B

C

D

E

10 | *Finsterer's Test*

Procedure: The patient is seated with the hand pronated and in a fist. Observe the hand for the normal prominence of the third metacarpal. Further, strike the area of the third metacarpal just distal to the center of the wrist and record the patient's response (Figs. A–D).

Rationale: The third metacarpal is the most prominent bony landmark on the dorsum of the hand. It should not be tender to percussion.

Classical Significance: Absence of a prominent third metacarpal or the elicitation of pain on percussion is significant for Kienböck's disease (Fig. E).

Clinical Significance: Any acute fracture of the area will also present with findings similar to those above (see Classical Significance).

Follow-up: Perform the tuning fork test or refer the patient for radiography.

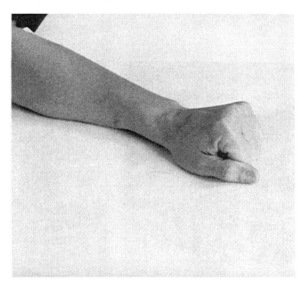

A

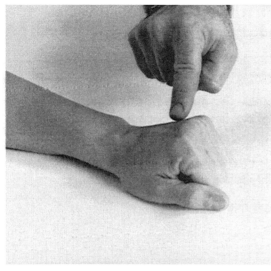

B

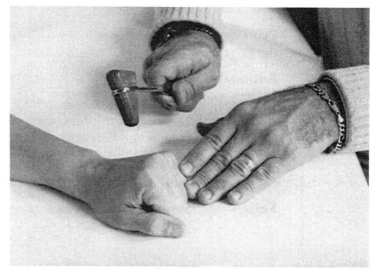

C

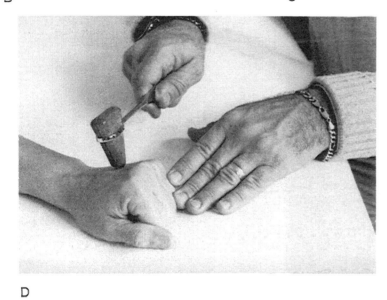

D

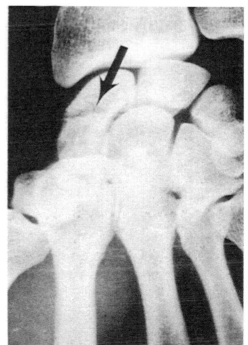

E

11 | *Fist Making Test*

Procedure: The patient is seated with the hand supinated. Ask the patient to flex all the fingers of the hand into a fist (Figs. A & B).

Rationale: An inability to perform this maneuver is indicative of median nerve lesion.

Classical Significance: Inability to flex the index and middle fingers as well as the thumb is caused by a paresis of the radial half of the flexor digitorum profundus and flexor pollicis longus and brevis, and indicates a median nerve lesion (Figs. C & D).

Clinical Significance: Patients with a history of osteoarthritis or rheumatoid arthritis may have difficulty performing this test but will show a good contractile effort.

Follow-up: Perform the pronation test or wrist flexion test.

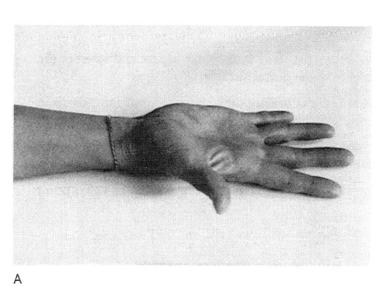

A

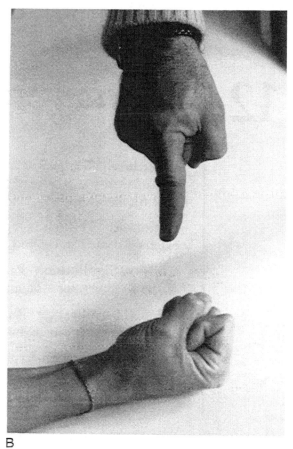

B

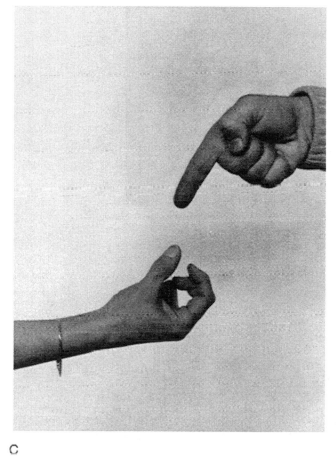

C

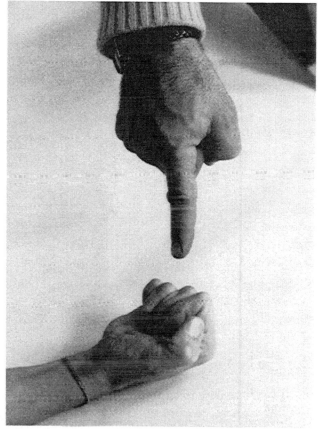

D

12 | *Flexion Stress Test*

Procedure: The patient is seated with the hand pronated. Grasp the forearm just proximal to the wrist and force the wrist into flexion with your other hand (Figs. A & B).

Rationale: This test compresses the wrist joint at its volar aspect and stresses the extensor compartment and ligaments of the dorsal surface.

Classical Significance: Pain over the dorsal surface of the wrist is significant for strain of the wrist extensors or sprain of the ligaments (Fig. C).

Clinical Significance: Pain over the volar surface of the joint may be significant for carpal tunnel syndrome (median nerve entrapment) (Figs. D & E).

Follow-up: Perform Kaplan's test (see Ch. 5), Phalen's test, or Dellon's two point discrimination test.

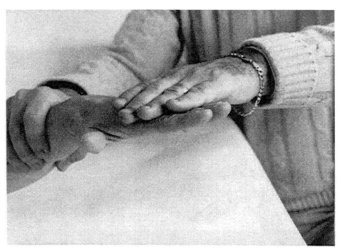

A

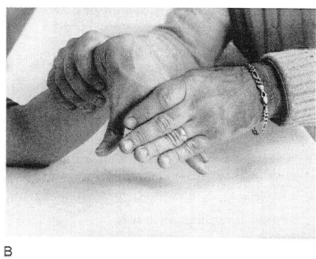

B

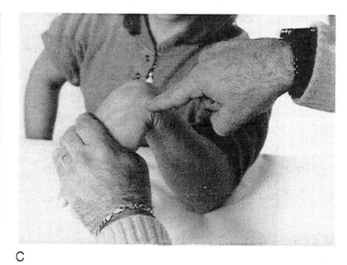

C

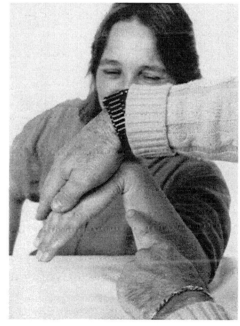

D

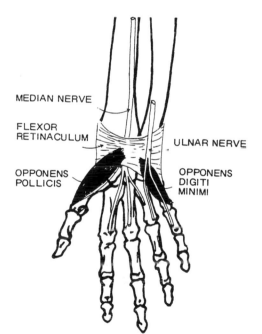

MEDIAN NERVE

FLEXOR
RETINACULUM

ULNAR NERVE

OPPONENS
POLLICIS

OPPONENS
DIGITI
MINIMI

E

13 | *Froment's Cone Test*

Procedure: Before doing this test, the integrity of the T1 nerve root must be determined. Next, with the patient seated, instruct the patient to form a cone by touching the fingertips to the thumb (Fig. A). Perform this test bilaterally.

Rational: The ability to perform this maneuver is dependent on the opponens muscle group, which requires an intact ulnar nerve.

Classical Significance: The inability to perform this maneuver is significant for an ulnar nerve lesion (Fig. B).

Clinical Significance: Inherent to this maneuver is the functionality of the intrinsic muscles of the hand. The integrity of the T1 nerve root must be tested before doing this test.

Follow-up: Perform Froment's sign or the needle threading pinch test.

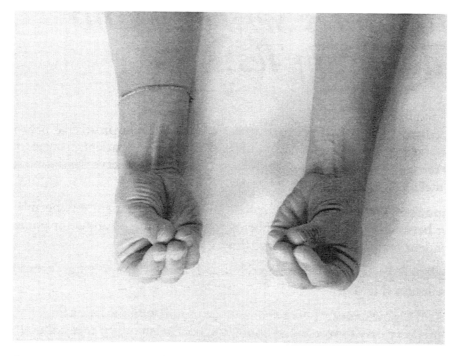

A

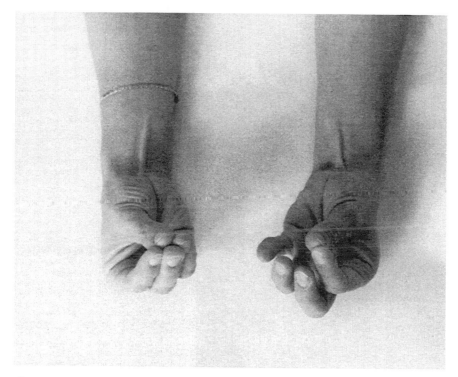

B

14 | *Froment's Sign (Thumb Adduction Test)*

Procedure: The patient is seated with the hand either supinated or pronated. Place a piece of paper between the thumb and index finger of the patient. Instruct the patient to hold the paper while an attempt is made to remove it. Observe the thumb for flexion at the interphalangeal (IP) joint (Figs. A & B).

Rationale: If the adductor pollicis is functional, the patient will be able to hold the paper between the digits without bending the thumb. The adductor pollicis muscle is dependent on an intact ulnar nerve (Fig. C).

Classical Significance: Bending the thumb at the IP joint is significant for an ulnar nerve lesion (Fig. D).

Clinical Significance: Be sure to align the thumb with the index finger because, if it is not, it is very easy to recruit the opponens mechanism when true adduction is sought.

Follow-up: Perform Froment's cone test or the needle threading pinch test.

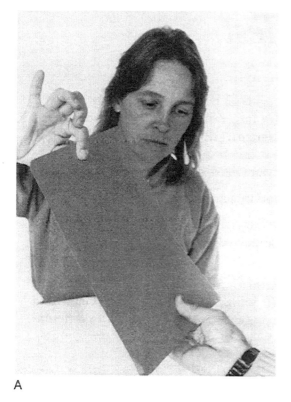

A

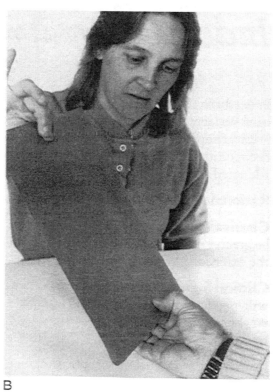

B

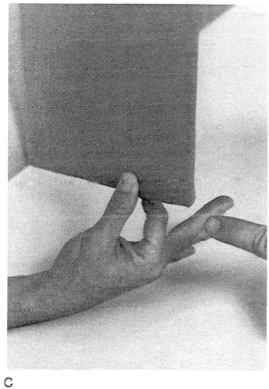

C

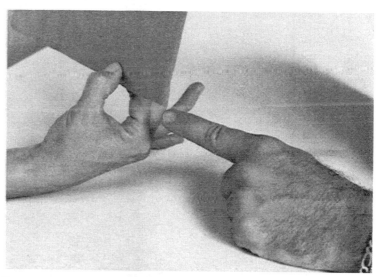

D

15 | *Index Extension Test*

Procedure: The forearm of the patient is prone with the hand completely flat on a hard surface. Ask the patient to abduct the index finger fully and then extend it at the metacarpophalangeal (MCP) joint and interphalangeal (IP) joint. Measure the distance between the fingertip pad and the table. Repeat this test with the index finger fully adducted and extended in the same fashion. Measure the distance as above (Figs. A–D).

Rationale: This test requires a functioning and intact radial nerve.

Classical Significance: The distance from the fingertip pad to the flat surface should be greater in the adducted position than in the abducted position. If this is not the case the extensor indicis is weak (Fig. E).

Clinical Significance: In patients with osteoarthritis or rheumatoid arthritis, this test will produce pain at the MCP joint or the IP joint. This may be interpreted as a weakness, resulting in a false-positive test. The presence of pain is the key for differentiation.

Follow-up: Perform the supination test or the wrist extension test.

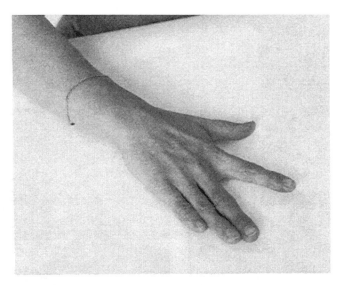

A

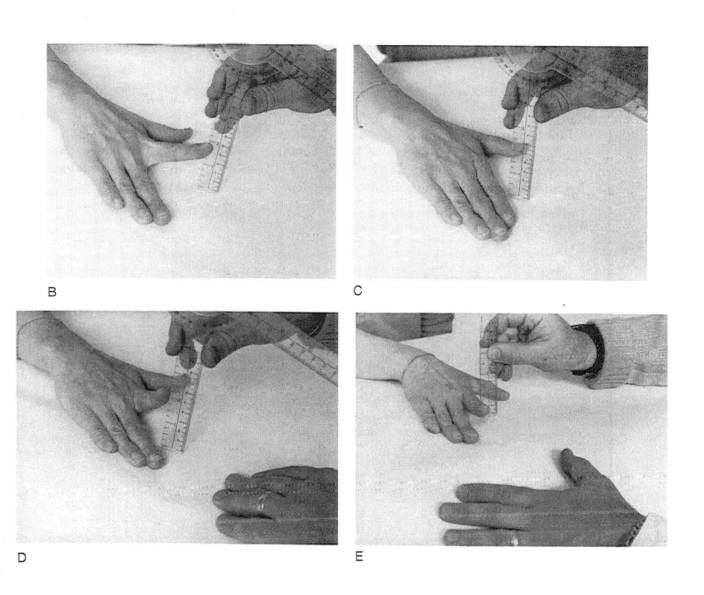

B

C

D

E

16 | *Maisonneuve's Test*

Procedure: The patient is seated. Instruct the patient to extend the arms at the elbow and to extend the wrists. Compare the degree of extension at the wrists (Figs. A–C).

Rationale: Hyperextension of the wrist can be due to trauma or muscle contracture, or both.

Classical Significance: Marked hyperextensibility is a sign of Colles fracture (Fig. D).

Clinical Significance: The wrist should be inspected for other deformities because this type of angulation may not be due to trauma. In addition, the patient history is important to be able to determine the proper diagnosis (Fig. E: complicated Colles fracture; 1, radial fracture; 2, slight dislocation of radial and ulnar junction).

Follow-up: Perform the tuning fork test or refer the patient for radiography.

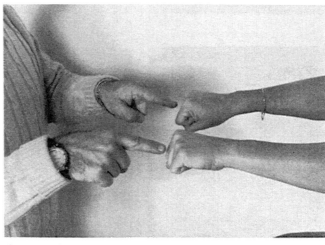

A

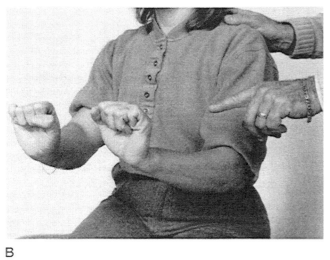

B

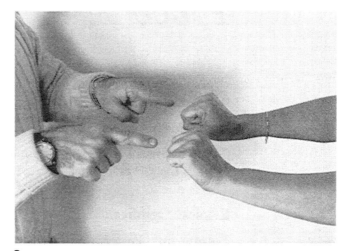

C

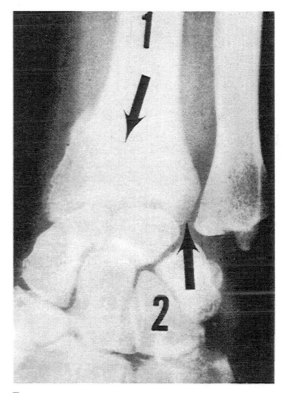

D

E

17 | Needle Threading Pinch Test

Procedure: The patient is seated. Ask the patient to pinch your index finger with the finger pads of the thumb and index finger of the suspected hand (Figs. A & B).

Rationale: This test requires an intact and functioning ulnar nerve.

Classical Significance: If the patient flexes the interphalangeal joint of the thumb and extends the metacarpophalangeal joint, suspect paresis of the adductor pollicis brevis. This is due to a lesion of the deep terminal branch of the ulnar nerve (Fig. C).

Clinical Significance: This test is similar to Froment's sign (Fig. D).

Follow-up: Perform Froment's sign or the palm sweeping test.

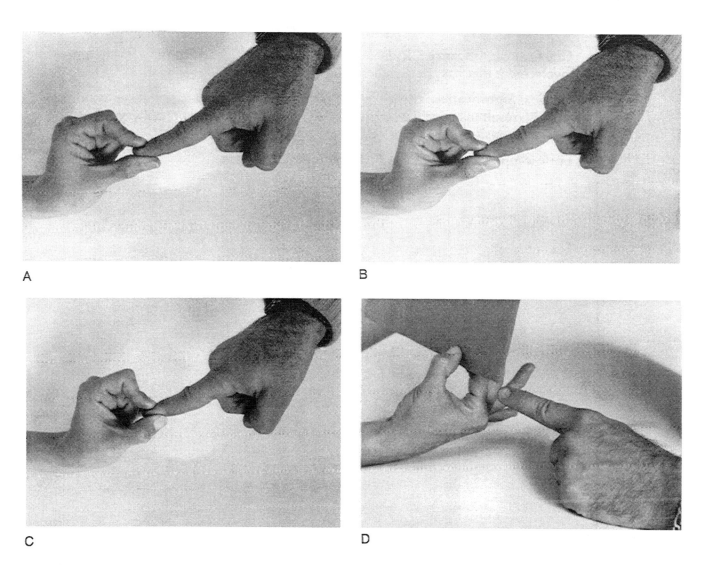

A

B

C

D

18 | *Oschner's Test*

Procedure: The patient is seated. Instruct the patient to clasp the hands together with the digits interlocking. Note the symmetry of the digits (Figs. A & B).

Rationale: Normally the digits interlock evenly.

Classical Significance: If one or more digits are extended consider median nerve involvement that has affected the flexor digitorum profundus (Fig. C).

Clinical Significance: Stenosing tenosynovitis that causes a trigger finger condition will also result in an inability to flex the digit. This finding does not always occur and will be inconsistent with repeated testing (Fig. D).

Follow-up: Perform Phalen's test or the pinch grip test.

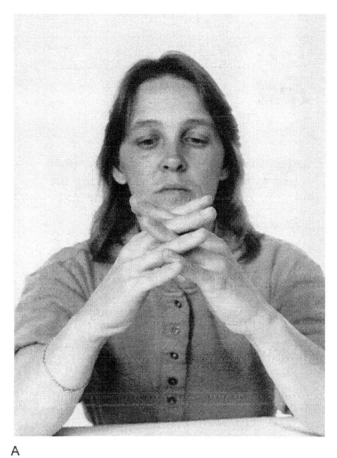

A

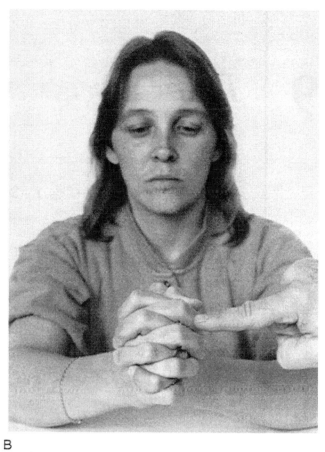

B

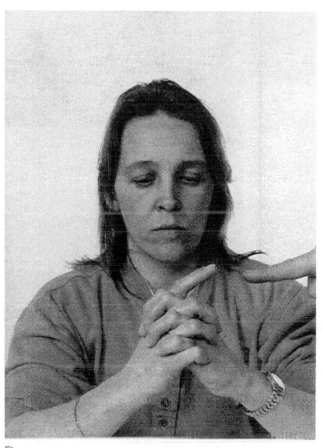

C

D

19 | *Palm Sweeping Test*

Procedure: The patient is seated. Ask the patient to sweep the thumb slowly to each metacarpophalangeal (MCP) joint of the second to fifth fingers without flexing the interphalangeal (IP) joint (Figs. A–D).

Rationale: This test requires an intact and functioning ulnar nerve.

Classical Significance: The inability to sweep the thumb across the MCP joint, without flexing the IP joint indicates a lesion of the deep terminal branch of the ulnar nerve (Fig. E).

Clinical Significance: The abductor pollicis brevis is properly functioning if the thumb pulls away from the palm during this test (Fig. F).

Follow-up: Perform the thumb and index circle test.

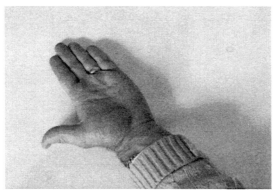

A

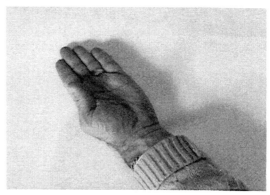

B

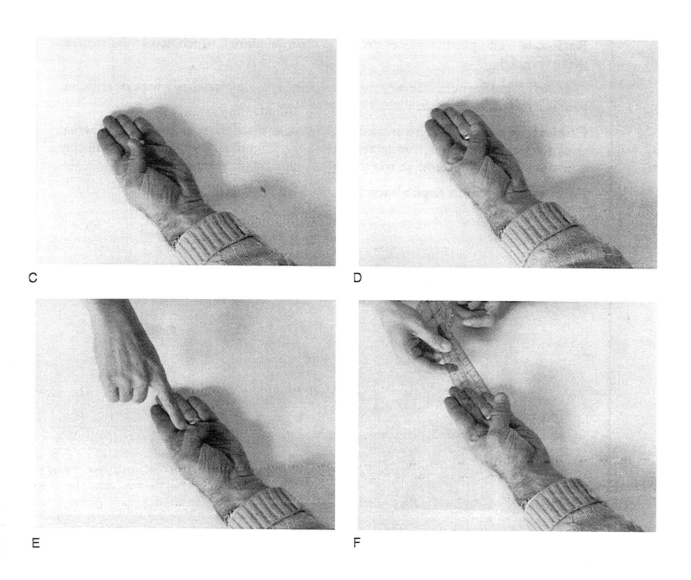

C

D

E

F

20 | *Phalen's Test*

Procedure: The patient is seated. Instruct the patient to place the hands back to back, elevate them to the level of the sternum, and maintain the position for about 1 minute (Figs. A & B).

Rationale: This position places stress on the carpal tunnel, which houses the median nerve (Fig. D).

Classical Significance: Sensory numbness, tingling, or paresthesia with or without pain is significant for median nerve entrapment (Fig. C).

Clinical Significance: This maneuver may cause discomfort in the involved wrist that is not a result of median nerve entrapment. Compare the discomfort with the uninvolved wrist to determine whether nerve entrapment is the cause (Fig. E).

Follow-up: Perform Kaplan's test (see Ch. 5) or Tinel's test.

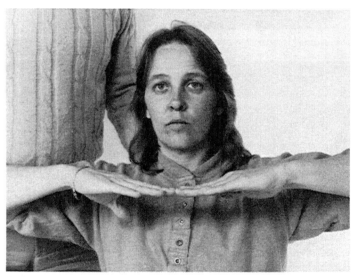

A

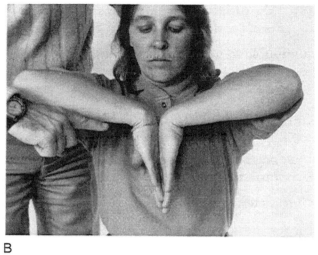

B

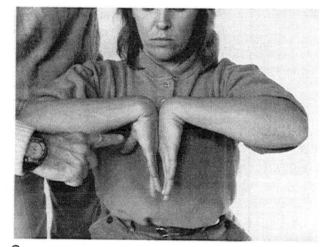

C

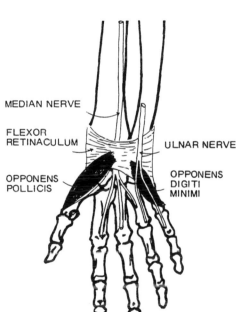

MEDIAN NERVE

FLEXOR
RETINACULUM

ULNAR NERVE

OPPONENS
POLLICIS

OPPONENS
DIGITI
MINIMI

D

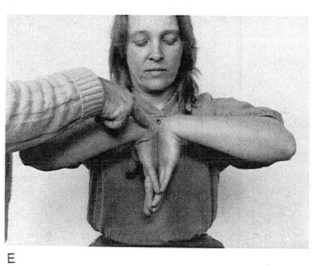

E

21 | *Pinch Grip Test*

Procedure: The patient is seated. Instruct the patient to pinch the tips of the index finger and thumb together. Observe the patient's performance (Figs. A & B).

Rationale: The normal individual will be able to touch tip to tip. A median nerve lesion will cause a pulp to pulp grip. This is due to entrapment of the median nerve by the pronator muscle group (Fig. D).

Classical Significance: The inability to perform a tip to tip grip is significant for a median nerve lesion (Fig. C).

Clinical Significance: Deformity of the fingers and the hands must be established before testing since this may hinder the normal tip to tip grip.

Follow-up: Perform Phalen's test or Tinel's test.

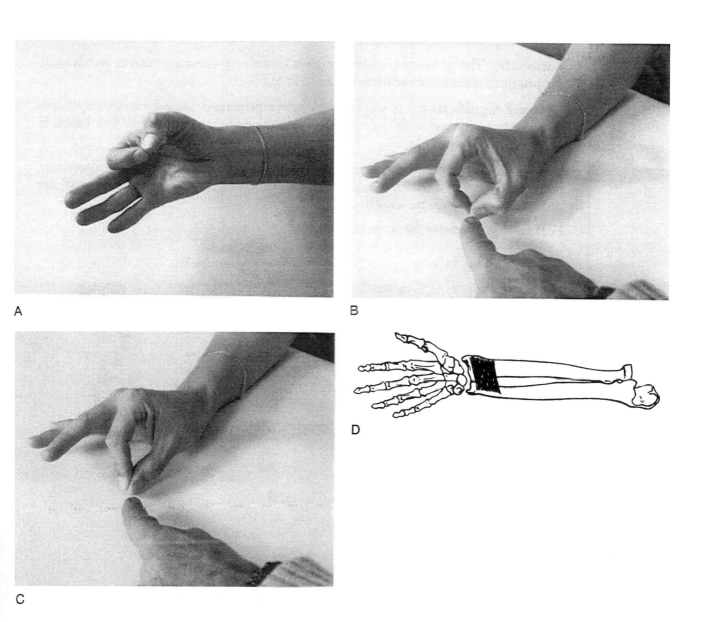

A

B

C

D

22 | *Pronation Test*

Procedure: The patient is seated with the forearms supinated on a flat surface. Ask the patient to pronate the forearms first alone and then against resistance (Figs. A–C).

Rationale: The presence of a median nerve lesion may cause a paresis or paralysis of the pronator muscles of the forearm (Figs. D & E).

Classical Significance: A weakness in active pronation against resistance of one forearm as compared with the other indicates a median nerve lesion. The lesion is usually at the elbow (Fig. F).

Clinical Significance: If the lesion to the median nerve is distal to the elbow, the patient may be able to actively pronate the forearm against resistance because the pronator teres muscle remains functional.

Follow-up: Perform the wrist flexion test.

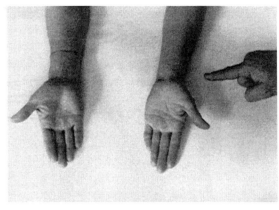

A

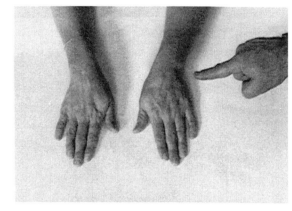

B

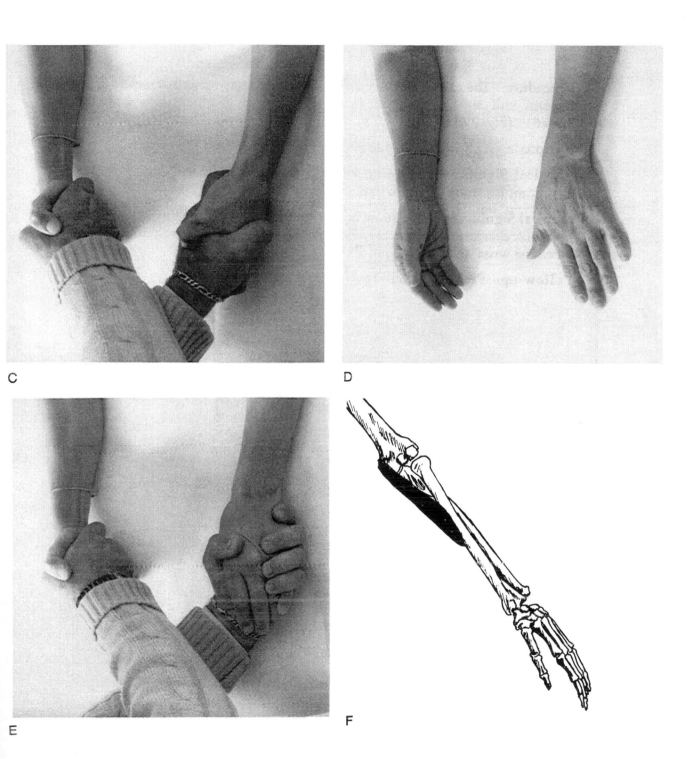

C

D

E

F

23 | *Radial Stress Test*

Procedure: The patient is seated with the hand in the anatomic position. Stabilize the forearm with one hand, grasp the hand with the other, and force the wrist into radial deviation (Figs. A–C).

Rationale: This stresses the ulnar side of the wrist.

Classical Significance: Reproduction of pain over the ulnar side of the wrist is significant for strain or sprain injury at the site of pain (Fig. D).

Clinical Significance: If a strain or sprain injury is present on the radial side, symptoms may decrease. This is because the ligamentous and tendinous bands are shortened when the wrist is forced into radial deviation (Fig. E).

Follow-up: Perform Finkelstein's test or the ulnar stress test.

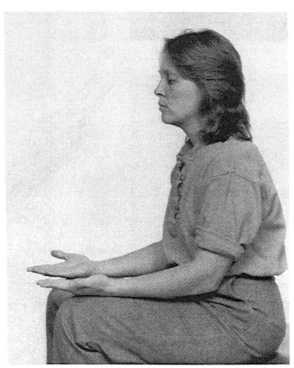

A

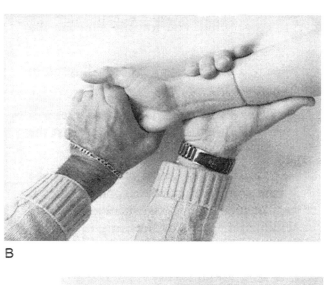

B

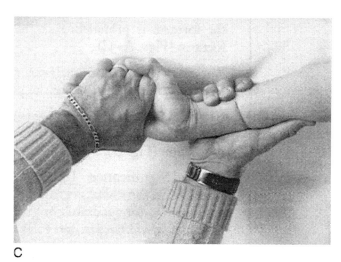

C

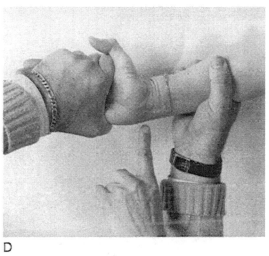

D

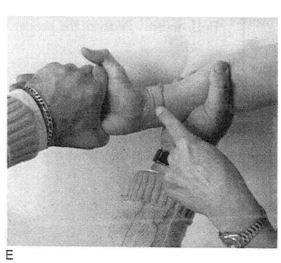

E

24 | *Resisted Passive Supination Test*

Procedure: The patient is standing with the elbow at the side and flexed 90 degrees, the forearm is pronated. Ask the patient to resist while you forcibly supinate the forearm (Figs. A–C).

Rationale: Pronator quadratus weakness due to a median nerve lesion will result in weak or absent resistance to the passive supination.

Classical Significance: In some cases of median nerve lesion, the pronator teres will be weak in addition to the pronator quadratus, resulting in an inability to resist the supination (Fig. D).

Clinical Significance: In cases in which the pronator teres is intact, the patient will be able to resist somewhat even though paresis of the pronator quadratus is present (Figs. E & F [E: pronator quadratus; origin, distal fourth of volar surface of ulna; insertion, distal fourth of lateral border, and volar surface of radius] [F: pronator teres; origin, humeral head, medial epicondylar ridge and common flexion tendon; ulnar head, medial side of coronoid process of ulna; insertion, middle of lateral surface of radius]).

Follow-up: Perform the pronation test or wrist flexion test.

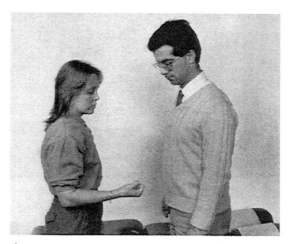

A

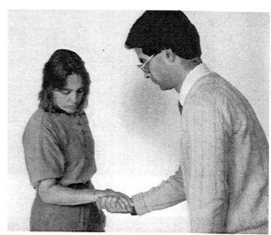

B

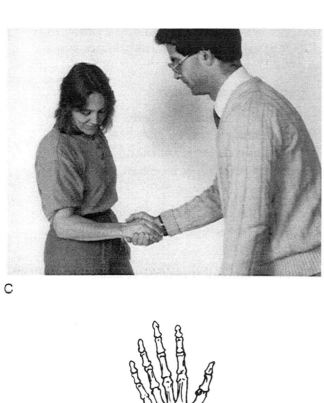

C

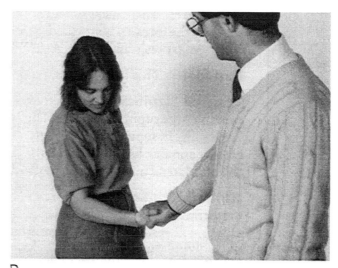

D

E

F

25 | *Supination Test*

Procedure: The patient is seated with the elbow flexed 90 degrees and held firmly to the side, the forearm is pronated. Ask the patient to supinate the forearm first alone and then against resistance (Figs. A–D).

Rationale: This test requires a functioning and intact radial nerve.

Classical Significance: Weakness or the inability to supinate the forearm indicates paresis of the supinator muscle. This muscle is supplied by the deep branch of the radial nerve (Fig. E: supinator; origin, lateral condyle of humerus, radial collateral ligament of elbow, annular ligament of radius, and supinator crest of ulna; insertion, upper one-third of lateral anterior surface of radius).

Clinical Significance: Be sure the forearm is not flexed more than 90 degrees when performing this test. If it is, the biceps muscle will be recruited to aid in supination, which will result in a false-negative test (Fig. F).

Follow-up: Perform the wrist extension test or thumb joint extension test.

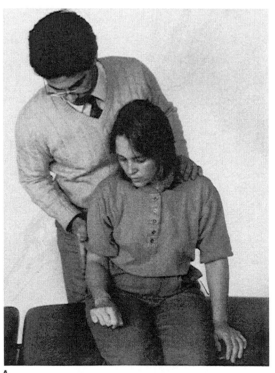

A

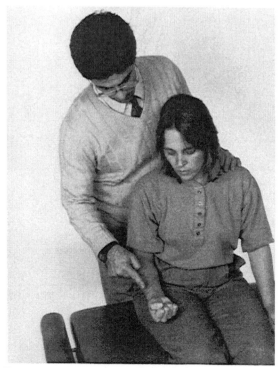

B

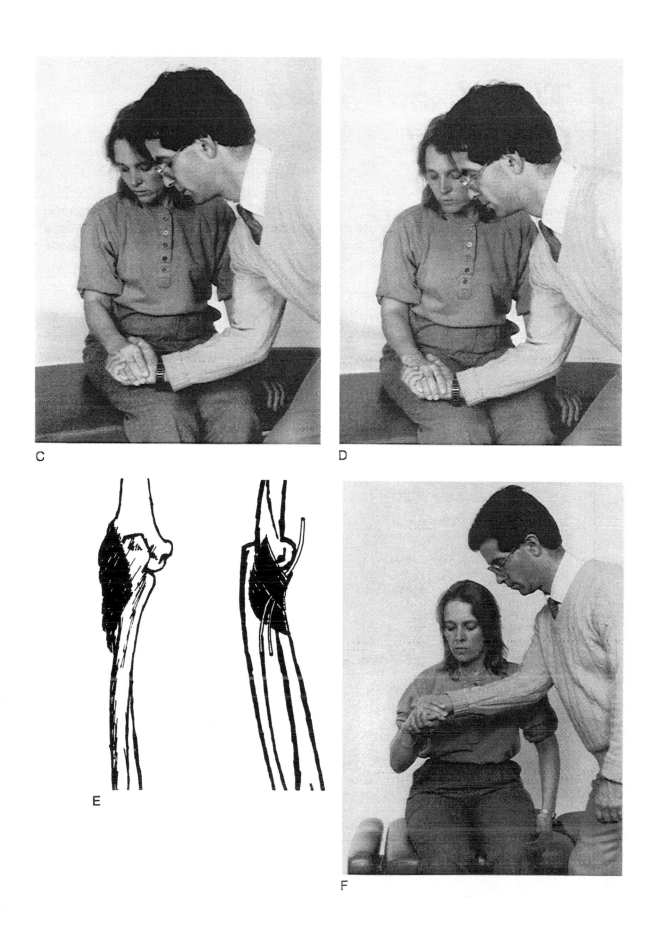

C

D

E

F

26 | *Thumb and Index Circle Test*

Procedure: The patient is seated. Ask the patient to make a circle with the thumb and index finger. The fingertips should touch one another. (If unable to touch tip to tip, a pulp to pulp grip is acceptable.) Then, try to break the circle while the patient resists the attempt (Figs. A–E).

Rationale: This test requires intact and functioning ulnar and median nerves.

Classical Significance: The inability to resist the circle being pulled open indicates an ulnar nerve lesion, which will be in the deep terminal branch of the ulnar nerve (Fig. F).

Clinical Significance: The inability to form the circle by pinching the thumb and index finger tip to tip is evidence of a median nerve lesion.

Follow-up: Perform Froment's sign or the palm sweeping test.

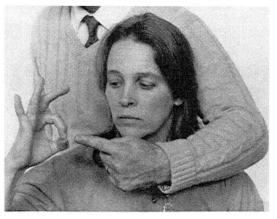

A

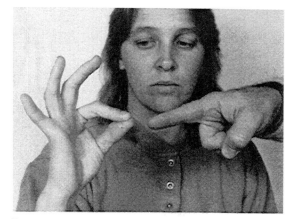

B

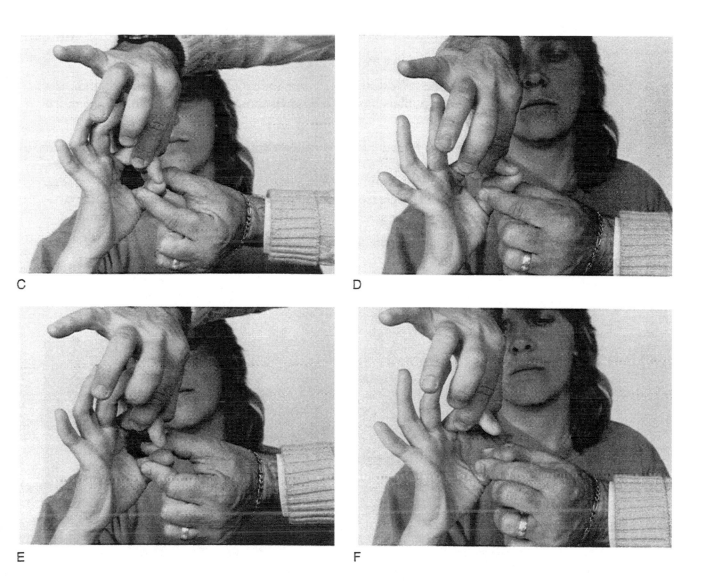

C

D

E

F

27 | *Thumb Joint Extension Test*

Procedure: The patient is seated with the patient's hand held by the examiner. Push the thumb into adduction. Then ask the patient to extend the metacarpophalangeal (MCP) and interphalangeal (IP) joints of the thumb (Figs. A–D).

Rationale: This test requires a functioning and intact radial nerve.

Classical Significance: Weakness or the inability to extend the thumb indicates paresis of the extensor pollicis longus and brevis muscles due to a lesion of the radial nerve (Fig. E).

Clinical Significance: In patients with osteoarthritis or rheumatoid arthritis, this test will produce pain at the MCP or IP joints. This may be interpreted as a weakness, resulting in a false-positive test. The presence of pain is the key for differentiation (Fig. F: rheumatoid arthritis; 1, decreased density between trabeculae; 2, decreased interarticular spacing; 3, periarticular swelling; 4, exostosis; 5, osteophyte; 6, subluxation).

Follow-up: Perform the supination test or wrist extension test.

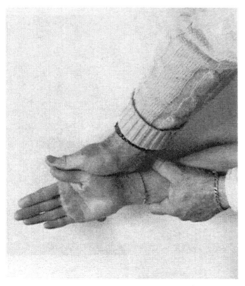

A

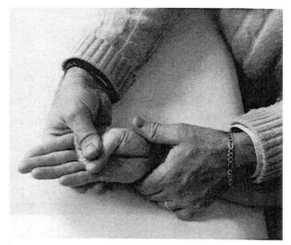

B

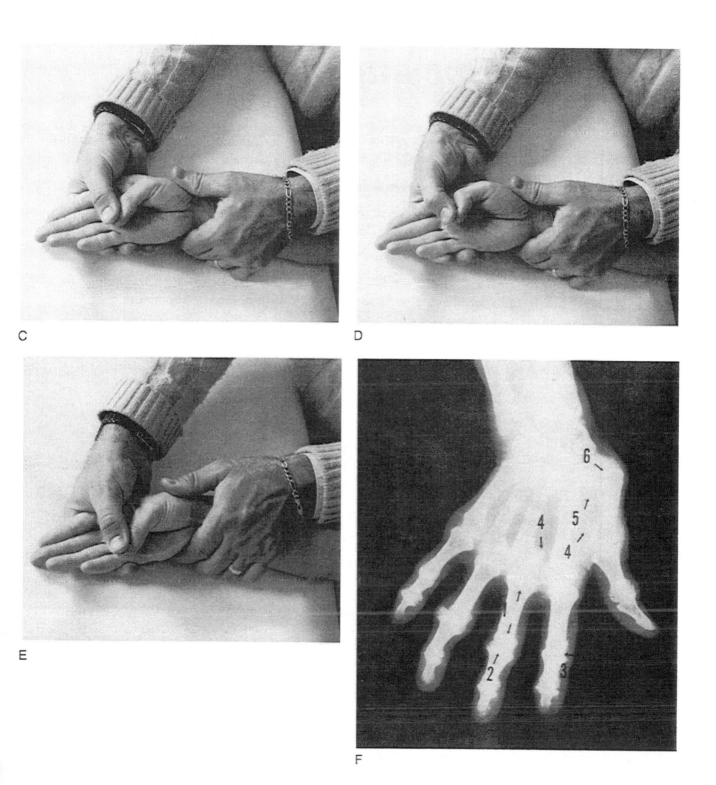

C

D

E

F

28 | *Thumb Tip to Fingertips Test (Opposition Test)*

Procedure: The patient is seated. Ask the patient to touch in this order the tips of the index, middle, ring, and little fingers with the tip of the thumb (Figs. A–D).

Rationale: This test requires an intact and functioning median nerve.

Classical Significance: The inability to perform this test is usually caused by paralysis of the opponens pollicis muscle (Fig. E).

Clinical Significance: Examine the palm for atrophy and test the other thenar muscles to check the function of the median nerve (Fig. F).

Follow-up: Perform the wrist flexion test or resisted passive supination test.

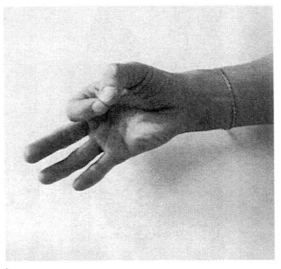

A

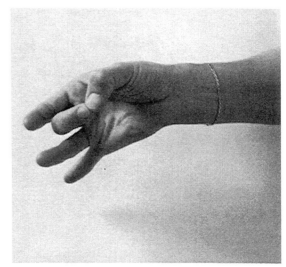

B

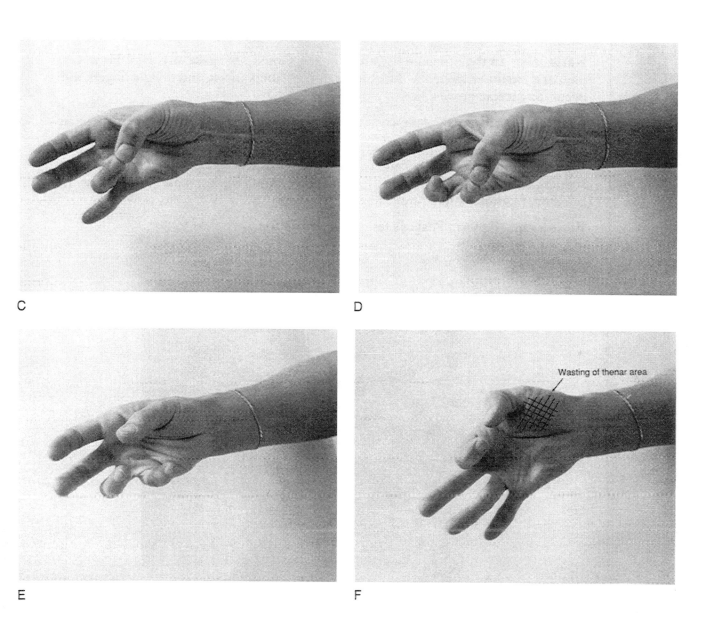

C

D

E

F

Wasting of thenar area

29 | *Tinel's Test*

Procedure: The patient is seated with the hand supinated. Tap over the carpal tunnel with your finger. Note the response of the patient (Figs. A–C & E).

Rationale: In the normal wrist, this tapping should not cause any pain. However, pain or dysesthesia along the distribution of the thumb, index, and middle fingers will occur if a median nerve lesion is present.

Classical Significance: An increase in tingling distal to the tapping indicates median nerve involvement (Fig. D).

Clinical Significance: Be careful not to tap with excessive force. This can cause tingling distally along the pathway of the nerve, resulting in a false-positive test. In addition, repeated tapping can damage the nerve.

Follow-up: Perform Phalen's test or Oschner's test.

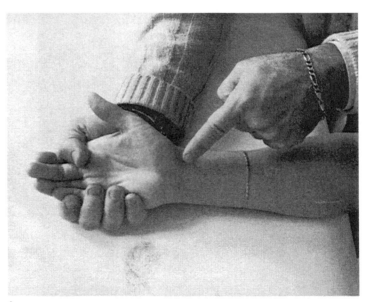

A

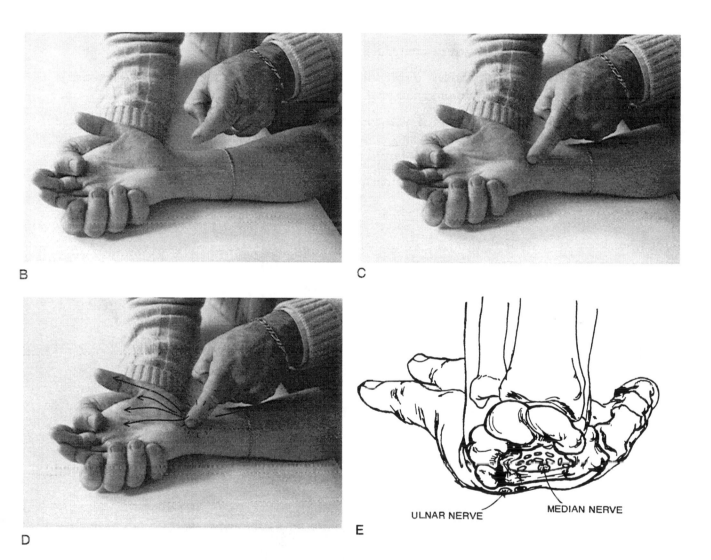

B

C

D

E

ULNAR NERVE   MEDIAN NERVE

30 | *Ulnar Stress Test*

Procedure: The patient is seated with the hand in the anatomic position. Stabilize the forearm with one hand, grasp the hand with the other, and force the wrist into ulnar deviation (Figs. A–C).

Rationale: This stresses the radial side of the wrist.

Classical Significance: Reproduction of pain over the radial side of the wrist is significant for strain or sprain injury at the site of pain (Fig. D).

Clinical Significance: If a strain or sprain injury is present on the ulnar side, the symptoms may decrease. This is because the ligamentous and tendinous bands are shortened when the wrist is forced into ulnar deviation (Fig. E).

Follow-up: Perform Finkelstein's test, the radial stress test, or the tuning fork test.

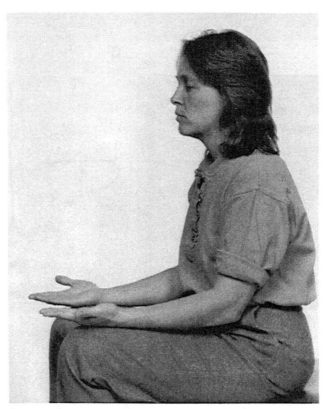

A

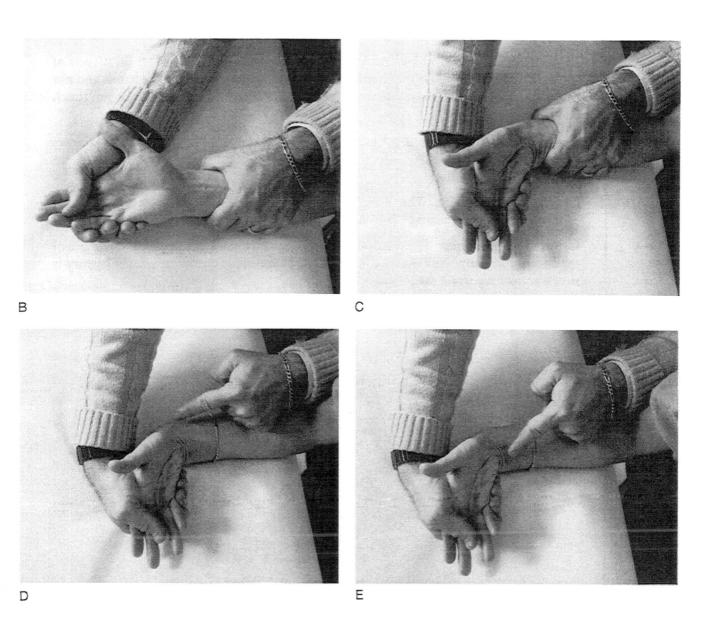

B

C

D

E

31 | *Wartenburg's Oriental Prayer Sign*

Procedure: The patient is seated. Ask the patient to extend and adduct the fingers of the hands while extending the thumbs. Then ask the patient to raise the hands and put them together palm to palm. Observe the hands to see whether the thumbs can touch and the fingers align (Figs. A–C).

Rationale: If the median nerve is functional, the thumb and the index finger of both hands will align perfectly. Failure of these areas to align indicates paralysis of the abductor pollicis muscle.

Classical Significance: The inability to align the thumbs and index fingers is significant for median nerve palsy (Figs. D & E).

Clinical Significance: Rheumatoid arthritis of the thumb will also limit the ranges of motion of the thumb and obstruct alignment. Therefore, a complete patient history is necessary for a correct diagnosis.

Follow-up: Perform nerve conduction velocity studies or refer the patient for electromyography.

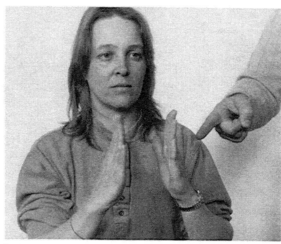

A

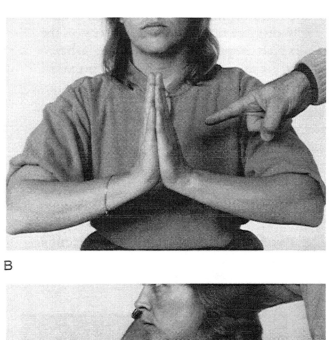

B

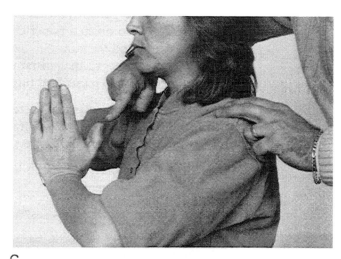

C

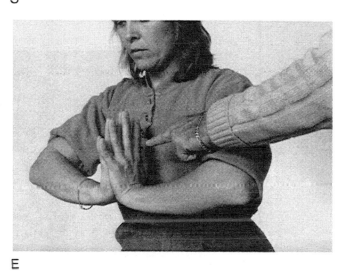

D

E

32 | *Weber Two Point Discrimination Test*

Procedure: The patient is seated with the hand supinated and resting on a hard surface. Using two opened paper clips, apply pressure to two adjacent points on the patient's palm. Find the minimal distance at which the patient can still distinguish two distinct stimuli. Record that distance. Repeat the above with the patient's proximal interphalangeal (PIP) joints and fingertips (Figs. A–F).

Rationale: This test is used to determine a baseline threshold of discrimination. The normal value for the palm is 5 to 8 mm (average, 6 or 7 mm); for the PIP joint, 4 to 8 mm (average, 6 mm); and for the fingertips, 2 to 6 mm (average, 4 mm).

Classical Significance: The inability to determine two distinct stimuli is an early sign of nerve lesion involvement.

Clinical Significance: See Classical Significance.

Follow-up: Perform Dellon's two point discrimination test or nerve conduction velocity studies, or refer the patient for electromyography.

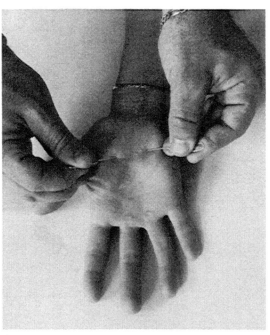

A

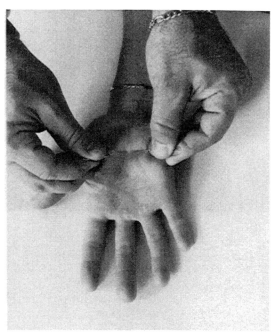

B

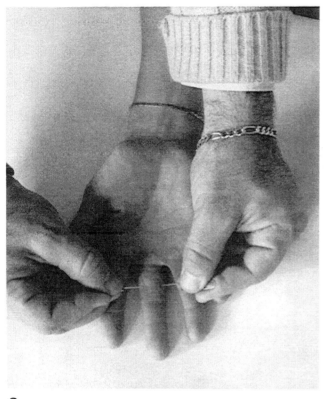

C

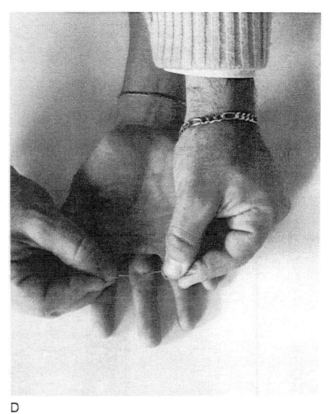

D

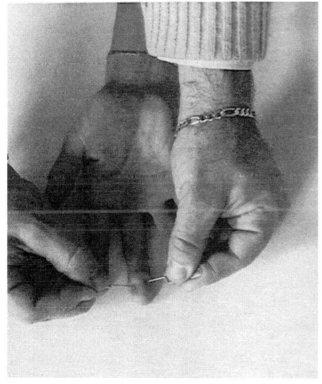

E

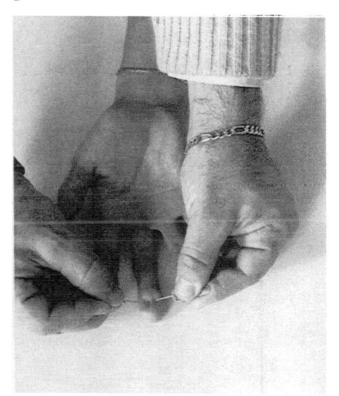

F

33 | *Wrinkle Shrivel Test*

Procedure: The patient is seated with the fingertips submerged in tepid water for 5 minutes. After the time has elapsed, observe the fingertips for wrinkling (Figs. A–D).

Rationale: Denervation of the area results in fingertips that do not wrinkle or shrivel.

Classical Significance: Failure of the pulp of the fingertips to shrivel in response to water hydration indicates denervation of the area (Fig. E).

Clinical Significance: This test is only valid for the first few months after an injury.

Follow-up: Perform nerve conduction velocity studies or refer the patient for electromyography.

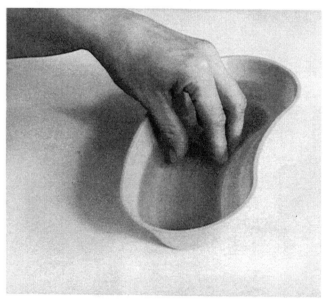

A

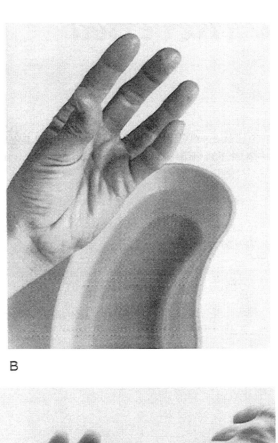

B

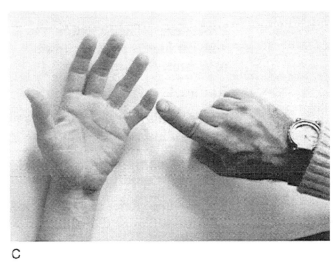

C

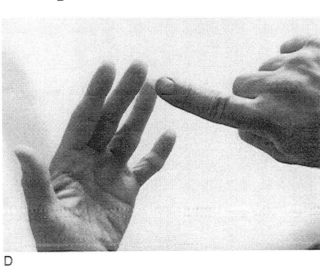

D

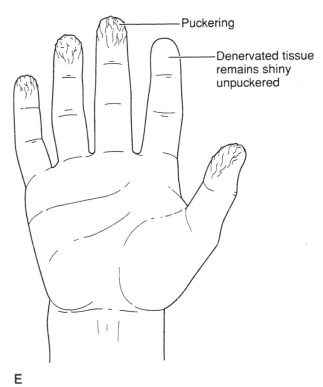

Puckering

Denervated tissue
remains shiny
unpuckered

E

34 | *Wrist Drop Test (Reversed Phalen's Test)*

Procedure: The patient is seated. Instruct the patient to place both palms together with the fingers pointing upward and both wrists fully extended. Then ask the patient to separate the hands, keeping the wrists extended (Figs. A & B).

Rationale: This maneuver requires an intact and functioning radial nerve.

Classical Significance: The inability to keep the wrist extended when the hands are separated indicates a radial nerve lesion due to compression entrapment (Fig. C).

Clinical Significance: This test will cause pain if the patient has a median nerve entrapment syndrome because of traction of the median nerve (Fig. D).

Follow-up: Refer the patient for electromyography, or perform nerve conduction velocity studies or Phalen's test.

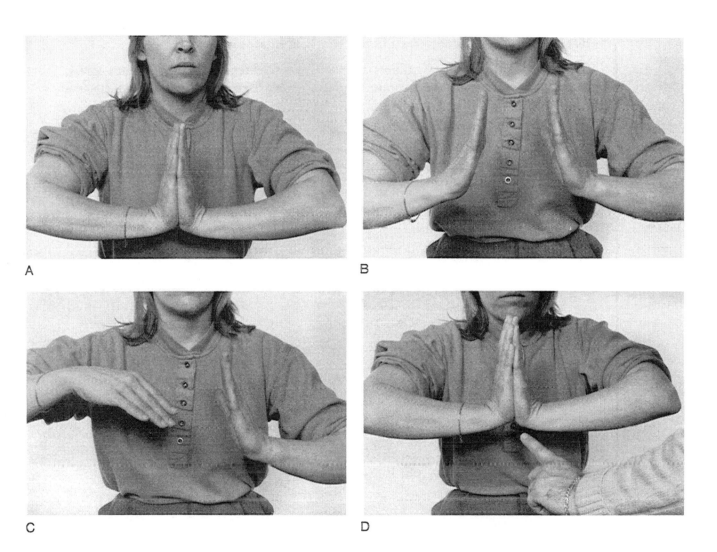

A

B

C

D

35 | *Wrist Extension Test*

Procedure: The patient is seated with the forearms pronated. Ask the patient to extend the wrists and then to supinate the forearms, first alone and then with resistance (Figs. A–D).

Rationale: This test requires a functioning and intact radial nerve.

Classical Significance: Weakness or the inability to extend the wrist indicates paresis of the extensor muscles, which are supplied by the deep branch of the radial nerve (Fig. E).

Clinical Significance: Extending the wrist against resistance is similar to the procedure in Cozen's test (see Ch. 5) and will cause pain in a patient with lateral epicondylitis. The reproduction of pain is a positive result for lateral epicondylitis but not for paresis of the extensor muscles. (Fig. F).

Follow-up: Perform the supination test or thumb joint extension test.

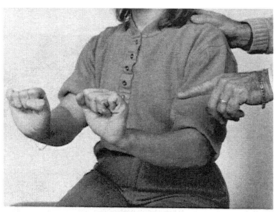

A

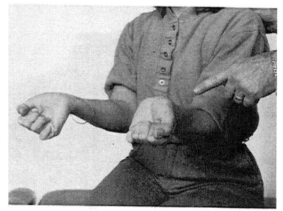

B

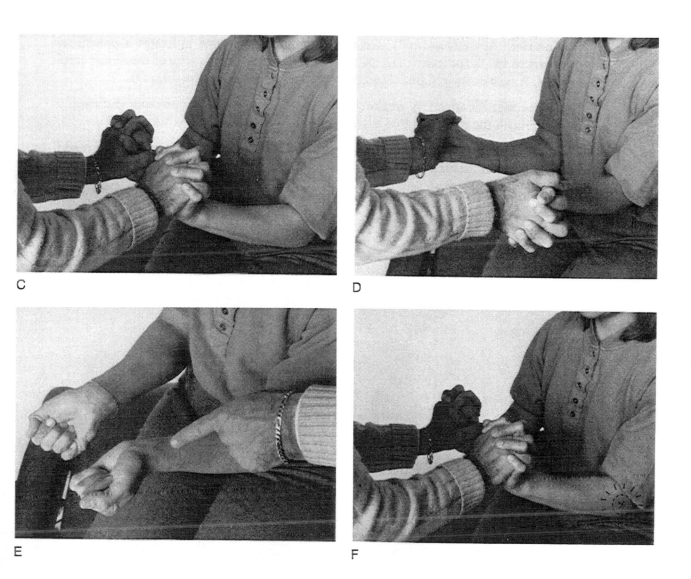

C

D

E

F

36 | *Wrist Flexion Test*

Procedure: The patient is seated with the forearms supinated. Ask the patient to flex the wrists first alone and then against resistance (Figs. A–C).

Rationale: A weakness in active flexion against resistance indicates a paresis or paralysis of the flexor muscles in the forearm. This is especially true of the flexor carpi radialis. A weakness without resistance indicates a true paralysis (Fig. D).

Classical Significance: A weakness in active flexion against resistance indicates a problem with the median nerve in or above the elbow.

Clinical Significance: A total inability to flex the wrist against resistance could indicate a lesion that is affecting the median and ulnar nerves (Fig. E).

Follow-up: Perform the thumb tip to fingertips test or the resisted passive supination test.

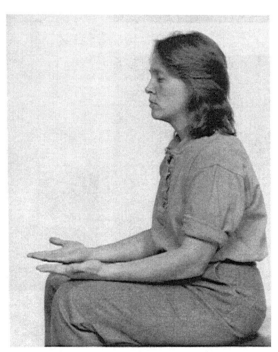

A

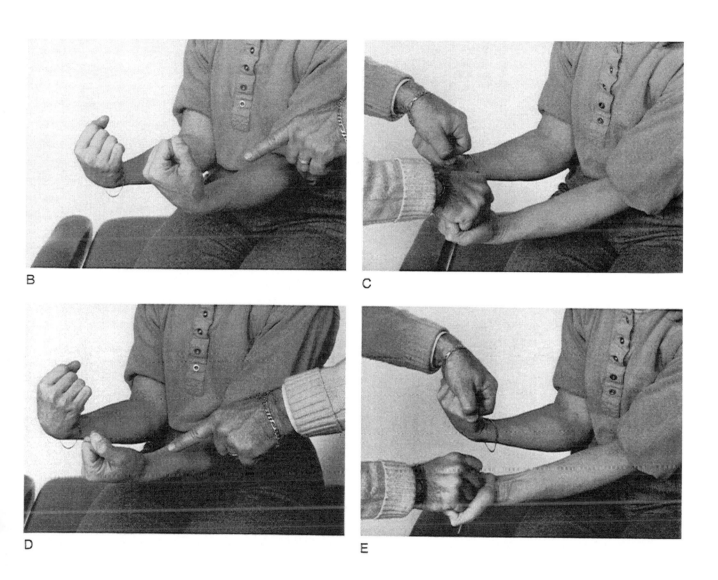

B

C

D

E

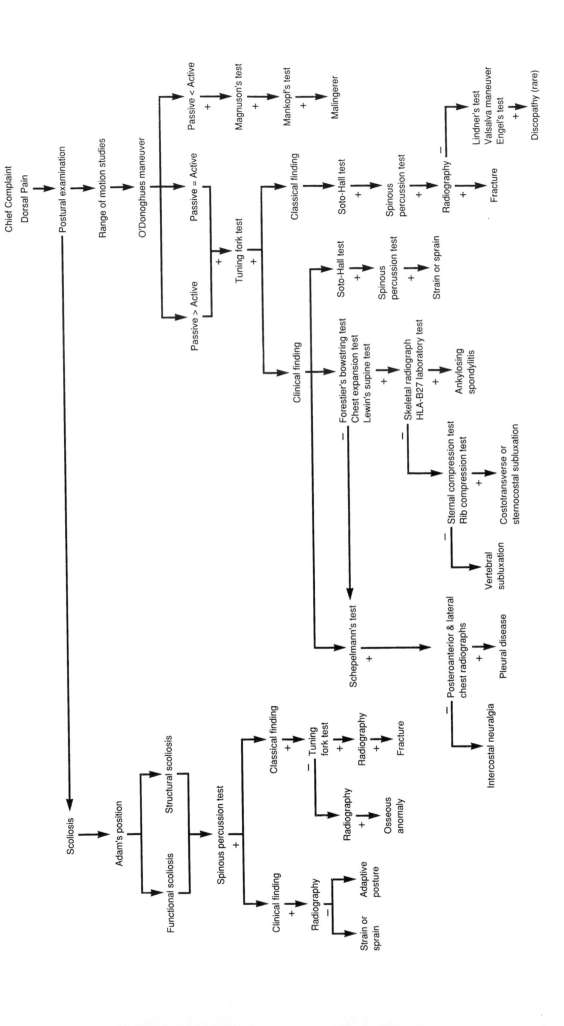

1 | *Range of Motion Studies*

When performing range of motion studies, it is important to use either an arthrodial protractor or an inclinometer. The *American Medical Association Guides for Impairment Ratings* now recommend the use of the inclinometer exclusively. It is impossible to separate the dorsal spine from the lumbar spine when performing ranges of motion. Therefore, the two are always recorded as dorsolumbar ranges of motion.

Flexion: Have the patient bend forward and touch the toes. Normal flexion is 80 to 90 degrees or the fingertips 4 to 6 inches from the floor. Flexion may be limited by such conditions as ankylosing spondylitis, degenerative disc disease, and osteoarthritis. However, the hamstring musculature restricts forward iliac rotation and tight hamstrings can result in loss of normal ranges of motion.

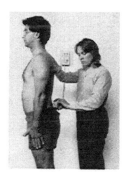 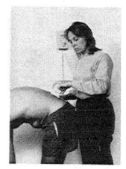 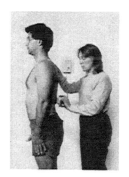 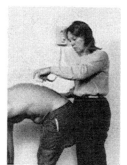

Extension: Have the patient bend at the waist as far back as possible. Normal extension is 20 to 30 degrees. Congenital anomolies such as facet tropism or knife clasp syndrome can significantly restrict dorsolumbar extension. Arthritic conditions, such as ankylosing spondylitis, degenerative disc disease, facet syndrome, and spondylolisthesis also result in loss of normal extension.

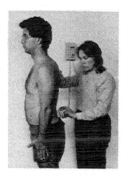 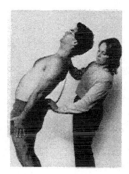 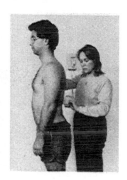 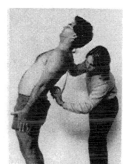

Rotation: Ask the patient to cross the arms or to place each hand on the opposite shoulder and to turn the torso as far right and left as possible. Normal rotation is 20 to 45 degrees.

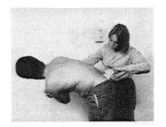 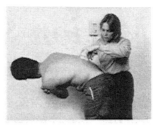 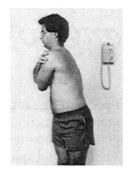 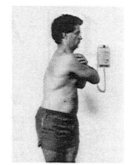

Lateral Flexion: With the patient's arms alongside the body, ask the patient to bend toward each side as if trying to reach the hand to the knee. Be sure the knees are locked. Check the fingertip level to see whether the bend is equal bilaterally. Normal lateral flexion is 20 to 35 degrees.

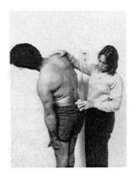 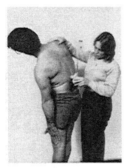 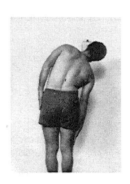 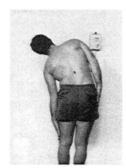

Quick Test: Perform the quick test if an inclinometer is unavailable. The patient is standing and bends backward from the waist as far as possible. Note whether a smooth C curve occurs in the lumbar spine. Next, ask the patient to bend forward from the waist (keeping legs straight) as if touching fingers to toes. Measure the distance between the fingers and the floor (normal is 4 to 6 inches).

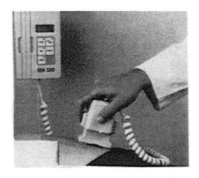 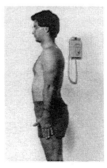 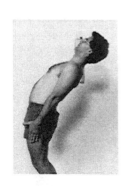 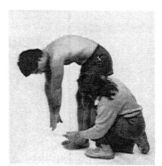

Classical Significance: The patient's ranges of motion should be within normal and the values should be equal bilaterally.

Clinical Significance: Acute or chronic injury may restrict ranges of motion bilaterally. If the ranges of motion are still within normal limits this is not normal. It is imperative to have good baseline ranges of motion on all patients.

Note: Active ranges of motion are largely a function of volition. An area that is strained is reactively guarded and any attempt to move will be restricted and discomforting. If the patient allows passive ranges of motion, they will be achieved to a greater degree and with less pain than with the active.

2 | *Adam's Position*

Procedure: The patient is either standing or seated. Stand behind the patient and ask the patient to bend forward at the waist (Figs. A–D).

Rationale: Perform this test on patients with visible scoliosis of unknown cause, or on patients with a family history of scoliosis, as part of a scoliosis screen.

Classical Significance: If forward flexion reducs the scoliosis angle, the scoliosis is one of functionality (Fig. E).

Clinical Significance: If the scoliosis angle does not change with flexion, the scoliosis is congenital (Fig. F).

Follow-up: Perform the spinous percussion test or Soto-Hall test.

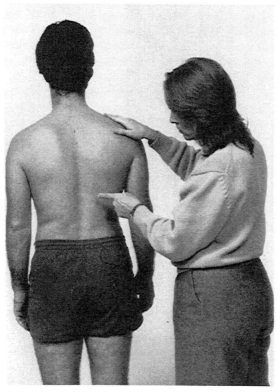

A

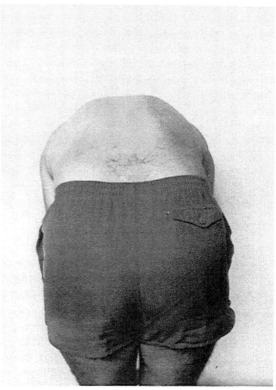

B

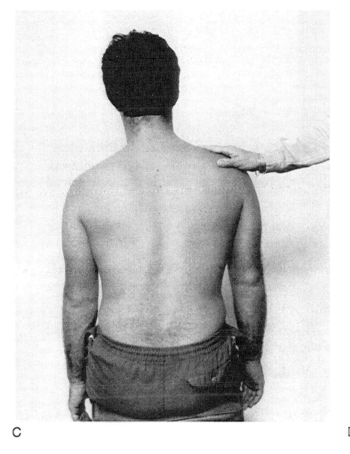

C

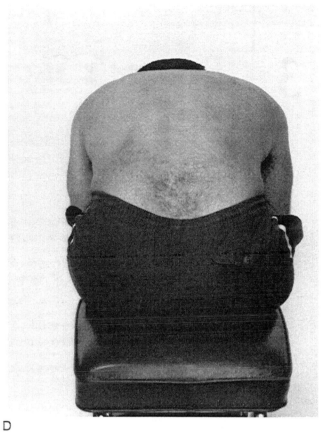

D

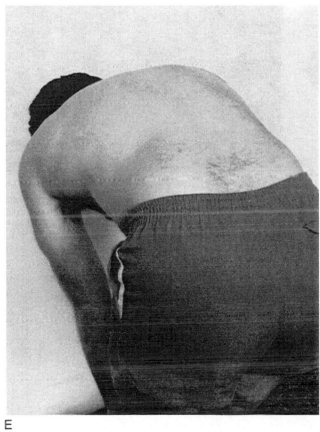

E

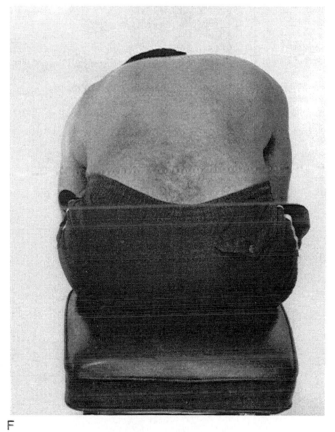

F

3 | *Beevor's Sign*

Procedure: The patient is supine. The abdomen is exposed for visualization of the umbilicus. Focus on the umbilicus as the patient sits partway up. If the patient has abdominal paralysis and cannot sit up this way, simply ask the patient to cough instead (Figs. A–E).

Rationale: Equal contraction of the abdominal musculature in the upper and lower quadrants results in the umbilicus remaining stationary.

Classical Significance: Paresis of the upper abdominals results in a downward pull of the umbilicus; paresis of the lower abdominals results in an upward pull of the umbilicus.

Clinical Significance: In total abdominal paralysis, the umbilicus will bulge instead of pulling up or down when the patient coughs (Fig. F).

Follow-up: Perform Lewin's supine test or the chest expansion test.

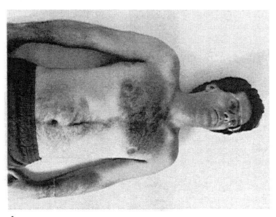

A

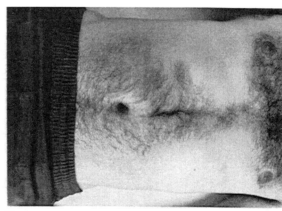

B

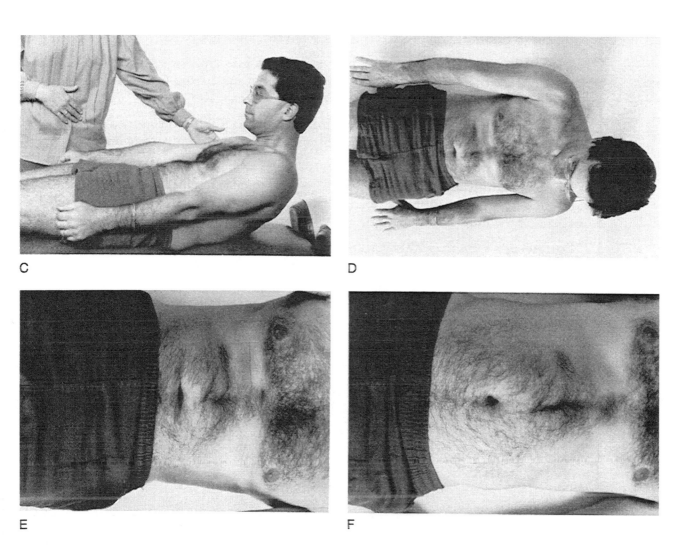

C

D

E

F

4 | *Chest Expansion Test*

Procedure: The patient is seated with the hands on hips or folded at shoulder level and parallel to the floor. Place a tape measure around the chest at the level of T4 or at the nipple line. Ask the patient to forcibly exhale. Record the measurement. Then ask the patient to breathe in deeply. Record this measurement (Figs. A–C).

Rationale: In certain conditions of the spine, such as ankylosing spondylitis and advanced degenerative osteoarthritis, or in advanced underlying lung pathology the amount of chest expansion that is normal will be decreased.

Classical Significance: The normal difference between the two recorded measurements is 1.5 to 2 inches (Figs. D & E [D: normal excursion; E: excursion of less than 1.5 inch]).

Clinical Significance: Normally this test is performed to test for ankylosing spondylitis or degenerative arthritis; however, remember that underlying lung pathology will also alter the normal expected measurements.

Follow-up: Perform Schepelmann's test, Lewin's supine test, or Forestier's bowstring test.

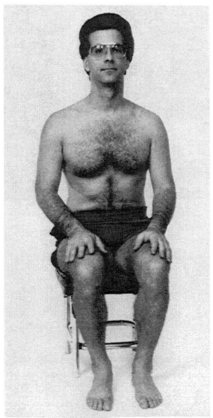

A

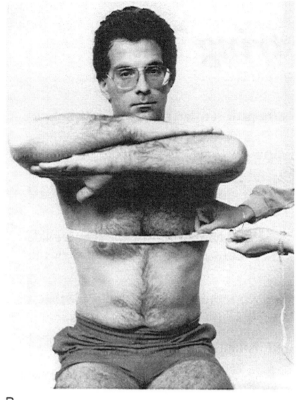

B

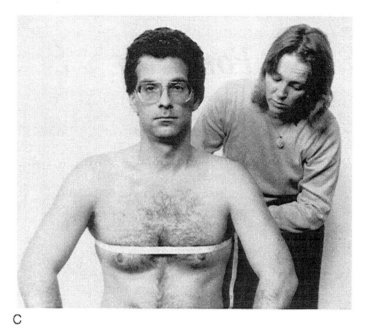

C

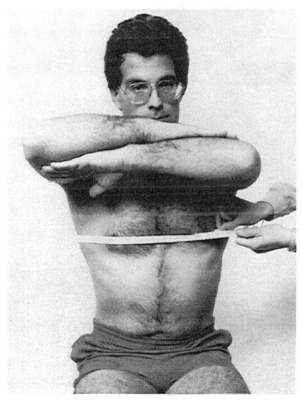

D

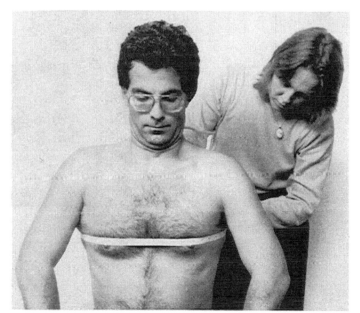

E

5 | *Forestier's Bowstring Test*

Procedure: The patient is standing. Instruct the patient to laterally flex the dorsolumbar spine (Figs. A–C).

Rationale: In the normal patient, lateral flexion causes the paraspinal muscles on the side being flexed to shorten and the contralateral paraspinal muscles to stretch. Any obstructive disease that prevents normal ranges of motion at the vertebral segmental motor unit will result in a positive Forestier's test.

Classical Significance: Shortening of the paraspinal musculature on the concave side and stretching of the contralateral musculature is normal (Fig. D). Failure for this to happen is a positive finding.

Clinical Significance: In pleuritic conditions, pain may be present on the side that is not being laterally flexed (Fig. E).

Follow-up: Perform Schepelmann's test, Lewin's supine test, or the chest expansion test.

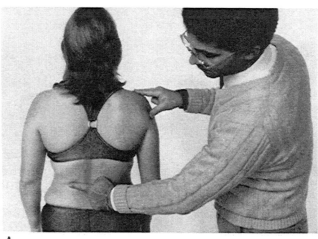

A

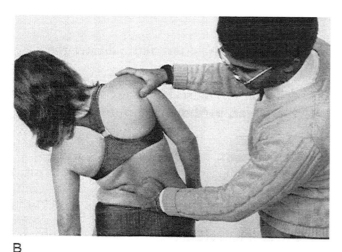

B

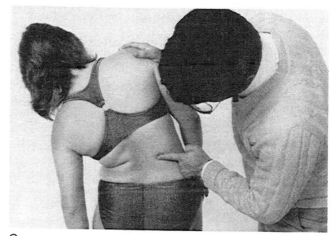

C

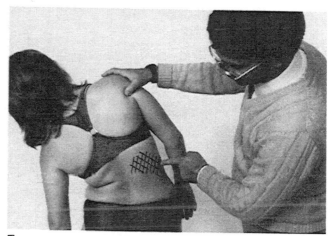

D

E

6 | *Lewin's Supine Test*

Procedure: The patient is supine. Stabilize the patient's legs at the ankles and instruct the patient to perform a sit-up without using the arms (Figs. A–C).

Rationale: If the spinal motor units are sound, the forward flexion from the dorso-lumbar spine will be free and unimpeded.

Classical Significance: The inability to sit up is a positive test and indicates the presence of ankylosing spondylitis (Fig. D).

Clinical Significance: If the patient has weak abdominal musculature or any disease affecting the motor integrity of the T8–T12 vertebrae, performing this test will be difficult (Fig. E).

Follow-up: Perform muscle testing on the abdominals, Beevor's sign, or Schepelmann's test.

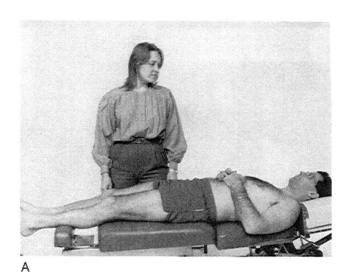

A

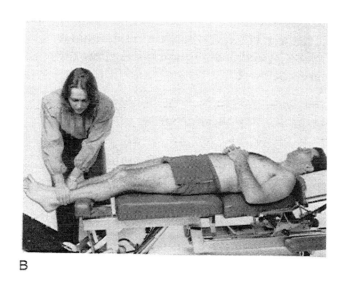

B

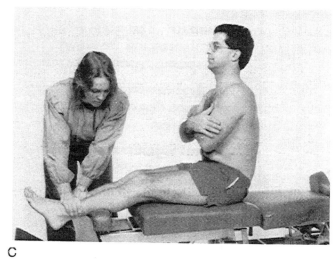

C

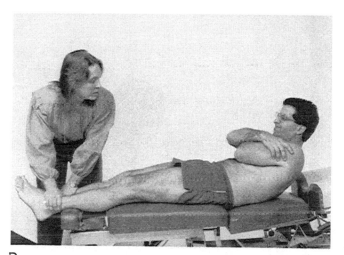

D

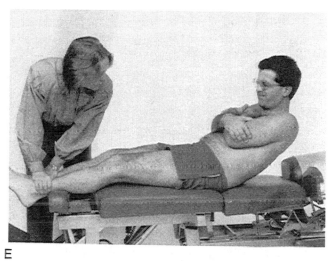

E

7 | *Lindner's Test*

Procedure: The patient is supine. Place both hands behind the patient's occiput and gently force the chin onto the chest while pushing and lifting the patient's upper body off the table to just past the shoulder blades (Figs. A–D).

Rationale: This test is similar to the Soto-Hall test. However, because the sternum is not stabilized and the patient is forced into a semiseated position, the forces along the supraspinous ligaments are transferred to levels below T7.

Classical Significance: An increase in radicular symptoms may indicate a discal protrusion that causes nerve root irritation (Fig. E). Intrathecal pressure will increase with this test.

Clinical Significance: Local pain below the level of T7 that extends into the lumbar spine indicates vertebral injury or ligamentous sprain at the level of the pain (Fig. F).

Follow-up: Perform the tuning fork test or the spinous percussion test.

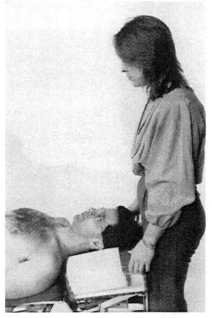

A

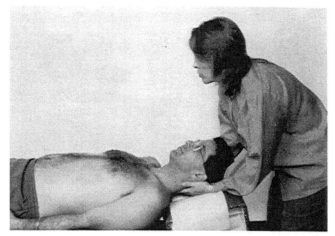

B

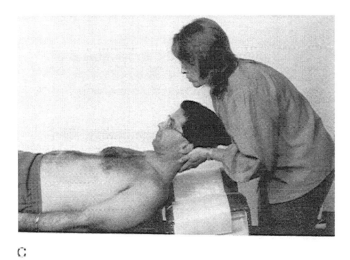

C

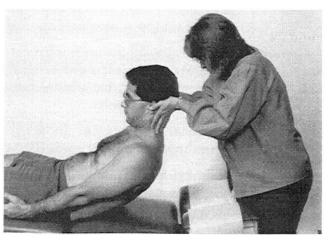

D

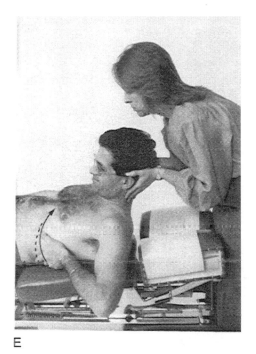

E

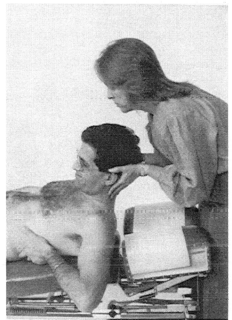

F

8 | O'Donoghues Maneuver

Procedure: The dorsolumbar spine of the patient is moved through its active and passive ranges of motion (Figs. A–C).

Rationale: In the normal patient or one with a muscle injury, the active ranges of motion are always less than or equal to the passive ranges of motion. This is because, to perform actively, the affected muscles must be used; passive performance will not aggravate the muscles.

Classical Significance: If the active ranges of motion are less than the passive, then active muscle involvement is the cause of the patient's pain (Fig. D).

Clinical Significance: If the active ranges of motion are greater than the passive, suspect a malingerer (Fig. E).

Follow-up: Perform Magnuson's test or Mankopf's test (see Ch. 14).

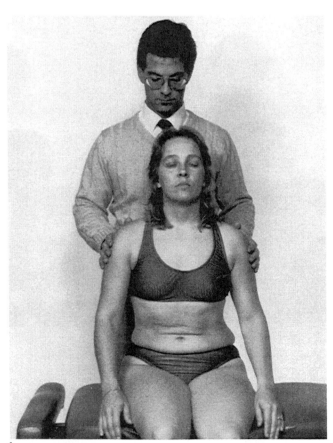

A

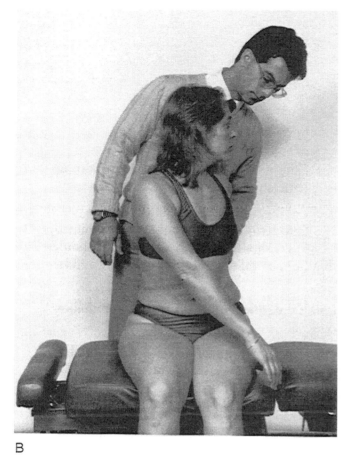

B

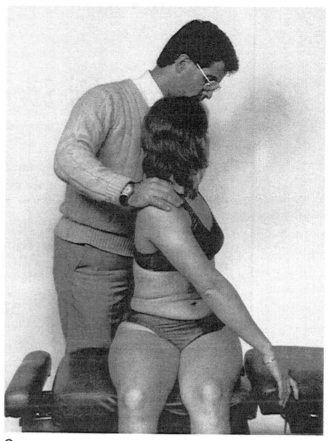

C

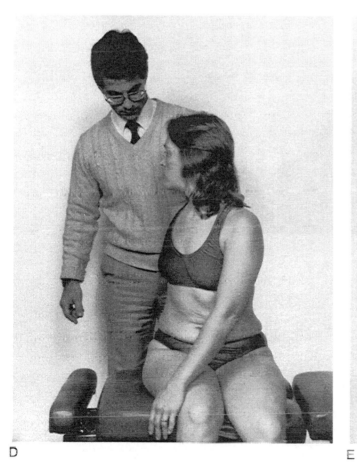

D

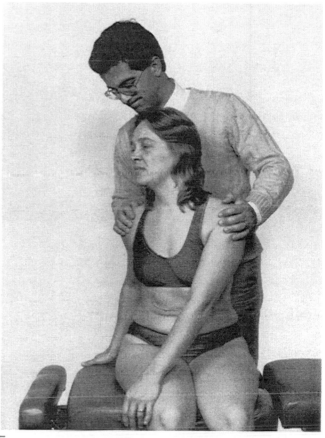

E

9 | *Pectoralis Stretch Test*

Procedure: The patient is supine. Instruct the patient to place the hands palm up behind the head, then to bring the elbows together, and then to let the arms relax to the table (Figs. A–D).

Rationale: The pectoralis muscle is primed into action when the elbows are adducted. After the muscle has been used, firing of the fibers should be inhibited and they should relax. The patient with a chronically spasmodic pectoralis muscle will be unable to relax the fired muscle.

Classical Significance: The test is positive if the patient is unable to release the elbow on the affected side back to the table (Fig. E).

Clinical Significance: The patient with a thoracic outlet syndrome that is caused by a pectoralis minor mechanism will complain of dysesthesia. Also the radial pulse will be absent. These findings are classical for thoracic outlet syndrome.

Follow-up: Perform Wright's test (see Ch. 2).

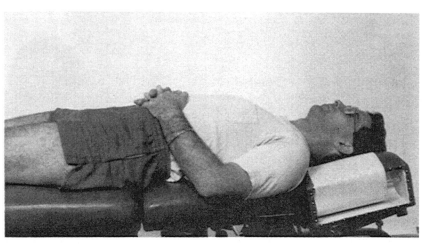

A

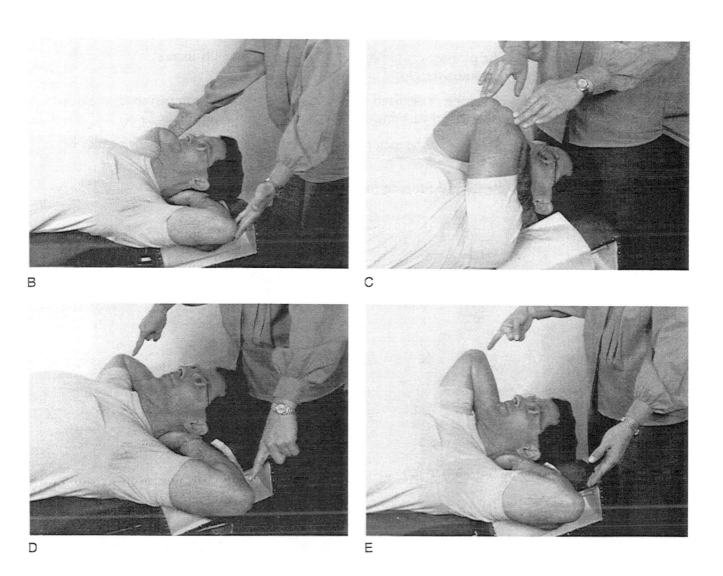

B

C

D

E

10 | *Rib Compression Test*

Procedure: The patient is seated. Place your forearms on either side of the lateral margins of the patient's rib cage. Apply pressure with the forearms, squeezing the patient's chest, to clasp your hands (Figs. A–D).

Rationale: The pressure caused by approximating the hands increases stress at the sternocostal, costotransverse, and costovertebral margins.

Classical Significance: Localized pain at the sternocostal, costotransverse, or costovertebral margins indicates a subluxated rib at the point of pain (Fig. E).

Clinical Significance: If the patient feels pain along the shaft of a rib, that rib may be fractured (Fig. F).

Follow-up: Perform the tuning fork test or the chest expansion test.

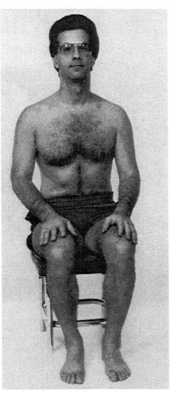

A

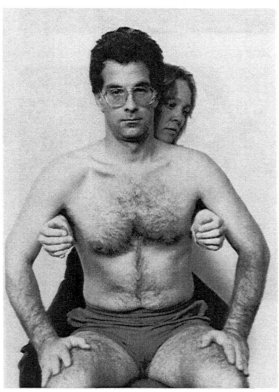

B

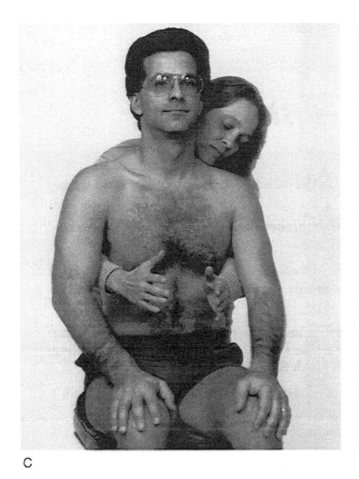

C

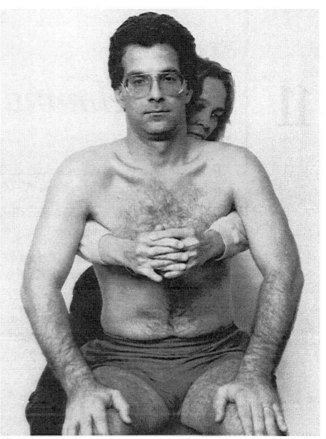

D

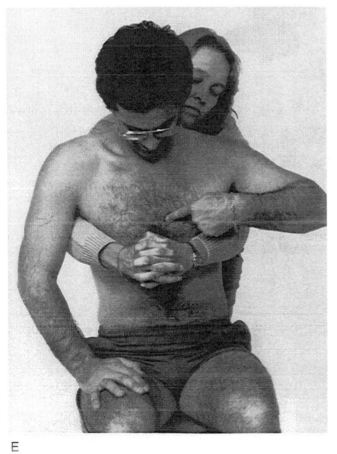

E

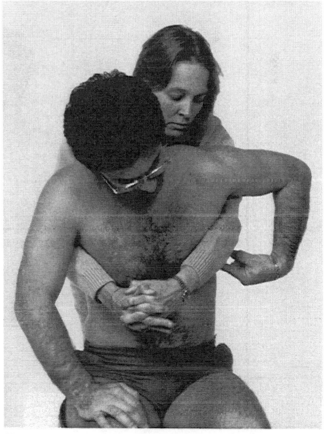

F

11 | *Schepelmann's Test*

Procedure: The patient is seated. Instruct the patient to laterally flex the spine to one side and then the other (Figs. A–C).

Rationale: This test is used to differentiate between intercostal neuralgia and underlying pleural inflammation.

Classical Significance: If pain is increased on the concave side, consider intercostal neuralgia. Pain occuring on the convex side indicates pleural inflammation (Figs. D & E).

Clinical Significance: This maneuver may result in a positive Forestier's bowstring test. This is an abnormal contracture response seen most commonly with ankylosing disease. However, usually no pain occurs with this response.

Follow-up: Perform Forestier's bowstring test, the chest expansion test, or Lewin's supine test.

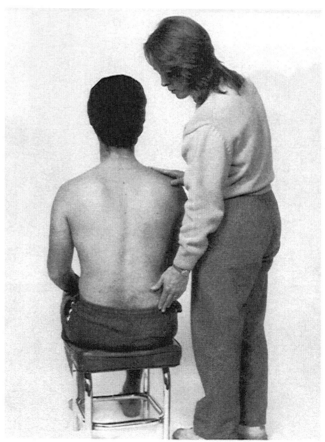

A

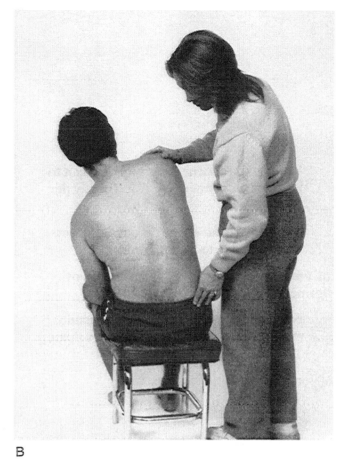

B

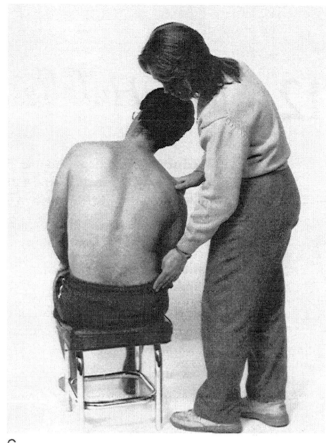

C

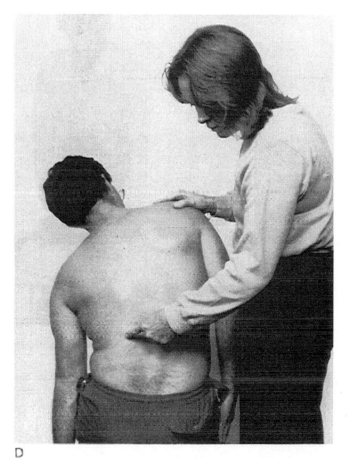

D

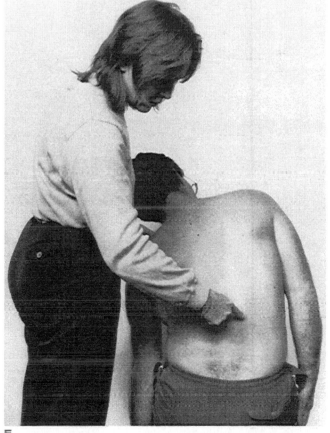

E

12 | *Soto-Hall Test*

Procedure: The patient is supine. Place one hand on the patient's sternum to affix it to the table. Cup the patient's head with your other hand along the occiput and gently flex the chin onto the chest (Figs. A–C).

Rationale: This test places traction along the posterior supraspinous ligaments. When the level of vertebral injury is reached, a noticeable local pain results.

Classical Significance: Local pain within the cervical or dorsal spine to the level of T7 may indicate fracture at that level, or a ligamentous sprain (Figs. D & E).

Clinical Significance: While not truly positive, an increase in pain at the cervicodorsal junction can be a result of trapezius spasm. If pain is reported below T7, re-evaluate the procedure (Fig. F).

Follow-up: Perform the spinous percussion test or the tuning fork test.

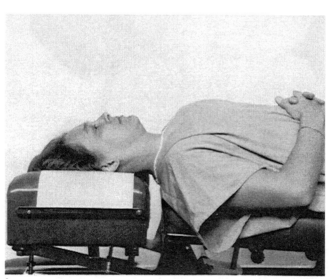

A

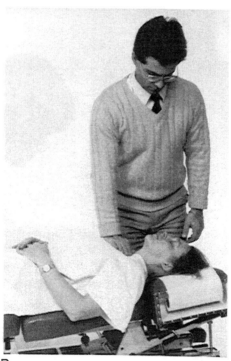

B

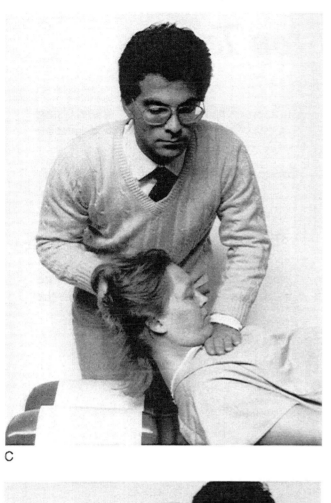

C

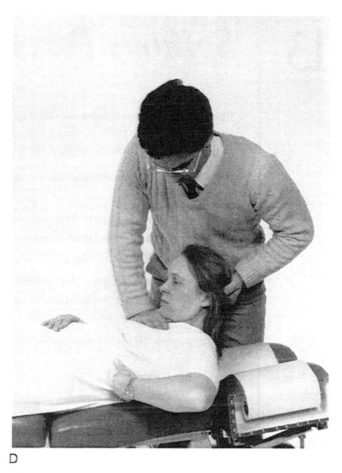

D

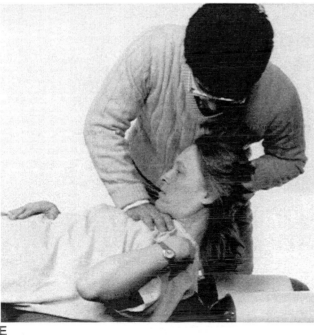

E

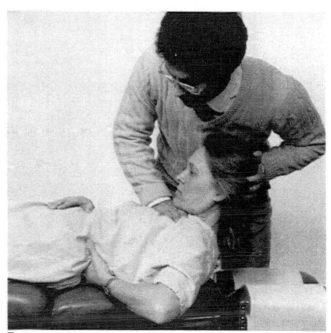

F

13 | *Spinous Percussion Test*

Procedure: The patient is seated with a slight forward bend to the dorsal spine. Using any neurologic hammer, strike the spinous processes of the dorsal vertebrae. Repeat by striking the paraspinal musculature (Figs. A–C).

Rationale: Any irritation of the spinous processes and surrounding tissue is exacerbated by this test.

Classical Significance: Localized pain may indicate a fractured vertebral segment. A disc lesion may be present if radicular pain increases; a ligamentous sprain will also cause a local nonradiating pain (Fig. D).

Clinical Significance: An increase in paraspinal pain on percussion may indicate muscular strain. Take care not to cause pain by the percussion alone, especially in the patient with a low pain threshold (Fig. E).

Follow-up: Perform the tuning fork test or the chest expansion test.

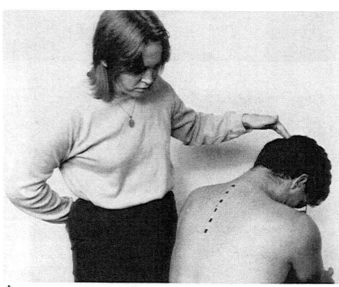

A

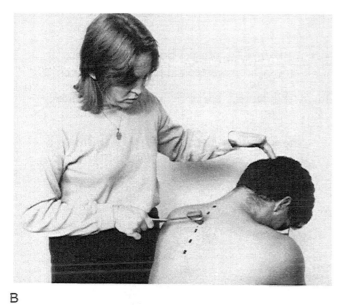

B

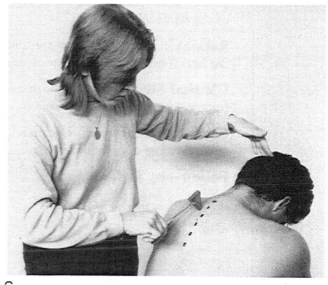

C

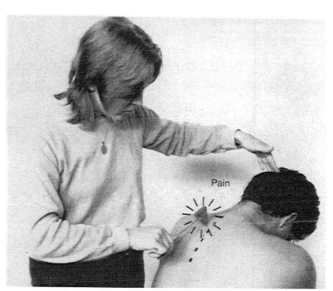

D

E

14 | *Sternal Compression Test*

Procedure: The patient is supine. Press down on the patient's sternum with the palms of the hands (Figs. A–C).

Rationale: Downward pressure on the sternum will increase a bowing of the ribs at the lateral margin. Also, separation of the rib along the sternocostal junction can occur.

Classical Significance: Localized pain in the lateral areas of a rib may indicate fracture at that point (Fig. D).

Clinical Significance: Localized pain at the sternocostal junction may indicate a subluxated or disarticulated rib (Fig. E).

Follow-up: Perform the chest expansion test or the tuning fork test.

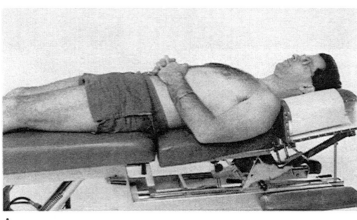

A

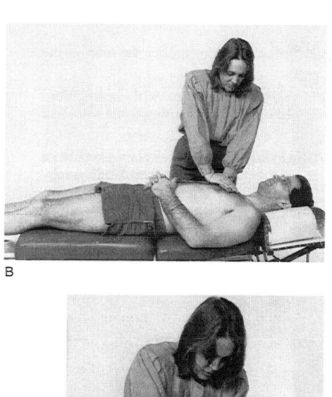

B

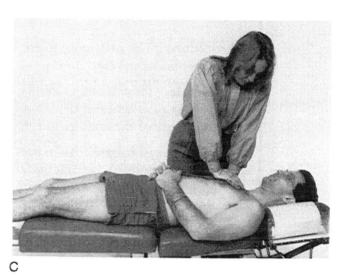

C

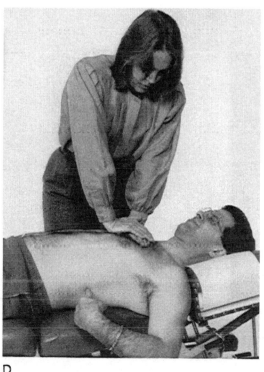

D

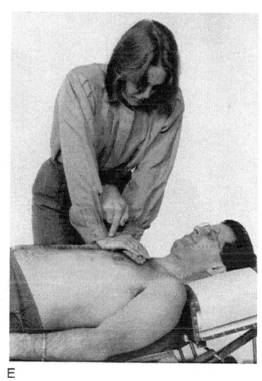

E

15 | *Tuning Fork Test*

Procedure: The patient is seated. Using a 128-cc tuning fork, place the stem on any bony prominence (Figs. A–D).

Rationale: The vibration caused by the tuning fork is transferred to the bony prominence being evaluated. If there is a fracture, the underlying vibrating tissue will cause the two ends of the fracture to rub.

Classical Significance: An increase in sharp pain at the area of the bony prominence being tested is positive for fracture. This is a good way to test for fracture if radiography is unavailable (Fig. E).

Clinical Significance: A subtle hairline fracture may cause only a slight increase in pain at the site being evaluated (Fig. F).

Follow-up: Perform the spinous percussion test.

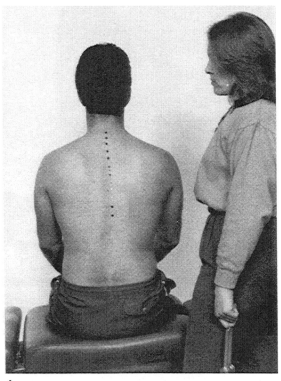

A

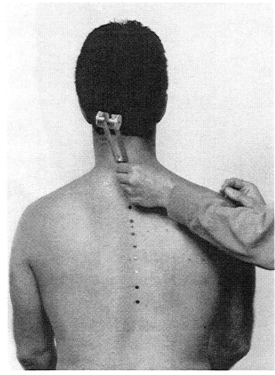

B

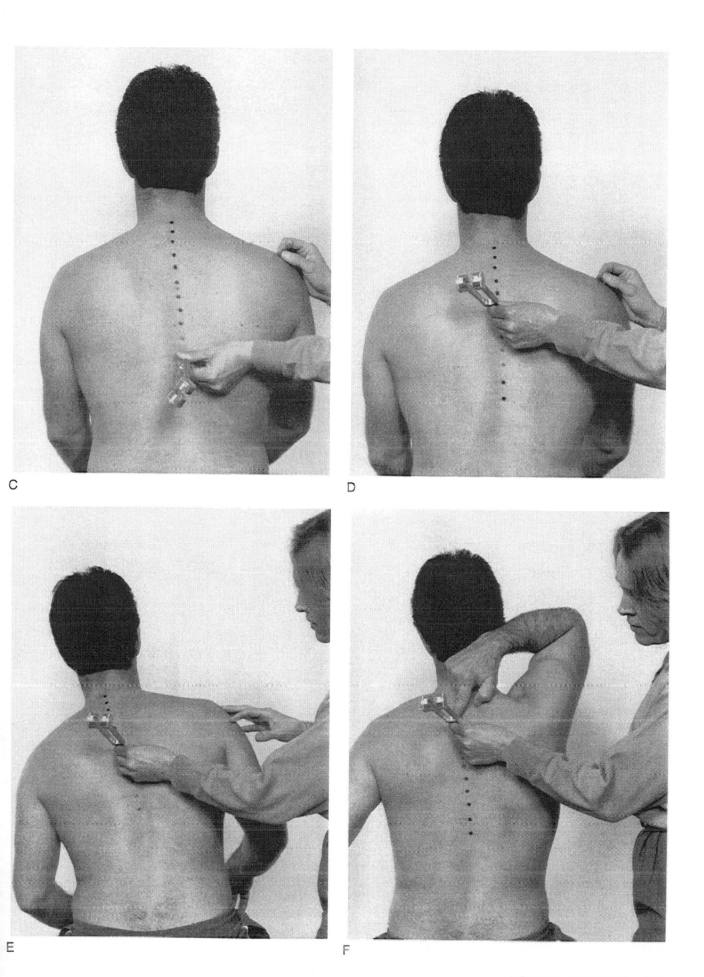

C

D

E

F

Lumbar and Sciatic Testing

1. Range of Motion Studies
2. Adam's Position
3. Adam's Sign
4. Advancement Test
5. Astrom Suspension Test
6. Bechterew's Test
7. Beery's Test
8. Belt Test
9. Bonnet's Sign
10. Bowstring Sign
11. Braggard's Test
12. Buckling Sign
13. Dejerine's Sign
14. Demianoff's Sign
15. Deyerle's Sciatic Tension Test
16. Double Leg Raise
17. Duchenne's Sign
18. Ely's Heel to Buttock Test
19. Ely's Sign
20. Engel's Test
21. Fajersztajn's Test
22. Femoral Nerve Traction Test
23. Goldthwait's Test
24. Heel Walk Test
25. Hyperextension Test
26. Jar Drop Test
27. Kemp's Test
28. Lasegue's Differential Test
29. Lasegue's Rebound Test
30. Lasegue's Straight Leg Test
31. Lewin's Punch Test
32. Lewin's Standing Test
33. Lindner's Test
34. McBride's Test
35. Milgram's Test
36. Minor's Sign
37. Murphy's Punch Test
38. Nachlas Test
39. Naffziger's Test
40. O'Connell Test
41. O'Donoghues Manuever
42. Petrin-Flip Test
43. Schober's Test
44. Seated Flexion Test
45. Sicard's Test
46. Spinous Percussion Test
47. Thomas Test
48. Toe Walk Test
49. Tripod Sign
50. Tuning Fork Test
51. Turyn's Test
52. Valsalva Manuever

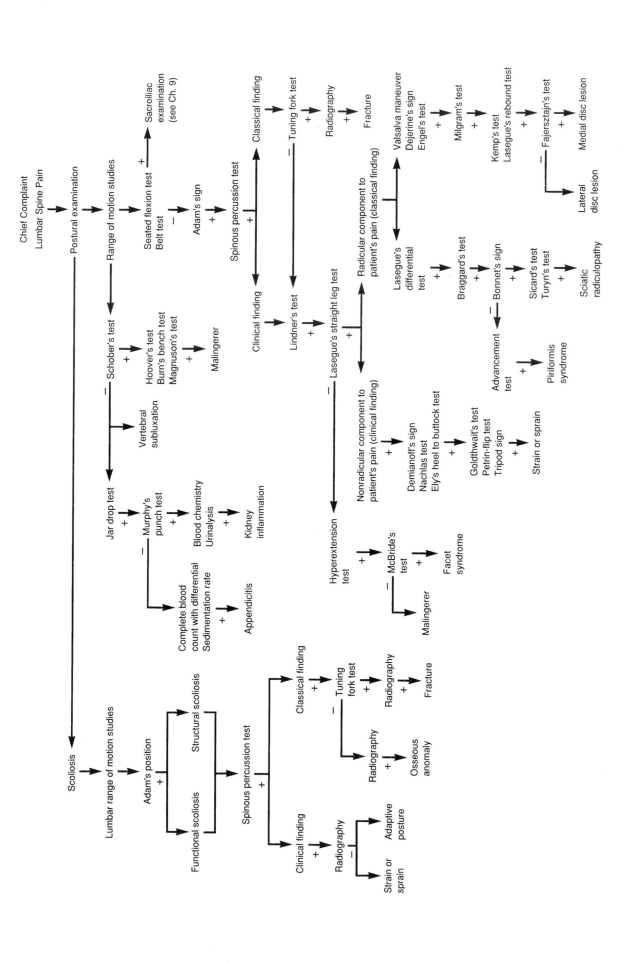

1 | *Range of Motion Studies*

When performing range of motion studies, it is important to use either an arthrodial protractor or an inclinometer. The *American Medical Association Guides for Impairment Ratings* now recommend the use of the inclinometer exclusively. It is impossible to separate the dorsal spine from the lumbar spine when performing ranges of motion. Therefore, the two are always recorded as dorsolumbar ranges of motion.

Flexion: Ask the patient to bend forward and touch the toes. Normal flexion is 80 to 90 degrees or the fingertips 4 to 6 inches from the floor. Flexion may be limited by such conditions as ankylosing spondylitis, degenerative disc disease, and osteoarthritis. However, the hamstring musculature restricts forward iliac rotation and tight hamstrings can result in loss of normal ranges of motion.

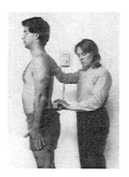 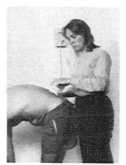 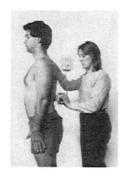 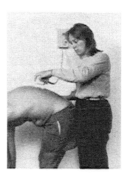

Extension: Ask the patient to bend at the waist as far back as possible. Normal extension is 20 to 30 degrees. Congenital anomalies such as facet tropism or knife clasp syndrome can significantly restrict dorsolumbar extension. Arthritic conditions such as ankylosing spondylitis, degenerative disc disease, facet syndrome, and spondylolisthesis also result in loss of normal extension.

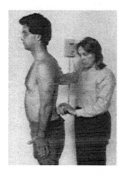 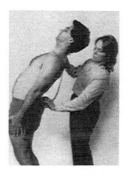 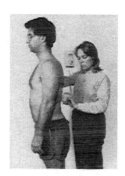 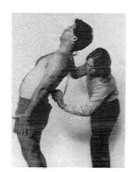

Rotation: Ask the patient to cross the arms or to place each hand on the opposite shoulder and to turn the torso as far right and left as possible. Normal rotation is 20 to 45 degrees.

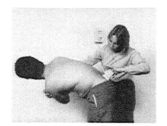 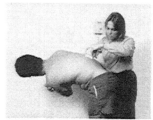 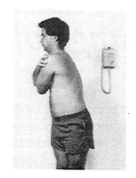 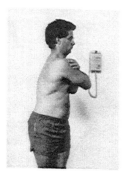

Lateral Flexion: With the patient's arms alongside the body, ask the patient to bend toward each side as if trying to reach the hand to the knee. Be sure the knees are locked. Check the fingertip level to see whether the bend is equal bilaterally. Normal lateral flexion is 20 to 35 degrees.

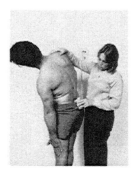 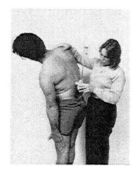 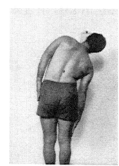 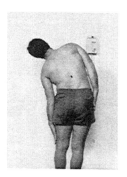

Quick Test: Perform the quick test if an inclinometer is unavailable. The patient is standing and bends backward from the waist as far as possible. Note whether a smooth C curve occurs in the lumbar spine. Next, ask the patient to bend forward from the waist (keeping legs straight) as if touching fingers to toes. Measure the distance between the fingers and the floor (normal is 4 to 6 inches).

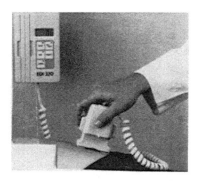 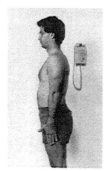 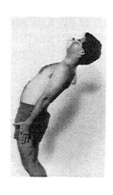 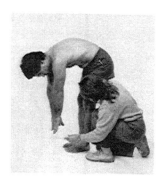

Classical Significance: The patient's ranges of motion should be within normal and the values should be equal bilaterally.

Clinical Significance: Acute or chronic injury may restrict ranges of motion bilaterally. If the ranges of motion are still within normal limits this is not normal. It is imperative to have good baseline ranges of motion on all patients.

Note: Active ranges of motion are largely a function of volition. In case of strain, the area is reactively guarded and any attempt to move will be restricted and discomforting. If the patient allows passive ranges of motion, they will be achieved to a greater degree and with less pain than with the active.

2 | *Adam's Position*

Procedure: This test is performed on patients who have either a visible or palpable scoliosis. The patient is standing. Stand behind the patient and ask the patient to bend forward, reaching for the toes. The severity of the scoliosis will either remain or reduce (Figs. A & B [B: idiopathic rotary scoliosis]).

Rationale: In a patient with functional scoliosis, the scoliosis should reduce due to stretching of the supraspinous ligaments as well as a reduction of axial compression. No visible change in severity will occur if the patient has structural scoliosis (Fig. E).

Classical Significance: If the angle of scoliosis reduces when the patient bends forward, the scoliosis is functional (Fig. C).

Clinical Significance: If no change in the scoliosis angle occurs, the scoliosis is structural in origin (Fig. D).

Follow-up: Perform postural analysis or the spinous percussion test.

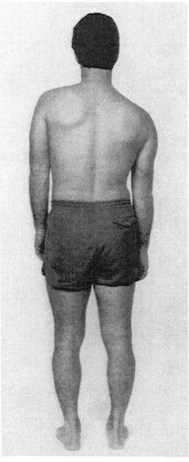

A

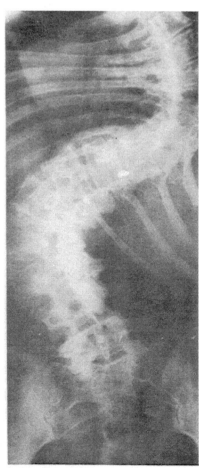

B

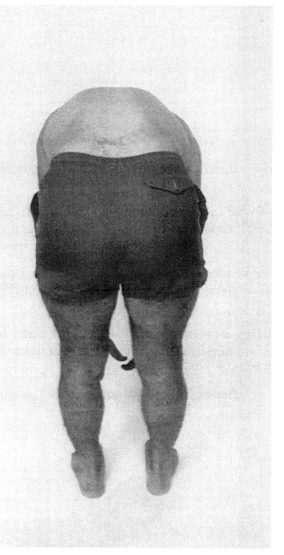

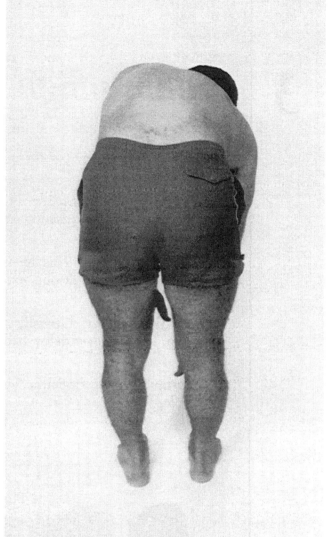

C   D

SCOLIOSIS TREATMENT[a]	
Curves	Mode of Treatment
<29°	Curvature is slow in progression Confine treatment to conservative means See the patient regularly for chiropractic adjustive technique & periodic evaluation of the curve at 3-month intervals until cessation of growth is evidenced by Risser of 4/5 (some authors believe that because one-third of the curves are 20–29° and do not progress, treatment may be withheld until progression of the curve is documented)
30–40°	Curvature is likely to increase Initiate treatment immediately and incorporate use of a brace Also, include chiropractic adjustive technique, physiotherapy, and aggressive exercises designed to derotate and laterally counterflex the curvature
>40°	In the adolescent, this degree of curve rarely responds to bracing Restore normomechanics using chiropractic adjustive technique; however, remember the limitations of physical matter In the case of acute deformation and/or debility, recommend a neurosurgical consultation

[a] The American Academy of Orthopedic Surgeons advise that the curve < 20° should not be treated but should be watched. It is our opinion, that any scoliotic deformity that is receptive to conservative management by chiropractic technique should be treated so that the curvature remains flexible and not rigid.

E

3 | *Adam's Sign*

Procedure: Observe the patient for pain produced when active dorsolumbar ranges of motion are performed.

Rationale: Flexion restriction is usually due to a discal lesion, extension restriction may be caused by facet irritation, and lateral flexion restriction is a result of strain or sprain injuries.

Classical Significance: This sign is positive when restriction or pain, or both, occurs in the following order: flexion, extension, lateral flexion, and finally rotation (Figs. A–F).

Clinical Significance: Generally, this sign is positive in the patient with acute low back pain. The patient with low back pain of nondiscal origin will not be restricted in flexion.

Follow-up: Perform the Petrin-flip test, Bechterew's test, Milgram's test, or Lasegue's straight leg test.

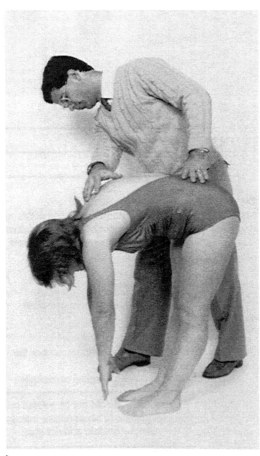

A

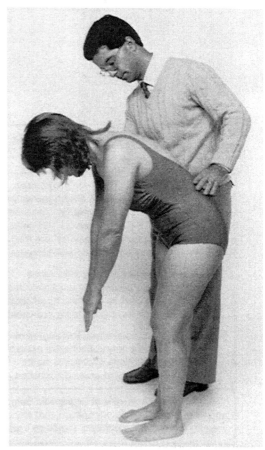

B

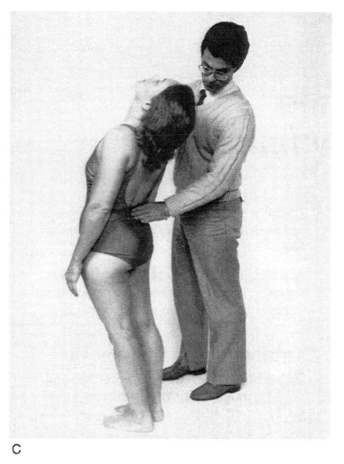

C

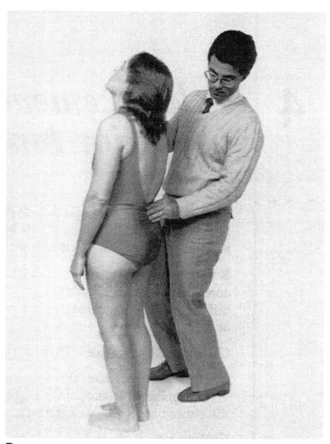

D

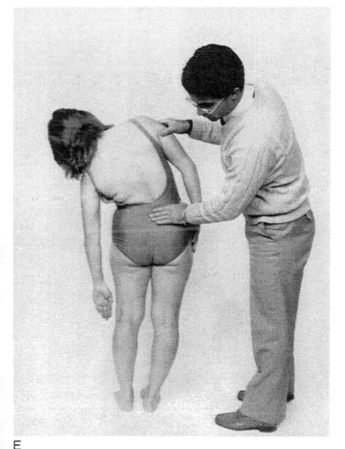

E

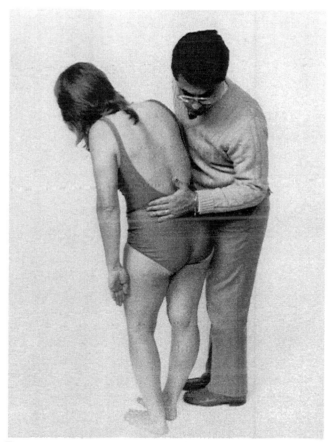

F

4 | *Advancement Test (Anterior Innominate Test)*

Procedure: The patient is standing upright. Ask the patient to place one foot forward and to bend from the waist to touch the toes of the front foot. Have the patient repeat the test with the other foot in front (Figs. A–E).

Rationale: This test puts extra strain on the sciatic nerve and should exacerbate this complaint in patients with known sciatic nerve radiculopathy. It is similar to Lasegue's differential test and Bechterew's test; if one is positive the other two should be positive as well.

Classical Significance: The test is positive if sciatic radicular pain is increased (Fig. F).

Clinical Significance: If the patient is able to perform this test without a problem and yet complains of sciatic pain during either Lasegue's straight leg test or Bechterew's test, the patient may be a malingerer.

Follow-up: Perform Lasegue's straight leg test, Bechterew's test, the Valsalva maneuver, or McBride's test.

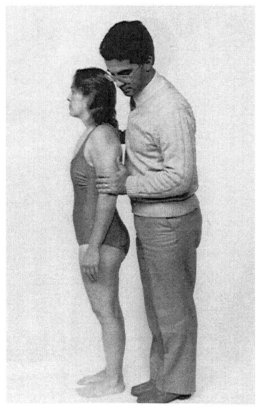

A

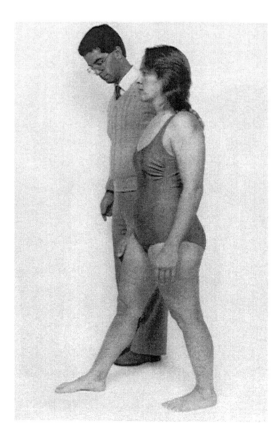

B

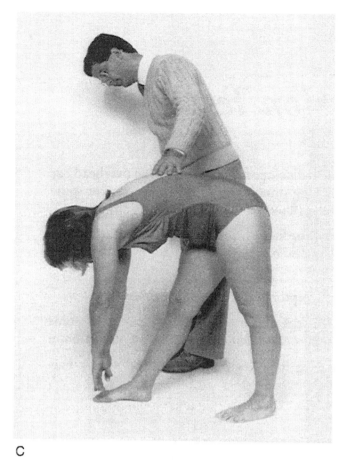

C

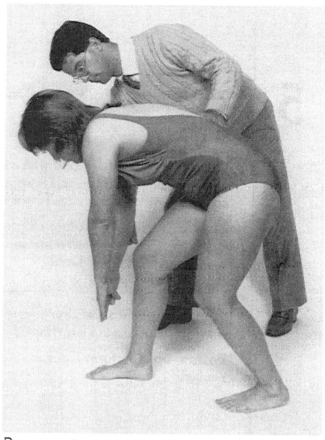

D

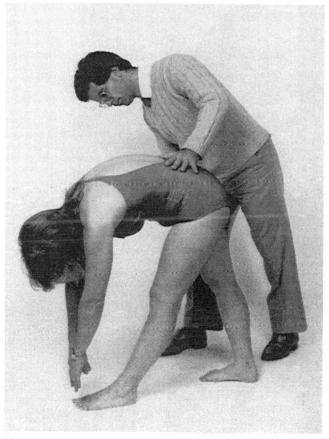

E

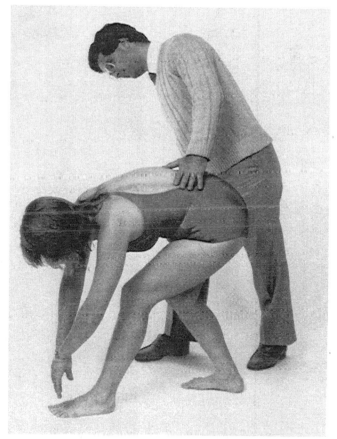

F

5 | *Astrom Suspension Test*

Procedure: Ask the patient with a sciatic radiculopathy to hold onto an overhead bar with the hands. The legs and lower torso hang straight down. Strike the lumbar spine and paralumbar area with a Taylor hammer (flat side only) (Figs. A–E).

Rationale: This procedure reduces axial loading on the vertebral column, thereby reducing pressure on individual discs. The disc bulge or herniation (protruded) discs will be significantly reduced.

Classical Significance: A reduction in symptoms indicates a discal lesion.

Clinical Significance: In patients with a scleratogenous referral of pain, symptoms may decrease because less strain is on the posterior elements of the vertebral column.

Follow-up: Perform Lasegue's straight leg test, Kemp's test, or the Valsalva maneuver.

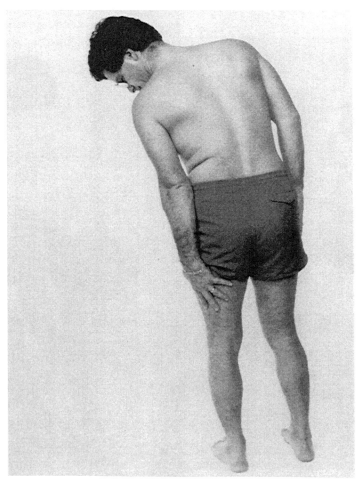

A

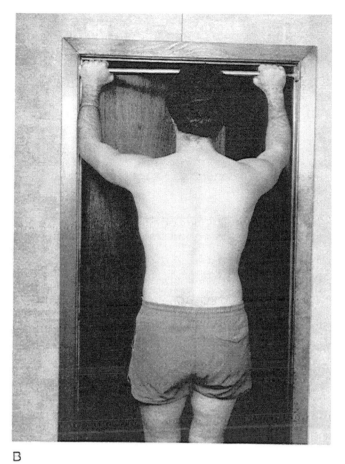

B

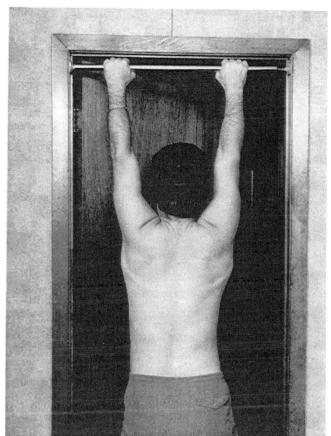

C

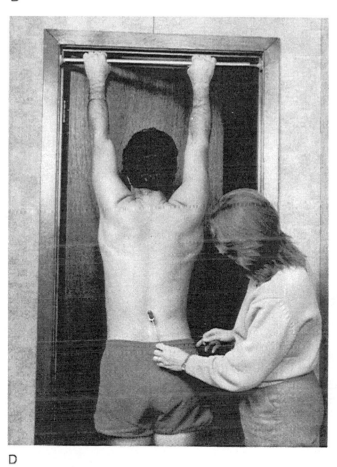

D

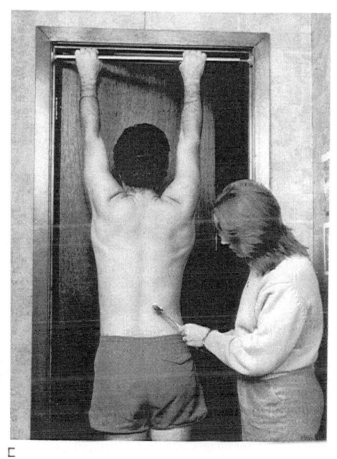

E

6 | *Bechterew's Test*

Procedure: The patient is seated. Instruct the patient to extend one knee at a time, and then both knees together (Figs. A–D).

Rationale: This test causes an increase in intrathecal pressure. The patient with a discal lesion will have difficulty performing this test. This is a good test for ruling out a malingerer, as it is really a sitting Lasegue test.

Classical Significance: An increase in sciatic radiculopathy when one knee is extended at a time indicates stretching of the sciatic nerve (Fig. E).

Clinical Significance: If this test produces an increase in radiculopathy only when both knees are extended, discal involvement is the more likely diagnosis because intrathecal pressure is increased (Fig. F).

Follow-up: Perform the Valsalva maneuver, Lasegue's straight leg test, or the advancement test.

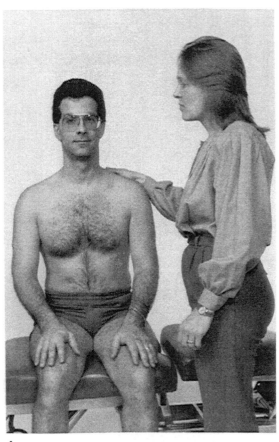

A

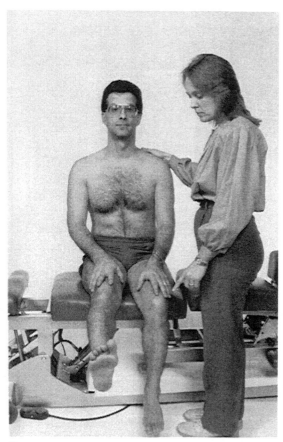

B

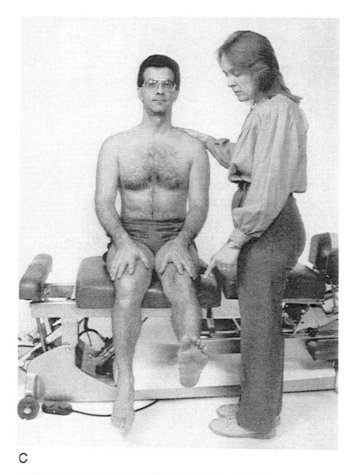

C

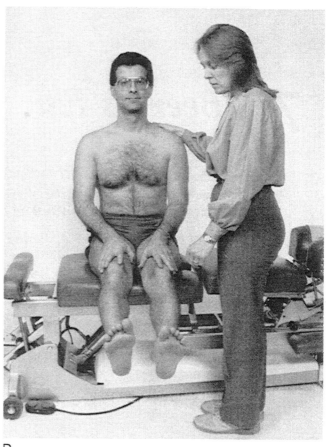

D

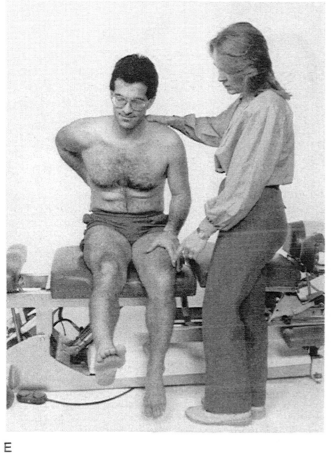

E

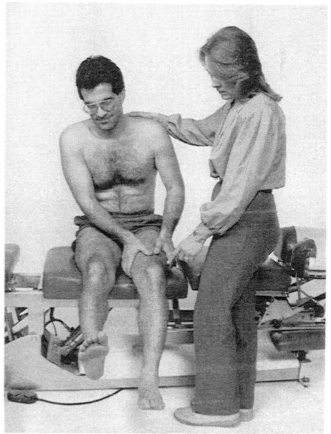

F

7 | *Beery's Test*

Procedure: Perform this test on the patient who complains of low back pain when standing. Ask the patient to sit and then to stand again, and to report the level and intensity of pain in both positions (Figs. A–C).

Rationale: Less strain is on the pelvis when the patient is sitting because the hamstrings are not pulled as tight.

Classical Significance: This test is significant if pain is reduced when the patient sits but not when the patient stands (Fig. D).

Clinical Significance: If pain is greater when the patient is seated, consider a discal problem because sitting increases intervertebral disc pressure. Standing will be easier than sitting if degenerative disc disease is present. This is the opposite of the classical finding (Fig. E).

Follow-up: Perform Dejerine's sign, the Valsalva maneuver, or the seated flexion test.

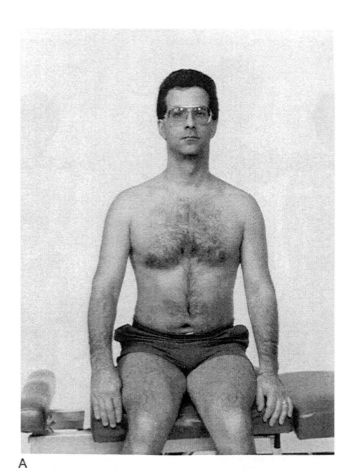

A

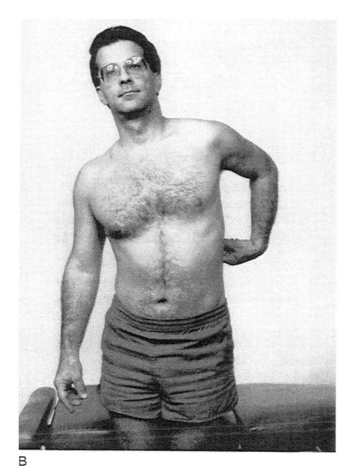

B

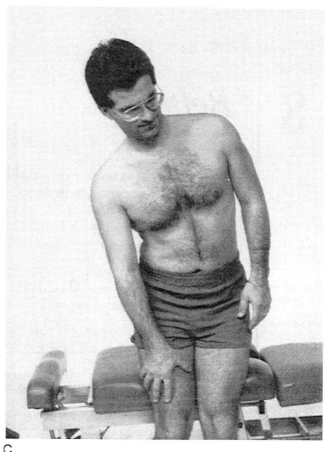

C

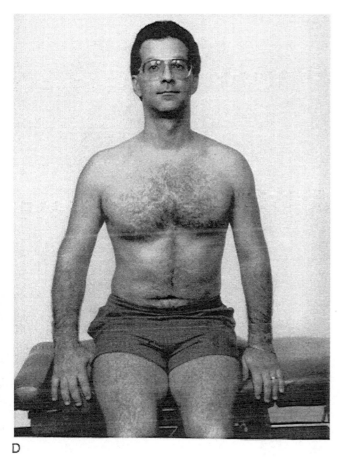

D

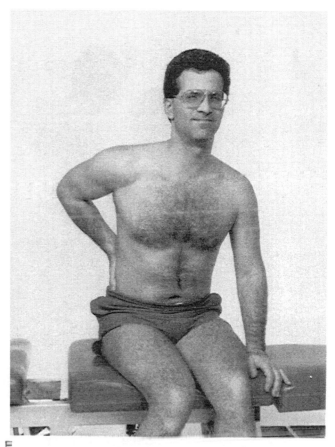

E

8 | *Belt Test*

Procedure: This test is performed only on patients who present with low back pain. The patient is standing, with the examiner behind the patient. Ask the patient to bend forward and to indicate the level at which pain occurs. Next, support the patient's sacrum with your hip while the patient again bends forward. Compare the level at which pain occurs (if any) (Figs. A–D).

Rationale: A properly functioning sacroiliac joint is necessary for forward flexion, as is lumbosacral and individual lumbar vertebral movement. The level of dysfunction is determined by comparing where the pain occurs with and without support.

Classical Significance: If pain occurs on forward flexion without support but is absent with support, the problem is at the sacroiliac joint (Fig. E).

Clinical Significance: If pain occurs on forward flexion with as well as without support, the problem is within the lumbar spine, including the lumbosacral junction (Fig. F).

Follow-up: Perform McBride's test, the seated flexion test, or Lasegue's straight leg test.

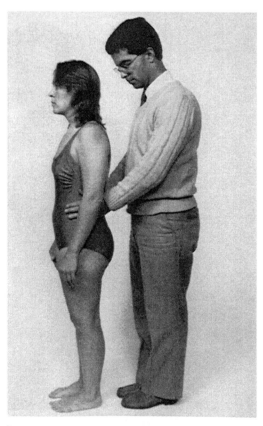

A

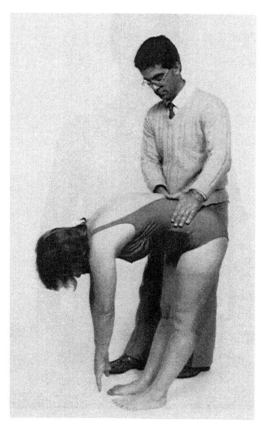

B

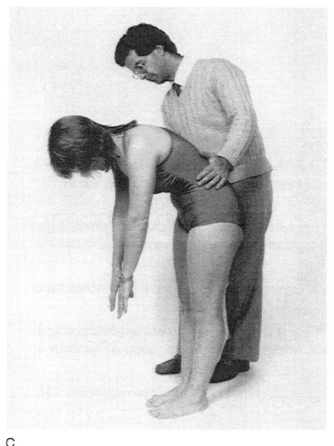

C

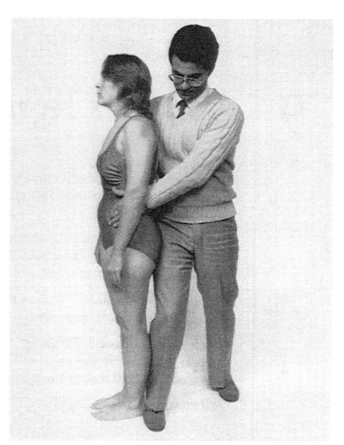

D

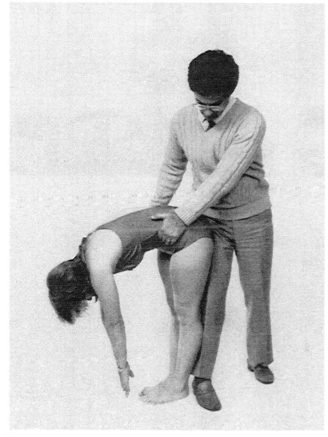

E

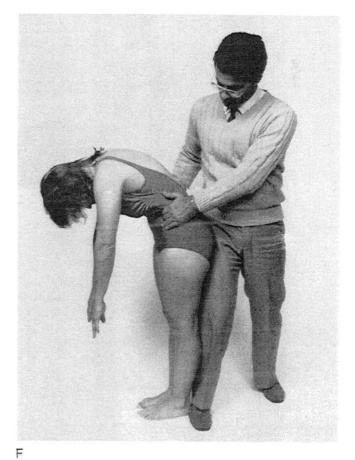

F

9 | *Bonnet's Sign*

Procedure: The patient is supine. Stabilize the leg at the ankle and knee while performing a straight leg raise and internally rotating and adducting the leg across the midline (Figs. A–D).

Rationale: It is our opinion that this version of Lasegue's straight leg test will help determine the cause of sciatic pain. Adduction and internal rotation of the limb cause a stretching of the piriformis musculature.

Classical Significance: Radicular pain into the limb indicates sciatic nerve root irritation due to piriformis entrapment (Fig. E).

Clinical Significance: If this test is positive then repeat it without the adduction and internal rotation. If the pain still exists, note the angle of the pain, to confirm a sacroiliac, lumbosacral, or lumbar lesion (Fig. F).

Follow-up: Perform Engel's test, Lasegue's differential test, or the advancement test.

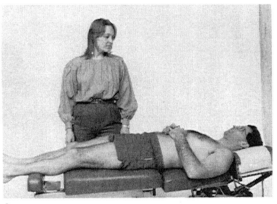

A

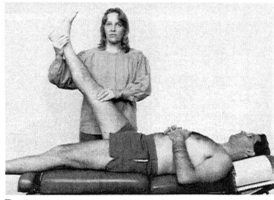

B

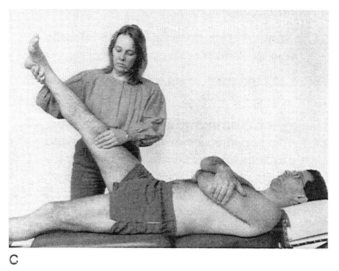

C

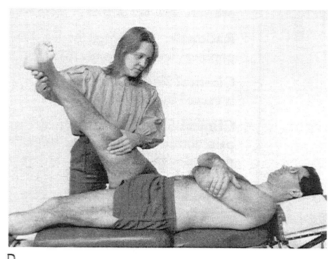

D

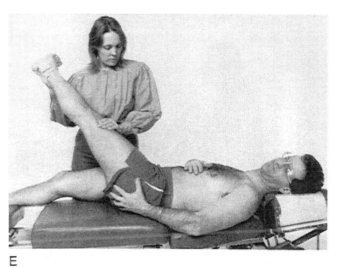

E

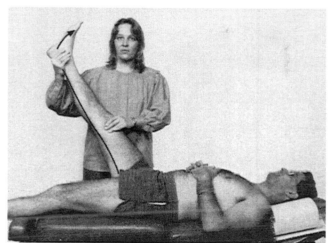

F

10 | *Bowstring Sign*

Procedure: The patient is supine. Sit on the table facing the patient and place the patient's leg on top of your shoulder. Then grasp the knee while applying digital pressure into the popliteal fossa with your thumbs (Figs. A–D).

Rationale: Elevating the leg stretches the sciatic nerve; pressing further into the popliteal fossa will exacerbate a sciatic condition even more.

Classical Significance: Pain is a positive test and indicates sciatic radiculopathy that is caused by nerve root compression (Fig. E).

Clinical Significance: Patients with very tight hamstrings may note nonradiating pain within the back of the thigh (Fig. F). If this happens, lower the leg slightly and proceed with pressing into the popliteal fossa. In addition, a Baker's cyst can cause leg pain on deep palpation of the posterior knee. When interpreting the results of this test, consider the direction of the pain. A retrograde direction indicates pain of a discal origin; pain beginning at the popliteal fossa that goes below the knee may be a result of entrapment of the popliteal nerve in the compartment of the knee joint.

Follow-up: Perform Kemp's test, Sicard's test, or Braggard's test.

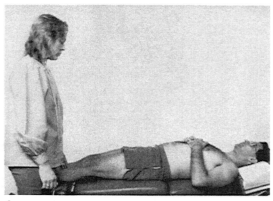

A

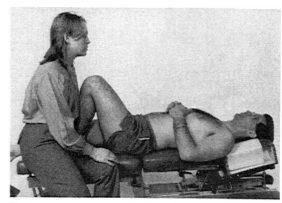

B

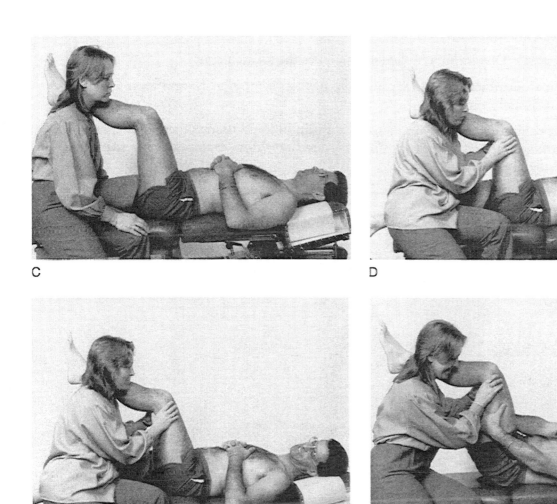

C

D

E

F

11 | *Braggard's Test*

Procedure: Perform this test only on patients with a positive Lasegue's straight leg test. The patient is supine. Raise the affected limb to the point of radicular pain. Then lower it 5 degrees or until the leg no longer causes radicular symptomatology and dorsiflex the foot (Figs. A–C).

Rationale: Dorsiflexion of the foot stretches the sciatic nerve.

Classical Significance: An increase in radicular symptoms is significant for sciatic nerve irritation (Fig. D).

Clinical Significance: Dull, nonspecific pain in the posterior thigh indicates tight hamstrings (Fig. E). Calf discomfort may indicate thrombophlebitis or spasmodic gastrocnemius musculature.

Follow-up: Perform Fajersztajn's test, the Valsalva maneuver, Sicard's test, or Homan's test (see Ch. 13).

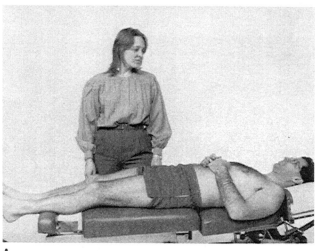

A

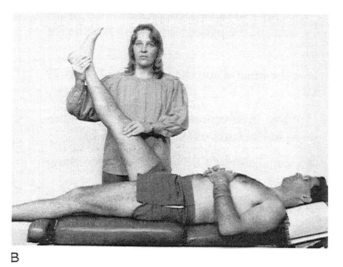

B

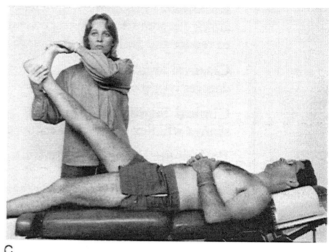

C

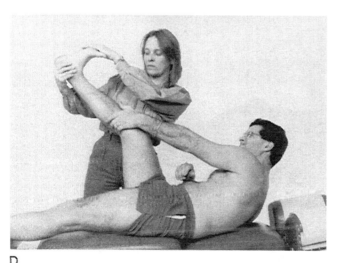

D

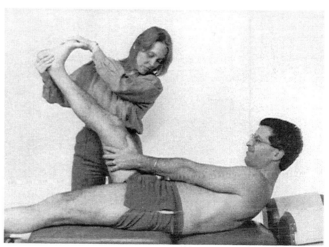

E

12 | *Buckling Sign*

Procedure: The patient is supine. Place one hand under the patient's ankle and the other on the knee. Raise the leg 90 degrees (Figs. A–C).

Rationale: In patients with sciatica, raising the leg will cause an increase in symptomatology at some point. In response to the discomfort, the patient will try to flex the leg to reduce the pulling on the nerve.

Classical Significance: Flexion of the leg at the knee when the leg is raised 30 to 70 degrees is positive for sciatica (Fig. D).

Clinical Significance: Patients without sciatic involvement but with tight hamstrings will flex the knee to reduce the pulling in the back of the thigh (Fig. E).

Follow-up: Perform Sicard's test, Turyn's test, Lasegue's differential test, or Braggard's test.

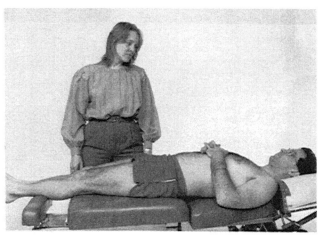

A

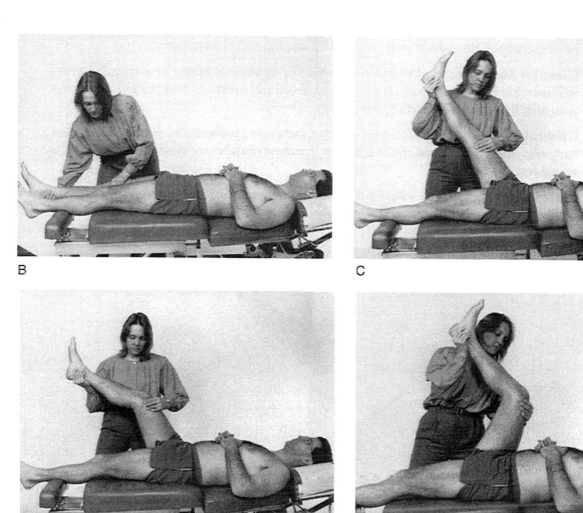

B

C

D

E

13 | *Dejerine's Sign*

Procedure: The patient is seated. Instruct the patient to cough hard, to sneeze, and then to bear down. These three components comprise Dejerine's triad (Figs. A–C).

Rationale: All three of these maneuvers raise the intra-abdominal pressure and have a jarring component, which puts mechanical stress on the lower back.

Classical Significance: Protrusion of a disc or of a spinal tumor or a spinal fracture will increase lower back pain. If a disc is involved and pressure is on the nerve root the pain will have a radicular component (Figs. D–F).

Clinical Significance: Local pain without radicular involvement, may indicate lumbar paraspinal musculature involvement, since these muscles are used in performing the above tests.

Follow-up: Perform the Valsalva maneuver, Lindner's test, Lasegue's straight leg test, or Bechterew's test.

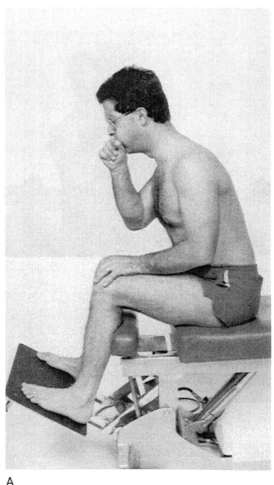

A

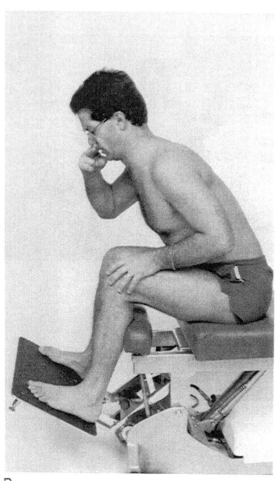

B

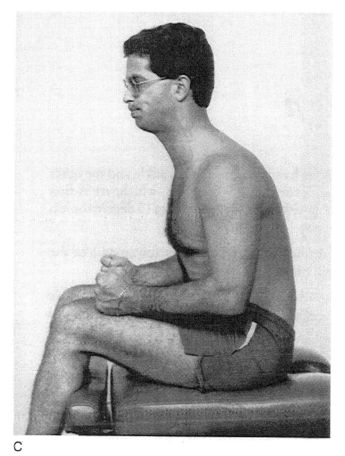

C

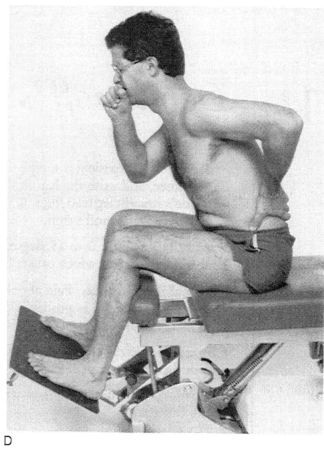

D

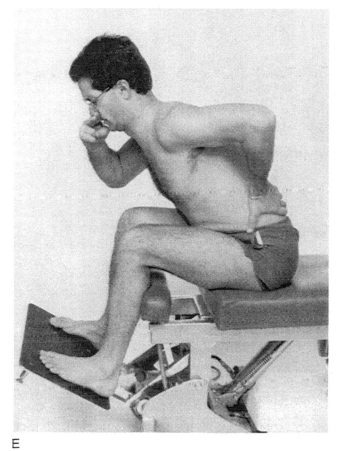

E

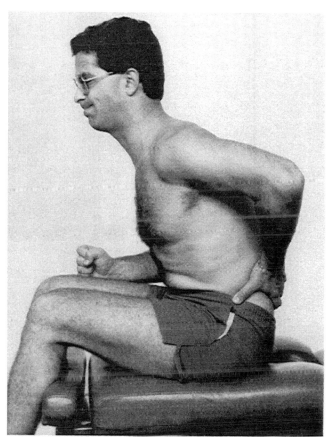

F

14 | *Demianoff's Sign*

Procedure: The patient is supine. Place one hand on the patient's ankle and the other on the knee, and raise the leg until pain occurs or to 90 degrees, whichever is first (Lasegue's straight leg test) (Figs. A–C). A positive finding at a level of 15 degrees or less is a positive Demianoff's sign.

Rationale: Pain at 0 to 15 degrees indicates active recruitment (or spasm) of the lumbar musculature, which causes limited lift power.

Classical Significance: Pain at or below 15 degrees of passive leg raising is a positive Demianoff's sign and is probably due to myospasm of the erector spinae group of muscles (Fig. D).

Clinical Significance: A severe disc lesion will also produce a positive Demianoff's sign in the patient with antalgia due to reactive muscle guarding (Fig. E).

Follow-up: Perform the Valsalva maneuver, Bechterew's test, the advancement test, or the belt test.

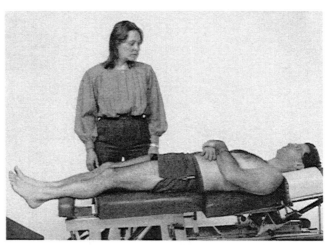

A

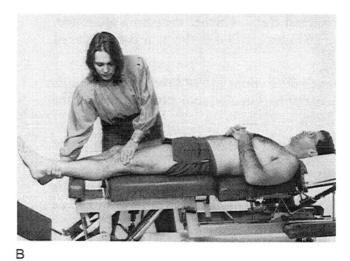

B

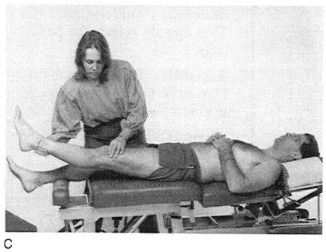

C

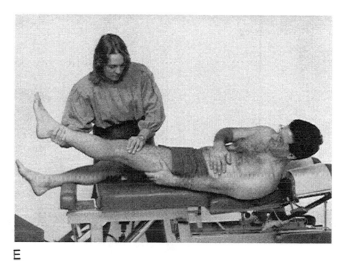

D

E

15 | *Deyerle's Sciatic Tension Test*

Procedure: The patient is seated with the legs dangling off the table. Extend the leg that causes a painful sciatica. Flex the knee and check whether the pain is alleviated. Then directly palpate the popliteal fossa and check whether the pain is reproduced (Figs. A – E).

Rationale: This test is similar to Lasegue's differential test and the bowstring sign. Flexion of the knee removes pressure on the hamstrings, and pressure within the popliteal fossa irritates the sciatic nerve.

Classical Significance: If flexion of the knee reduces pain and compression of the popliteal fossa re-creates the radicular pattern, the test is positive (Fig. F).

Clinical Significance: As with similar tests be sure to determine that the pain is retrograde and not from a local lesion in the popliteal fossa or from fibula head subluxation.

Follow-up: Perform the bowstring sign, Lasegue's differential test, or the belt test.

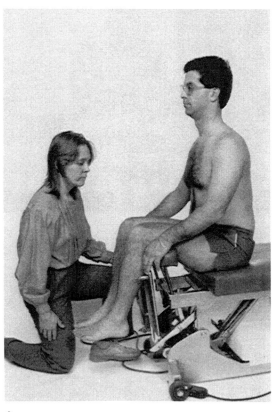

A

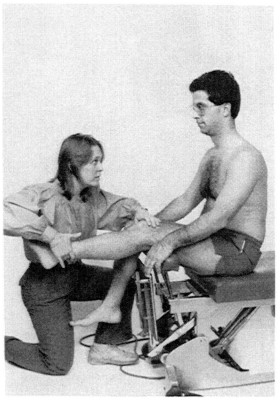

B

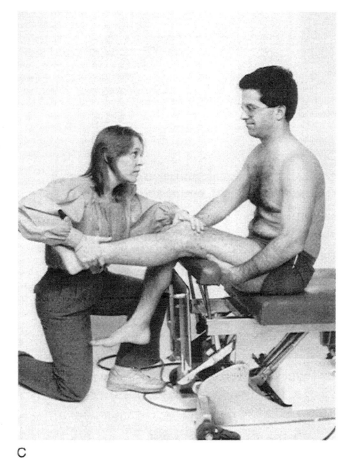

C

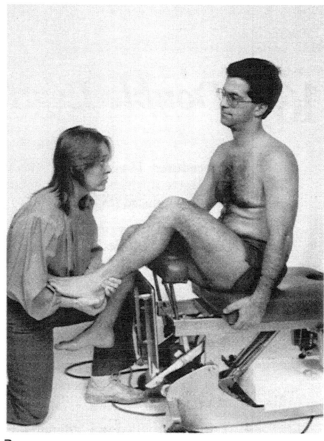

D

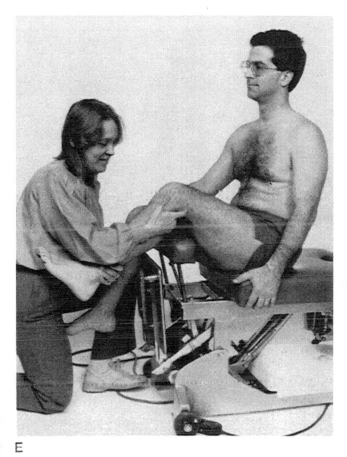

E

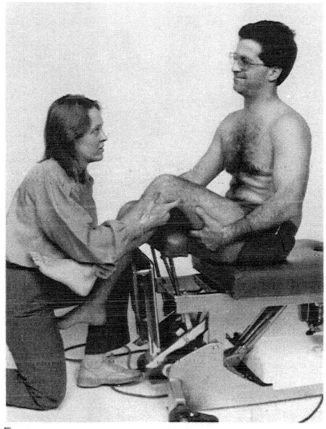

F

16 | *Double Leg Raise*

Procedure: The patient is supine. Perform a single straight leg raise on each leg noting the degree at which pain is produced. Then elevate both legs, noting the angle at which pain is produced (Figs. A–D).

Rationale: There is a greater degree of mobility at the sacroiliac joint and lumbosacral area when a single leg is raised. Raising the legs together puts more stress on the sacroiliac joint and the lumbosacral junction. It also increases the tractioning of the nerve roots that supply the posterior leg.

Classical Significance: Pain that is reproduced similar to that when one leg is elevated but that occurs at a lower level than when each leg is tested individually is a positive test (Fig. E).

Clinical Significance: Ensure that the patient's legs remain passive as these maneuvers are performed. Otherwise components of strain or sprain may contribute to the patient's response (Fig. F).

Follow-up: Perform Milgram's test, Sicard's test, or Braggard's test.

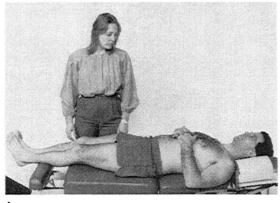

A

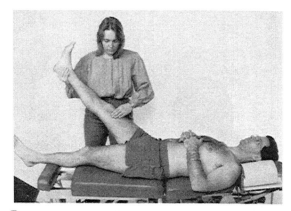

B

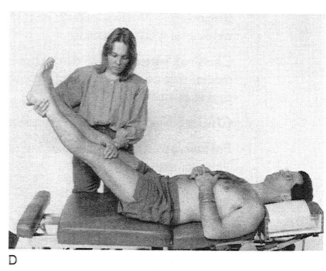

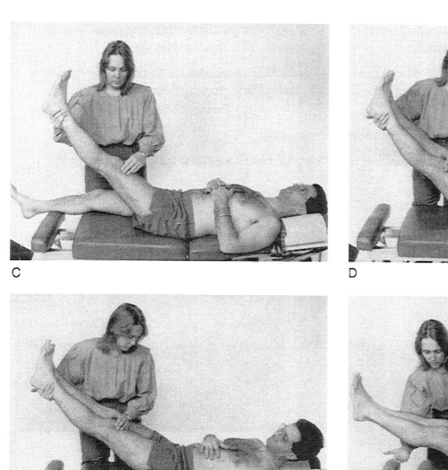

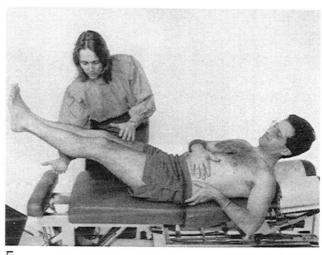

C

D

E

F

17 | *Duchenne's Sign*

Procedure: The patient is supine. Place cephalad pressure on the first metatarsal head of the foot with your finger and ask the patient to plantar flex the foot (Figs. A–E).

Rationale: Normal plantar flexion will not occur in patients with peroneus muscle weakness, which is usually due to S1 nerve root and L5 disc involvement.

Classical Significance: If the first metatarsal offers no resistance to the finger or the medial side of the foot dorsiflexes while the lateral side plantar flexes (inversion), the sign is positive (Fig. F).

Clinical Significance: See Classical Significance.

Follow-up: Perform the heel walk test, toe walk test, Lasegue's straight leg test, or the Valsalva maneuver.

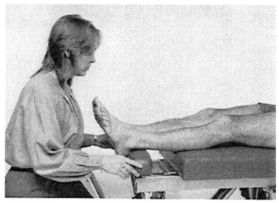

A

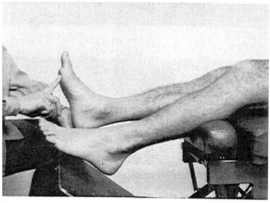

B

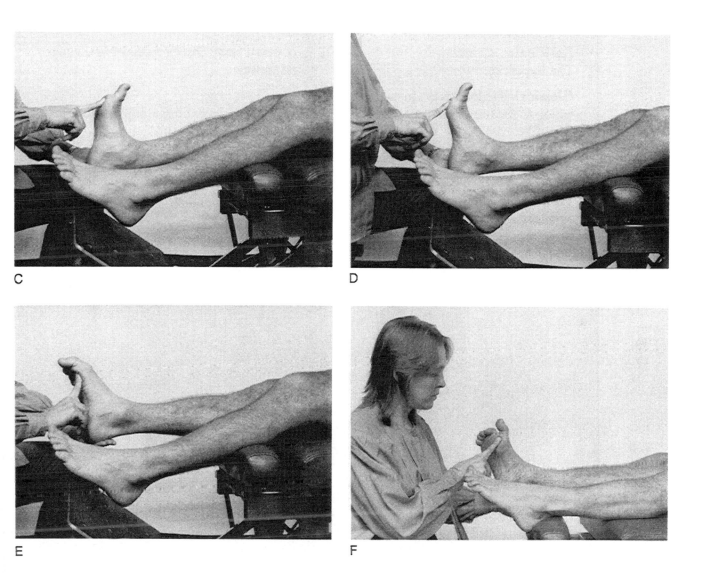

C

D

E

F

18 | *Ely's Heel to Buttock Test*

Procedure: The patient is prone. Flex the patient's knee, bringing the heel onto the contralateral buttock. If this can be performed then lift the flexed knee off the table to hyperextend the hip (Figs. A–D).

Rationale: Crossing the limb over causes a torsional stress that first occurs in the hip. The hyperextension adds a pull in the iliopsoas muscle.

Classical Significance: Inability to perform the above procedures can indicate aggravation of the lumbar nerve roots, lumbar adhesions, psoas irritation, or hip dysfunction (Fig. E).

Clinical Significance: Hyperextension of the knee will extend the lumbar spine and can aggravate a facet irritation, which will result in scleratogenous pain.

Follow-up: Perform the Nachlas test, Yeoman's test (see Ch. 9), or the hyperextension test.

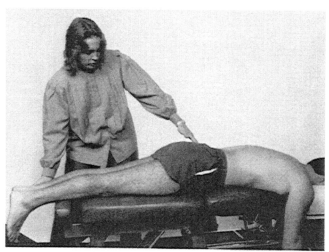

A

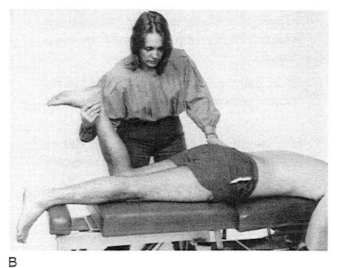

B

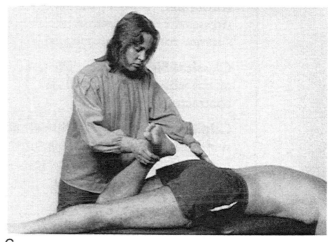

C

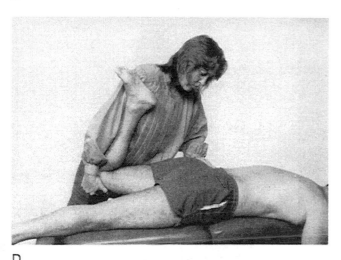

D

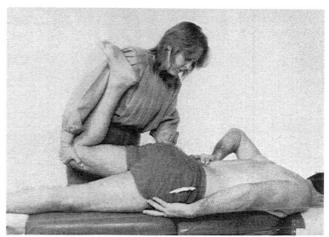

E

19 | *Ely's Sign*

Procedure: The patient is prone. Flex the patient's knee, bringing the heel to the ipsilateral buttock. Do not stabilize the pelvis (Figs. A–D).

Rationale: Bringing the heel to the ipsilateral buttock without stabilizing the buttock stresses the rectus femoris muscle, a part of the quadriceps group. This stress causes an anterior rotational torque within the pelvis (Fig. F).

Classical Significance: The test is positive if the pelvis on the side being tested raises off the table. The thigh will also abduct as a result of rectus femoris or tensor fascia lata contracture (Fig. E).

Clinical Significance: Hip pathology or limitation in hip ranges of motion due to subluxation can cause a false-positive result. It is important to test the hip joint ranges of motion for freedom of movement before doing this test.

Follow-up: Perform the Thomas test, Ober's test (see Ch. 10), or Mennell's test (see Ch. 9).

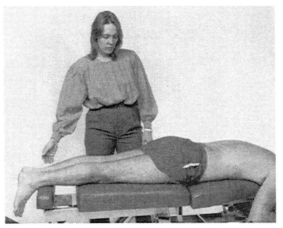

A

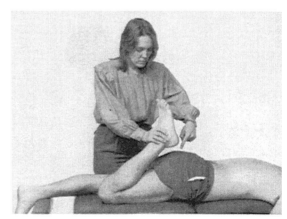

B

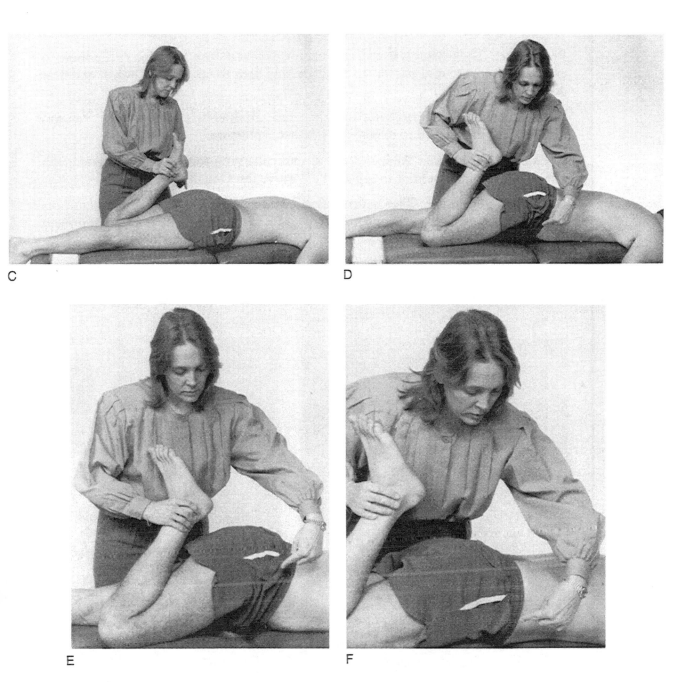

C

D

E

F

20 | *Engel's Test (Triangle Test)*

Procedure: The patient is seated. Instruct the patient to bring the chin to the chest, to extend both knees until parallel to the floor, and then to take a deep breath and bear down (Figs. A–D).

Rationale: This test combines Lindner's test, Bechterew's test, and the Valsalva maneuver. It is designed to maximize intrathecal pressure.

Classical Significance: An increase in the radicular symptomatology associated with a space-occupying lesion of the spine is a positive test (Fig. E).

Clinical Significance: This maneuver will exacerbate any low back complaint because intrathecal pressure is maximized (Fig. F). Localized back pain may represent strain or sprain injury or facet problems and should be investigated.

Follow-up: Perform Dejerine's sign, Lasegue's straight leg test, or Lasegue's differential test.

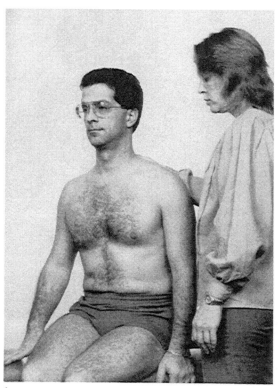

A

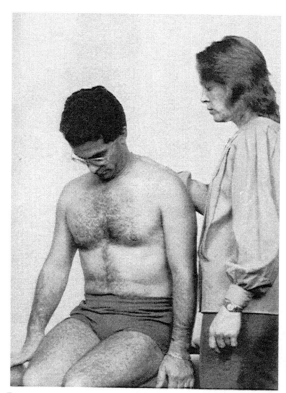

B

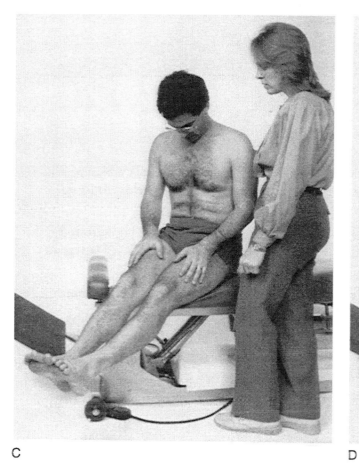

C

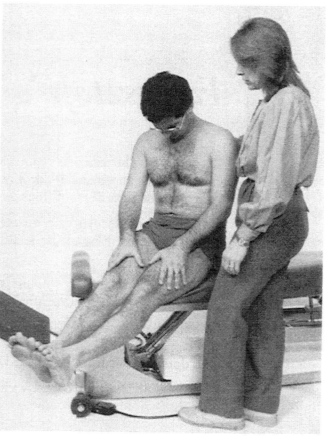

D

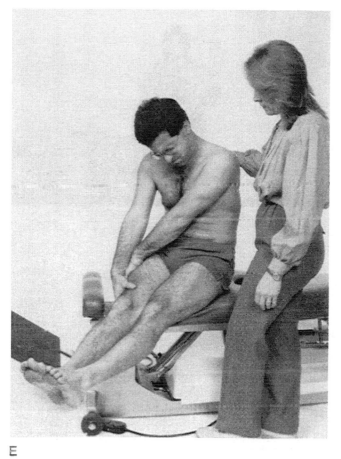

E

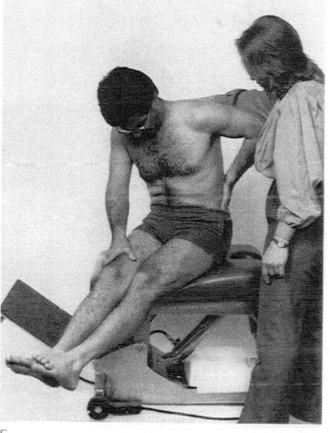

F

21 | *Fajersztajn's Test*

Procedure: The patient is supine. Raise the unaffected leg to the point at which pain is created on the contralateral side. Lower the leg 5 degrees or to slightly below the level of pain and dorsiflex the foot (Figs. A–D).

Rationale: Radicular pain on the affected leg when the unaffected leg is tested is caused by tractioning of the sciatic nerve from pelvic rotation and by irritating an inflamed disc.

Classical Significance: The test is positive if radicular symptomatology increases in the affected leg when the unaffected leg is tested (Fig. E).

Clinical Significance: Tight hamstrings will cause pain in the unaffected limb (the side being tested) and should not be considered positive for sciatic radiculopathy when pain does not occur in the affected leg (Fig. F).

Follow-up: Perform Bechterew's test, the advancement test, or the Valsalva maneuver.

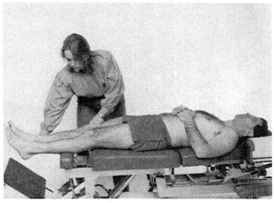

A

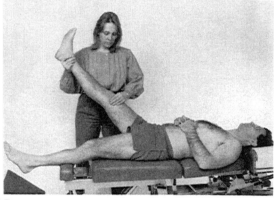

B

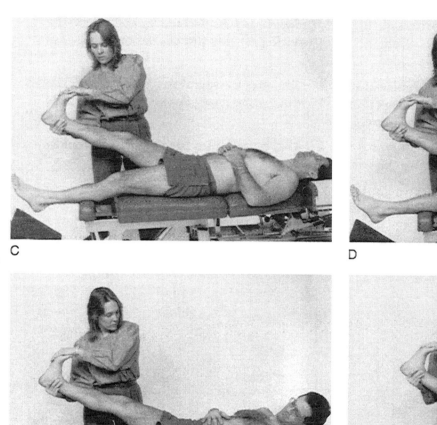

C

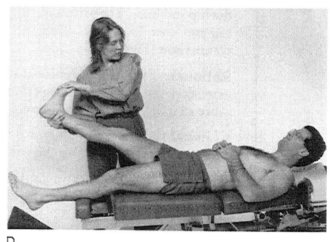

D

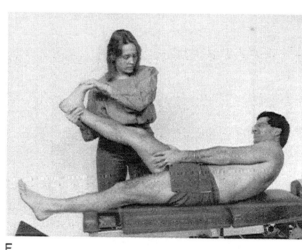

E

F

22 | *Femoral Nerve Traction Test*

Procedure: The patient lies on the unaffected side with the lower leg slightly flexed at the hip and knee. The back is not hyperextended. Grasp the affected leg and extend the hip and knee 15 degrees. Then, flex the knee. Repeat this test on the other side for comparison (Figs. A–D).

Rationale: This test is similar to Ely's heel to buttock test and the Nachlas test. The extension of the hip and the leg causes stress through the roots; flexion of the knee adds more stretch to the femoral nerve.

Classical Significance: Reproduction of radicular pain into the anterior thigh indicates a femoral nerve lesion (Fig. E).

Clinical Significance: Pain into the medial anterior groin and hip indicates a lesion of the L3 nerve root (Fig. F).

Follow-up: Perform the Nachlas test or Lasegue's straight leg test.

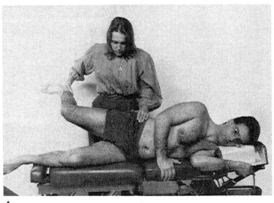

A

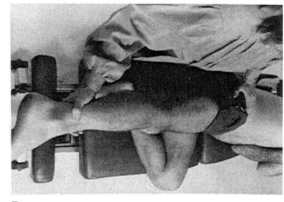

B

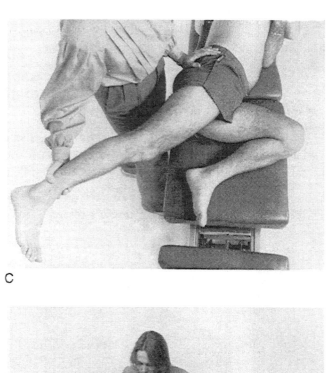

C

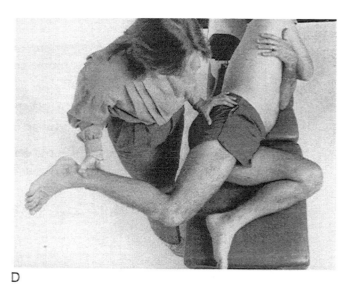

D

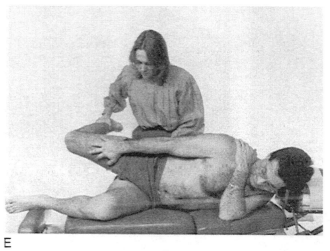

E

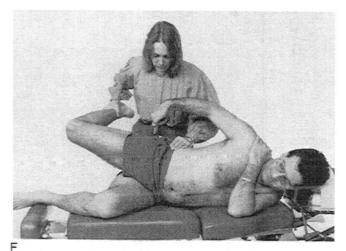

F

23 | *Goldthwait's Test*

Procedure: The patient is supine. Place one hand under the lumbosacral junction and the other hand under the heel of the patient. Raise the leg off the table. Repeat the test on the other side (Figs. A–F).

Rationale: In the normal patient, one should be able to raise the leg off the table about 90 degrees. In addition, the lumbosacral articulation should begin to open up without pain.

Classical Significance: If pain occurs when raising the leg before the lumbosacral junction opens, consider sacroiliac involvement.

Clinical Significance: If pain occurs when raising the leg after the lumbosacral junction begins to move, consider lumbosacral involvement, such as a strain or sprain or facet syndrome.

Follow-up: Perform Lasegue's straight leg test, Kemp's test, or Bechterew's test.

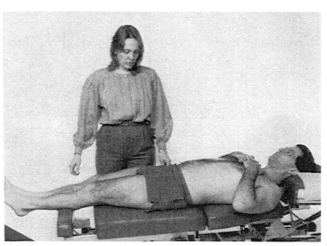

A

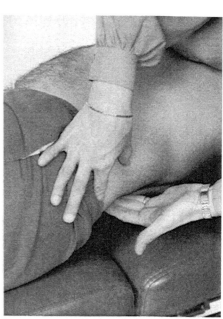

B

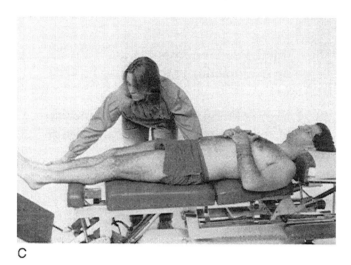

C

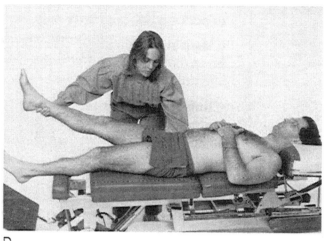

D

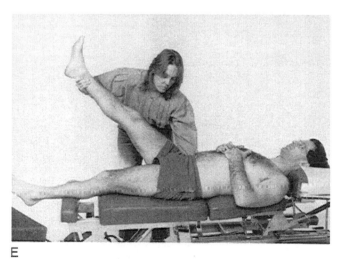

E

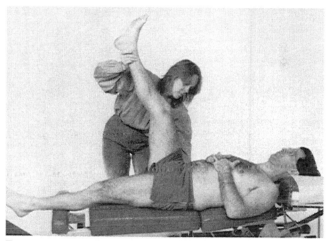

F

24 | *Heel Walk Test*

Procedure: Ask the patient to walk on the heels forward and then backward for at least 10 steps (Figs. A–D).

Rationale: The patient with intact motor power from the L5 nerve root should be able to perform this maneuver with ease.

Classical Significance: The inability to perform this test indicates a lesion at the L5 nerve root, such as an L4 disc protrusion or prolapse. The ability to toe walk will also be affected (Fig. E).

Clinical Significance: A patient with an L4 nerve lesion will also have difficulty performing the heel walk test. This is because the L4 nerve innervates the tibialis anterior muscle. In this case the toe walk test will be normal (Fig. F).

Follow-up: Perform Lasegue's straight leg test, Kemp's test, or the Valsalva maneuver.

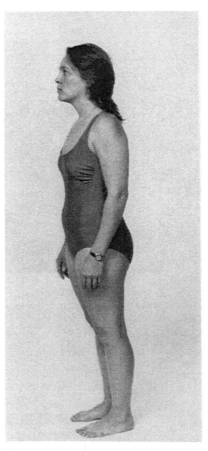

A

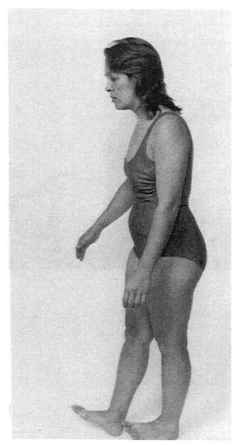

B

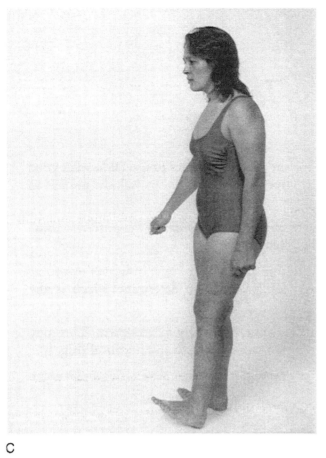

C

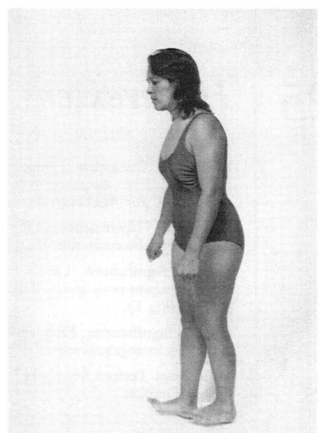

D

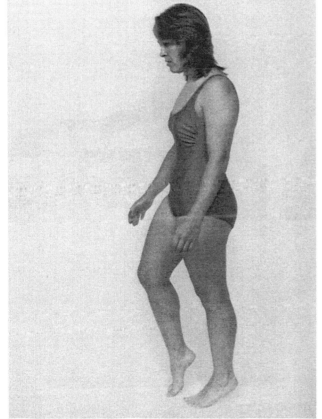

E

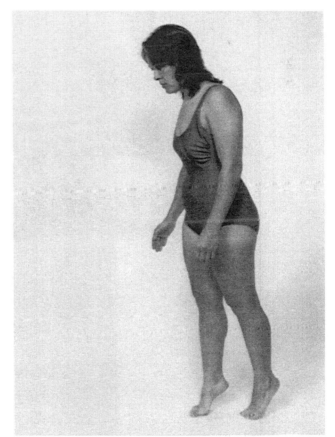

F

25 | *Hyperextension Test*

Procedure: The patient is prone. Anchor the patient's ankles to the table with your hands and instruct the patient to raise the upper torso off the table. Ask the patient to point to any pain that occurs (Figs. A–D).

Rationale: Hyperextension of the lumbar spine actively contracts the posterior musculature and also compresses the posterior elements.

Classical Significance: Localized pain within the lumbar spine indicates muscular strain or ligamentous sprain. Repeat this test passively to determine which is the problem (Fig. E).

Clinical Significance: Facet jamming can occur, especially in a tropism. This may result in scleratogenous referral of pain, which will be diffuse and nonlocal (Fig. F).

Follow-up: Perform Kemp's test, Lasegue's straight leg test, or the active and passive ranges of motion.

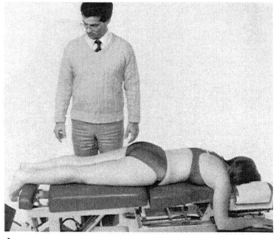

A

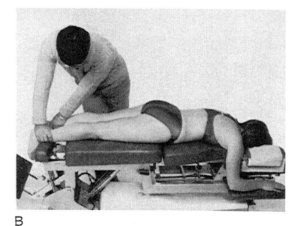

B

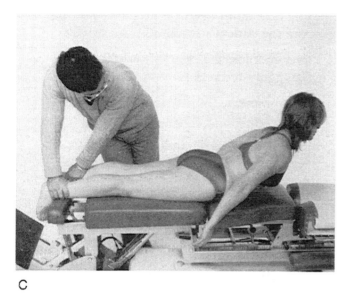

C

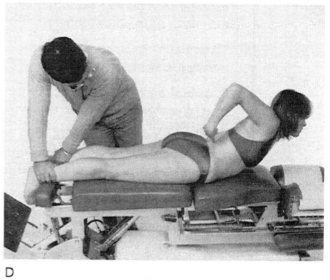

D

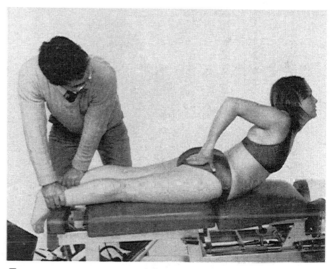

E

F

26 | *Jar Drop Test*

Procedure: The patient is standing upright. Ask the patient to go up on the toes to the extreme that plantar flexion allows. Once this maximum height is attained, ask the patient to drop abruptly onto the heels. Record the patient's response (Figs. A–C).

Rationale: In acute inflammation of the lower abdominal and posterior viscera, this jarring mechanism puts additional stress on the aggravated viscera, increasing the pain.

Classical Significance: The reproduction or an increase in the pain of the visceral-related problem is considered a positive test (Fig. D).

Clinical Significance: This test is designed to test the colon and for acute cases of appendicitis. Pain from a kidney or from lower back spasm may also occur. Local pain indicates a lower back spasm; radiating pain into the leg may indicate a lumbar disc problem (Figs. E & F).

Follow-up: Perform Lewin's punch test, Murphy's punch test, or the Astrom suspension test.

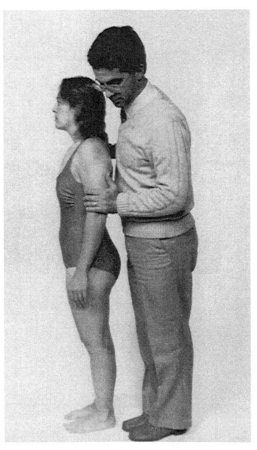

A

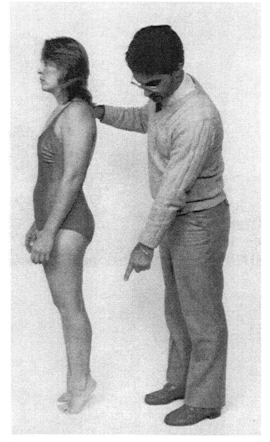

B

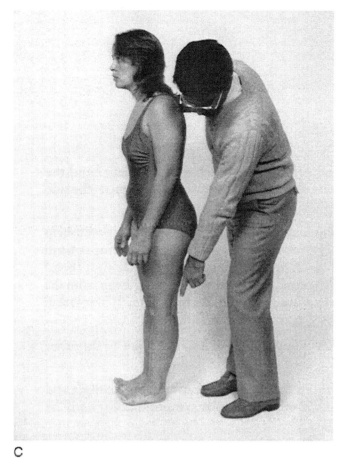

C

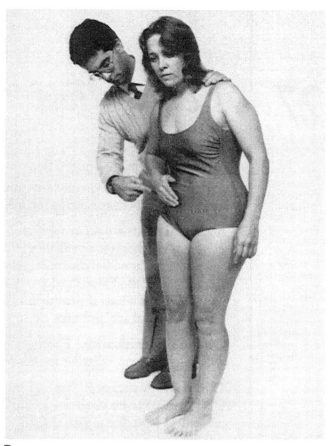

D

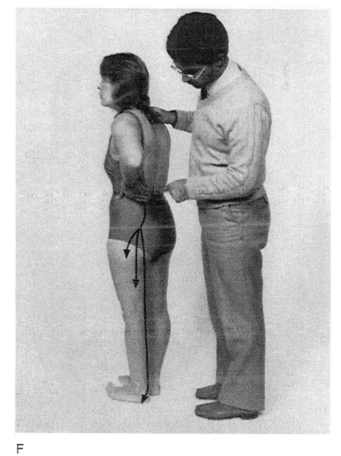

E

F

27 | *Kemp's Test*

Procedure: The patient is sitting. Stand behind the patient and obliquely bend the patient backward first to one side and then other. Record the patient's response (the side the patient is bent toward is recorded as the affected side) (Figs. A–C).

Rationale: In a patient with an antalgia due to a discal lesion, this test could help confirm whether it is a medial or lateral disc protrusion. If the patient is leaning toward the pain, it is a medial disc protrusion (Fig. D: posteromedial disc protrusion; 1, thecal impingement medial to the dorsal root ganglion). If the patient is leaning away from the pain then it is a lateral protrusion (Fig. E: posterolateral disc protrusion; 1, herniation lateral to dural sac and may cause stenosis at intervertebral foramen).

Classical Significance: Forcing the patient out of antalgia into one plane or the other will help confirm whether the disc is lateral or medial (Fig. F).

Clinical Significance: Severe unilateral lumbar myospasm can result in antalgia and what appears to be a positive Kemp's test. However, radicular symptomatology will be present in true discal pathology.

Follow-up: Perform Lasegue's straight leg test, the Valsalva maneuver, or Fajersztajn's test.

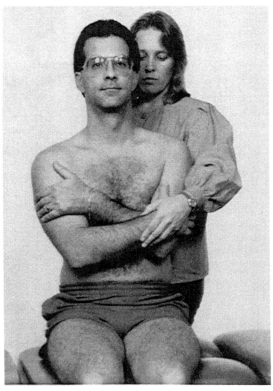

A

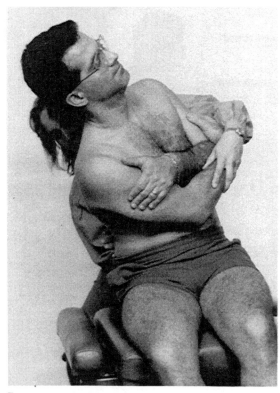

B

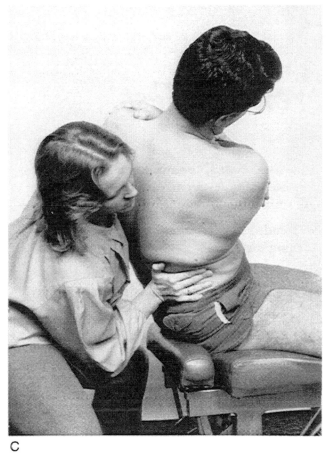

C

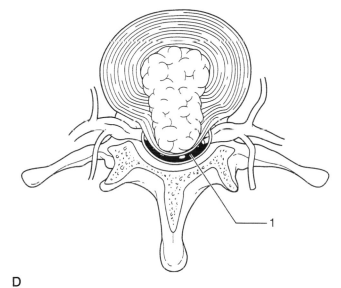

D

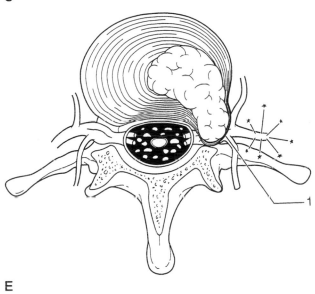

E

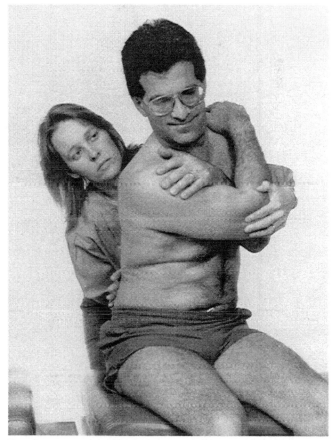

F

28 | *Lasegue's Differential Test*

Procedure: The patient is supine. Place one hand behind the ankle and the other on the knee; raise the leg to the point of pain. Note the type and angle of the pain. Next, raise the leg and flex the knee (Figs. A–D).

Rationale: Raising the leg with the knee extended stresses the sciatic nerve because it is stretched; the stretching is reduced by flexing the knee.

Classical Significance: The patient with true sciatic radiculopathy will have a decrease in pain when the knee is flexed. This finding rules out hip pathology and indicates the lumbar spine as the origin of pain (Fig. E).

Clinical Significance: If the sciatica is due to hip pathology, the pain will not lessen with knee flexion. This is called the buttock sign (Fig. F).

Follow-up: Perform Bechterew's test, the advancement test, or the Valsalva maneuver.

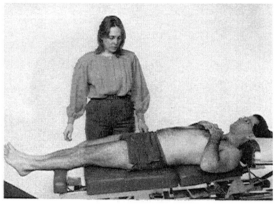

A

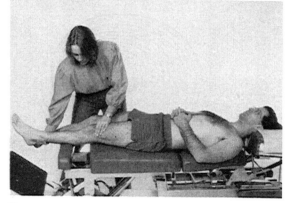

B

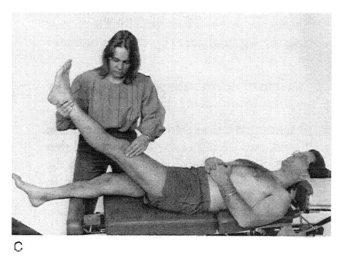

C

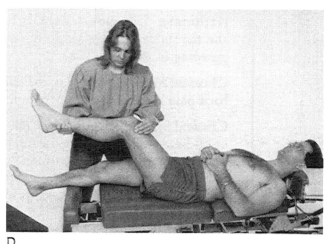

D

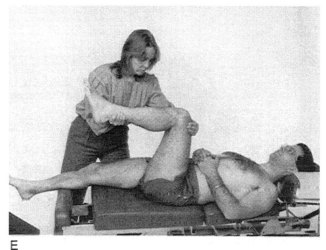

E

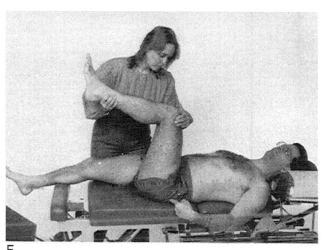

F

29 | *Lasegue's Rebound Test*

Procedure: The patient is supine and relaxed. Perform Lasegue's straight leg test to the point of muscle spasm or resistance or to the point of pain, whichever is first. Then drop the leg unexpectedly into a pillow or your other hand (Figs. A–D).

Rationale: Lasegue's straight leg test establishes the point of irritation for the patient and the sudden jarring motion from dropping the leg unexpectedly causes voluntary guarding of the lower back.

Classical Significance: Reproduction of pain into the leg or an aggravation of the low back pain is significant. It could indicate iliopsoas involvement (Fig. E).

Clinical Significance: Although the classical interpretation is for iliopsoas irritation or of disc conditions above the lumbosacral level, any jarring of the lumbar spine that induces reactive muscle contraction will reproduce lower back pain. The area of the radiating pattern or the location of the pain is the guide to the differential diagnosis. In addition, complaints of visceral pain, such as in appendicitis, may also be exacerbated by this test (Fig. F).

Follow-up: Perform Lasegue's straight leg test, Schober's test, the Thomas test, or the Valsalva maneuver.

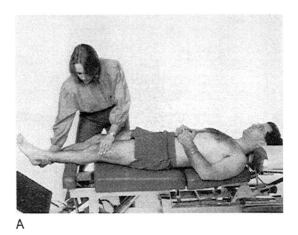

A

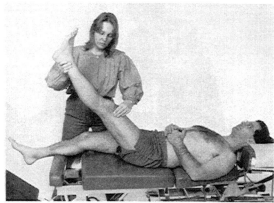

B

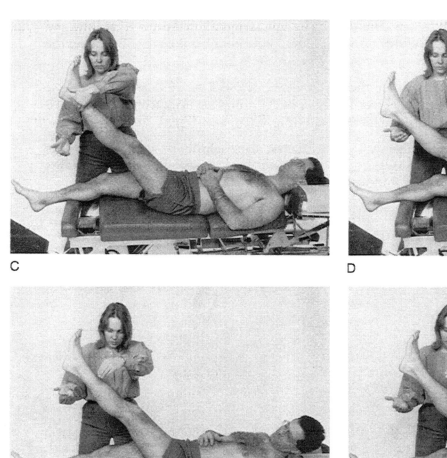

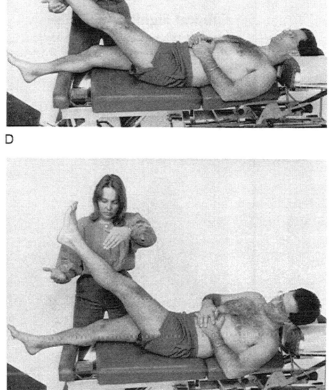

Lasegue's Straight Leg Test

Procedure: The patient is supine. Place one hand under the patient's ankle and the other hand on the knee and raise the leg 90 degrees (Figs. A–D).

Rationale: This test creates different biomechanical forces on the sacroiliac joint and lumbar nerve roots. Therefore, it is important to note not only the type of pain but the angle at which it occurs.

Classical Significance: A leg that can only be raised 0 to 30 degrees indicates a sacroiliac lesion; 30 to 60 degrees indicates lumbosacral involvement; and about 90 degrees indicates lumbar spine involvement (Fig. E).

Clinical Significance: Pain at 0 to 15 degrees, although rarely seen, may indicate lumbar muscle or psoas recruitment or spasm (see also Demianoff's Sign). Remember that tight hamstrings may be the cause of pain behind the thigh (Fig. F).

Follow-up: Perform Braggard's test, Fajersztajn's test, Bechterew's test, or Lasegue's differential test.

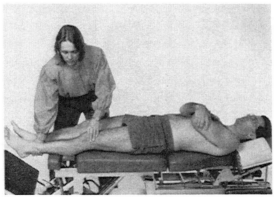

A

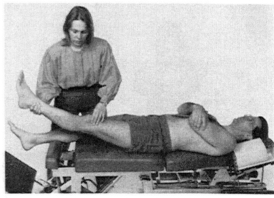

B

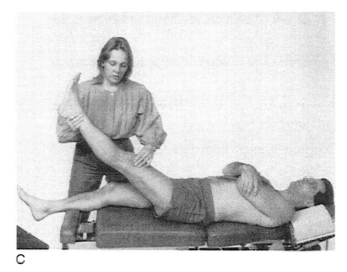

C

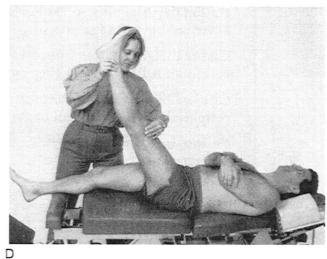

D

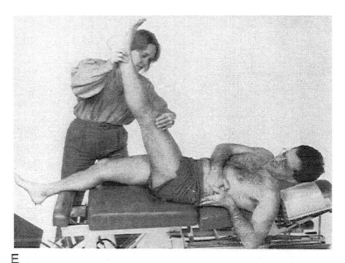

E

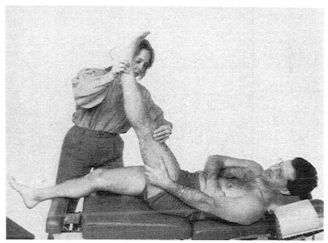

F

31 | *Lewin's Punch Test*

Procedure: The patient is standing. Stand behind and to one side of the patient and strike the buttocks of the affected side with the ulnar side of a closed fist (Figs. A–C).

Rationale: The jarring of the buttocks on the side of pain causes direct irritation of the lower lumbar and sacral roots.

Classical Significance: Discal lesion aggravation at a lower lumbar or upper sacral nerve root is a positive test (Fig. D).

Clinical Significance: Pain that occurs from the buttocks downward represents peripheral nerve entrapment of the sciatic nerve (Fig. E).

Follow-up: Perform Lasegue's straight leg test, Kemp's test, the advancement test, or Bechterew's test.

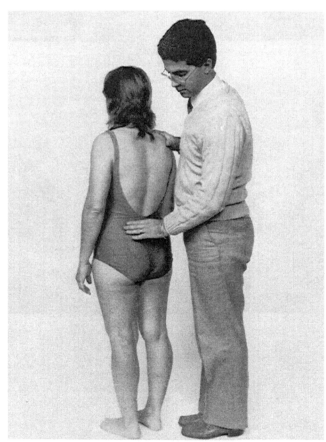

A

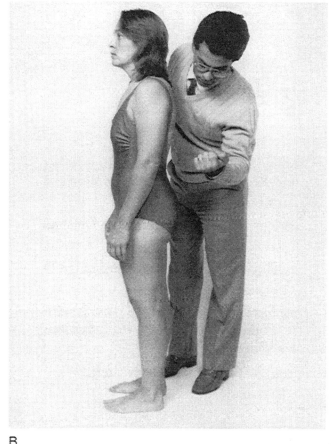

B

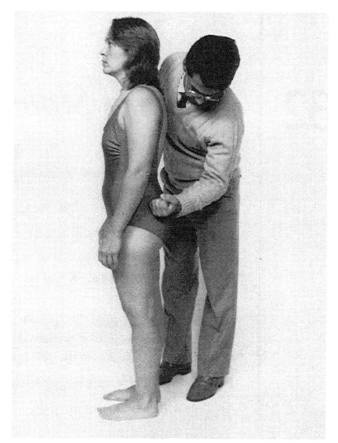

C

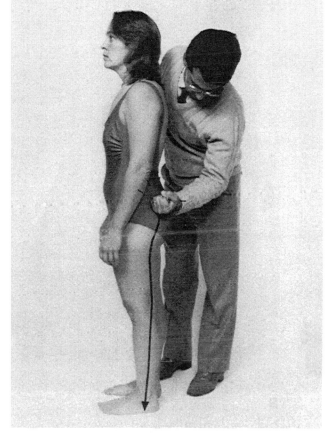

D

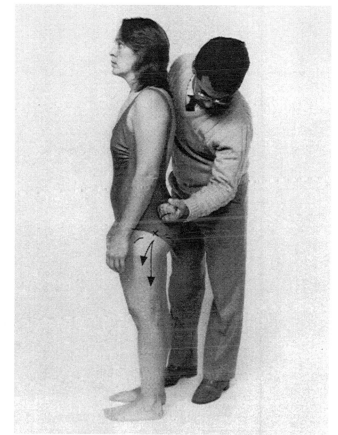

E

32 | *Lewin's Standing Test*

Procedure: The patient is standing. Stand behind the patient and, while supporting the patient's pelvis, force one knee into extension. Repeat the test on the other knee and on both knees together (Figs. A–C).

Rationale: This test will stretch tight hamstrings excessively, causing the knees to flex.

Classical Significance: Knees returning to flexion indicate tight hamstrings (Figs. D & E).

Clinical Significance: A patient with severe lumbar myospasm may present with buckled knees, because it is more comfortable for the patient. Forcing the knees into extension can exacerbate the patient's low back pain (Fig. F).

Follow-up: Perform Lasegue's straight leg test, Adam's sign, or Beery's test.

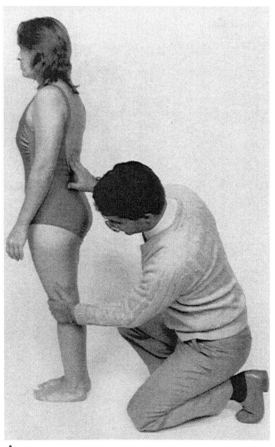

A

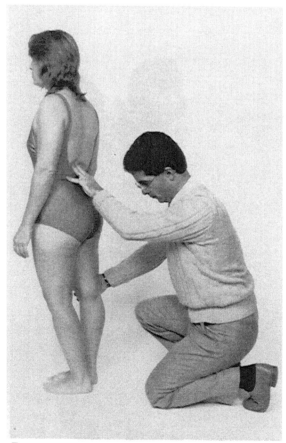

B

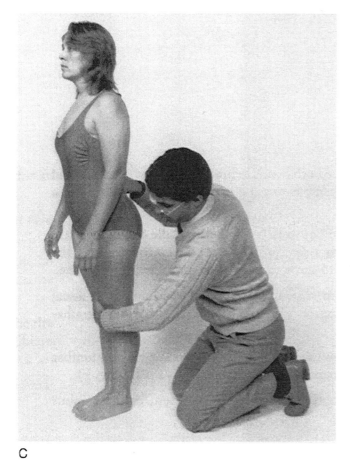

C

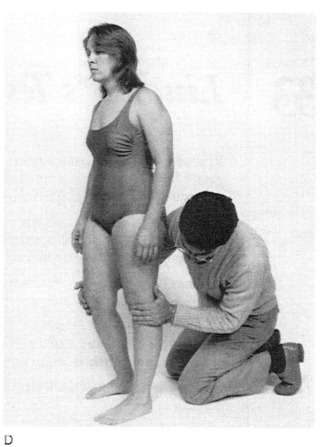

D

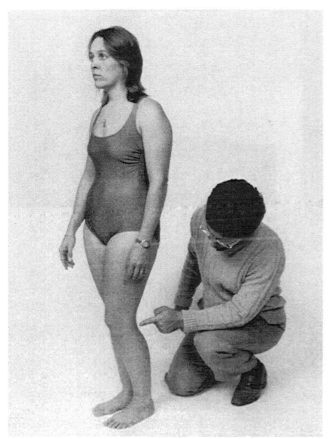

E

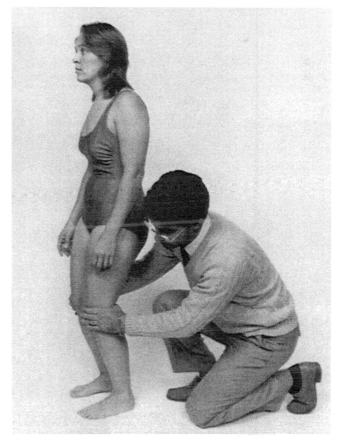

F

33 | *Lindner's Test*

Procedure: The patient is supine. Place both hands behind the patient's occiput and gently force the chin onto the chest while pushing the patient up off the table into a semiseated position (Figs. A–D).

Rationale: This test is similar to the Soto-Hall test. Because the sternum is not stabilized and the patient is forced into a semiseated position, the forces along the supraspinous ligaments are transferred to the levels below T7 into the lumbar spine.

Classical Significance. An increase in radicular symptoms may indicate a discal protrusion that is causing nerve root irritation (Fig. E). This test also increases intrathecal pressure.

Clinical Significance: Local pain below the level of T7 and extending into the lumbar spine indicates vertebral injury or ligamentous sprain at the level of pain (Fig. F).

Follow-up: Perform the Valsalva maneuver, the tuning fork test, or the spinous percussion test.

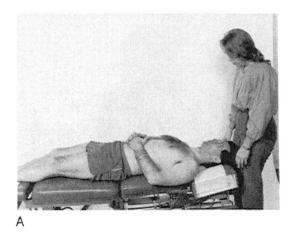

A

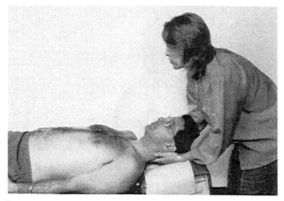

B

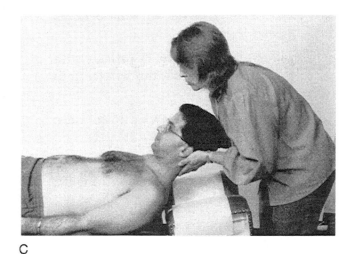

C

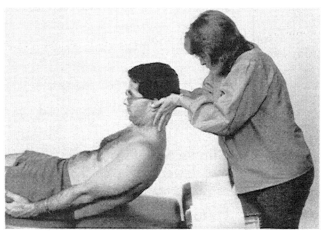

D

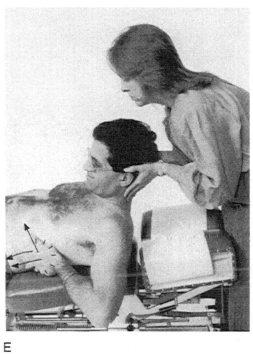

E

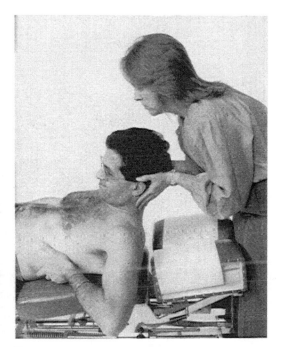

F

34 | *McBride's Test*

Procedure: The patient is standing. Ask the patient to stand on one leg while bending the other knee and bringing it toward the chest (Figs. A–C).

Rationale: This procedure causes a flattening of the lumbar curve. In patients with facet syndrome or irritation of the lumbar spine from hyperlordosis, this will result in less strain along the facet plane.

Classical Significance: A reduction in lower back symptomatology is a positive test (Fig. D).

Clinical Significance: This test is normally used as a malingering test. If the patient with lower back pain believes it will make the problem worse and refuses to do it, suspect a malingerer (Fig. E).

Follow-up: Perform Burn's bench test (see Ch. 14), Kemp's test, or Lasegue's straight leg test.

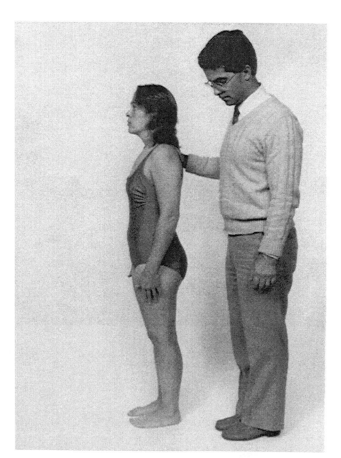

A

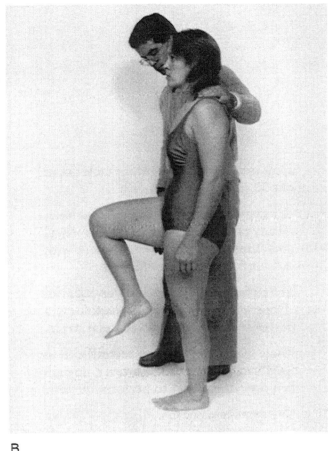

B

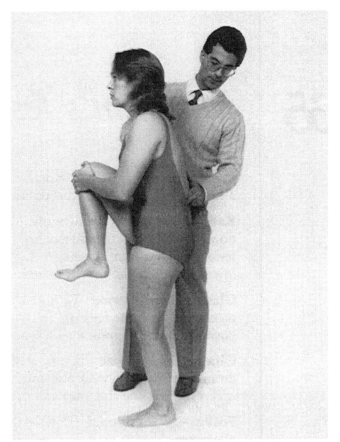

C

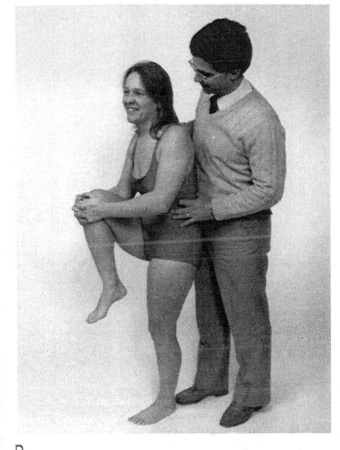

D

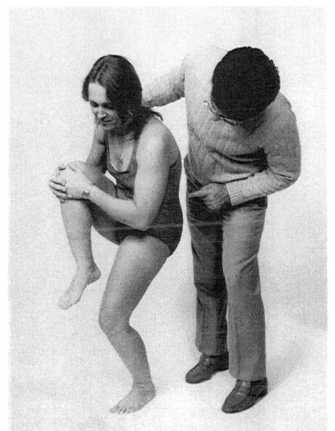

E

35 | *Milgram's Test*

Procedure: The patient is supine. Ask the patient to raise both legs off the table about 3 to 4 inches and to hold this position for about 30 seconds (Figs. A–E).

Rationale: A person with normal lower back integrity, including normal disc function, should be able to hold this position without any problem. In a patient with a discal lesion, this test increases intrathecal pressure and exacerbates pain; in the patient with low back strain, the stressed muscles must work harder to perform this test.

Classical Significance: The test is positive if the patient cannot perform this test at all or cannot hold the legs up for 30 seconds. Depending on the symptomatology, a positive result may indicate discal nerve irritation or increased lumbar muscular strain.

Clinical Significance: Patients with psoas muscle spasm may find this test difficult to do and patients with weak abdominals cannot perform the test at all. However, no pain will result and the abdomen will protrude when the patient tries to perform the test.

Follow-up: Perform the Thomas test, Lewin's supine test (see Ch. 7), or the Valsalva maneuver.

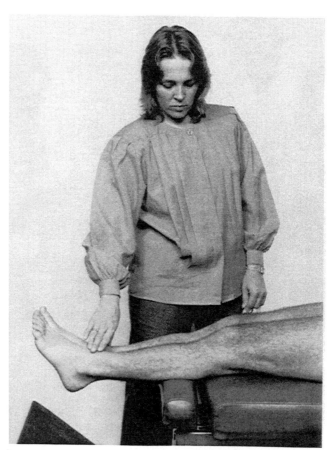

A

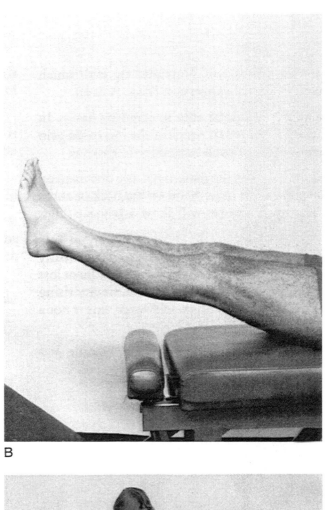

B

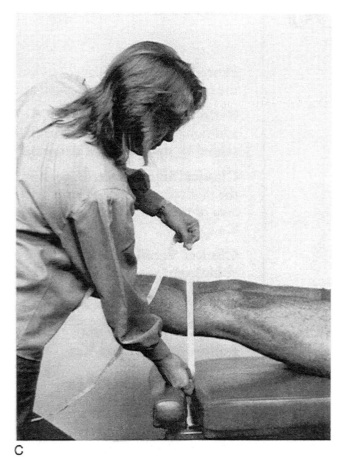

C

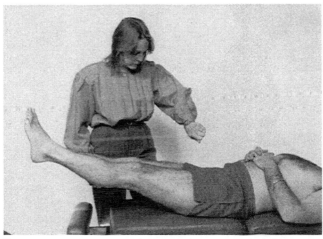

D

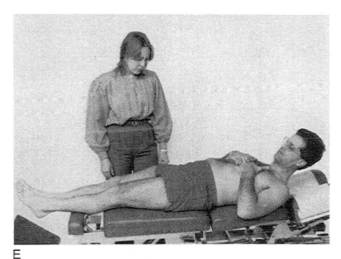

E

Minor's Sign

Procedure: Ask the patient to rise from a seated position. Note the ease with which the patient is able to rise as well as the patient's facial expression (Figs. A & B).

Rationale: The patient with low back pain will not be able to stand up easily. In addition, the patient's face should indicate discomfort as a result of the increased pain caused by standing up. The normal patient will have good lumbopelvic rhythm.

Classical Significance: A positive test is indicated by the patient placing one hand on the thigh opposite the affected side, while putting the other hand on the back or at the area of pain when attempting to stand. The facial features will show a grimace (Figs. C–E).

Clinical Significance: Patients with ankylosing spondylitis will also have difficulty rising from the seated position. This is due to stiffness in the spine, with subsequent loss of normal lumbopelvic rhythm. In addition, obese patients will have difficulty rising from a seated position because of weight imposed restrictions. However, this is not a significant finding.

Follow-up: Perform Kemp's test, Lasegue's straight leg test, or the Valsalva maneuver.

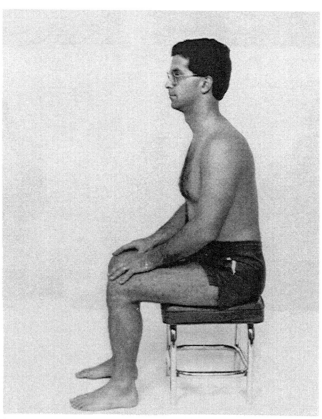

A

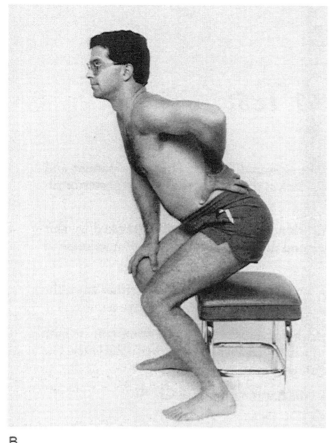

B

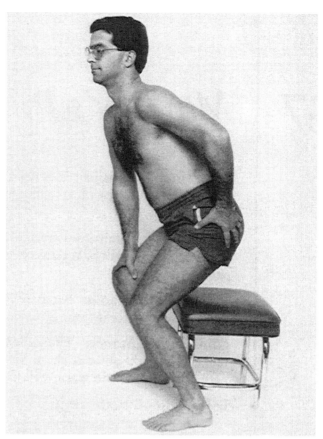

C

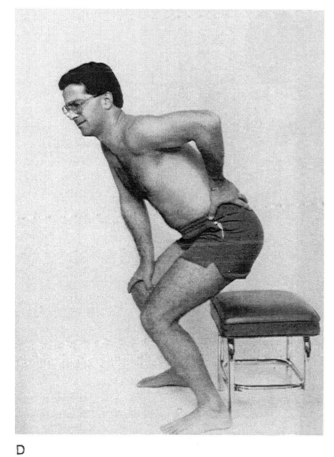

D

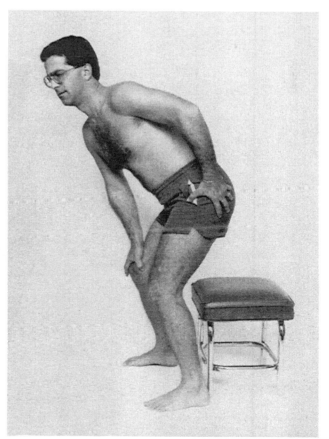

E

37 | *Murphy's Punch Test*

Procedure: The patient is either standing or seated. Stand behind the patient and deliver a short choppy blow to the patient's flank at the level of the twelfth posterior rib (Figs. A–C).

Rationale: Inflammation created by the kidney will be further aggravated by this jarring. The area will be reactively guarded and this irritation will cause an increase in pain.

Classical Significance: An increase of lancinating pain that radiates either from the flank to the anterior into the groin or around the lower rib cage is a positive test (Fig. D).

Clinical Significance: The patient with herpes zoster will also complain of pain radiation into the anterior chest. This pain will follow a specific dermatomal level. The patient with a muscle spasm will have increased local pain only (Fig. E).

Follow-up: Perform the jar drop test or the hopping test (see Ch. 9).

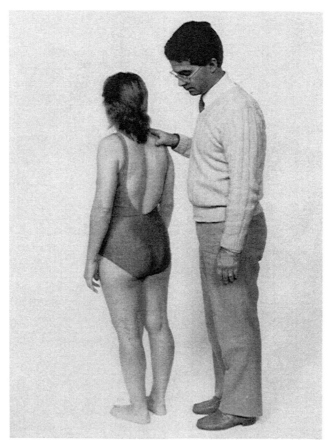

A

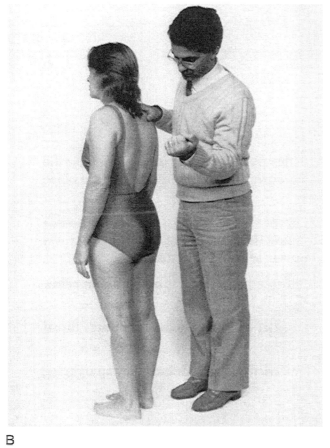

B

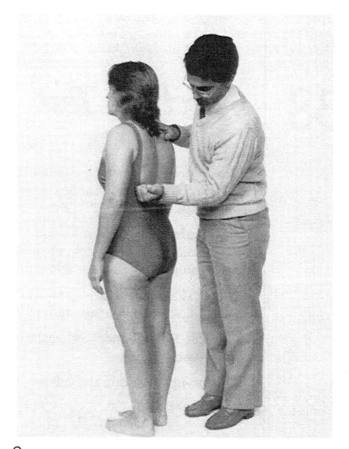

C

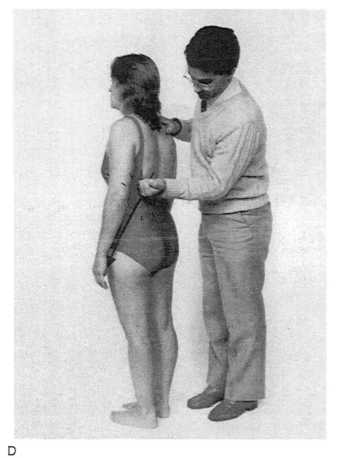

D

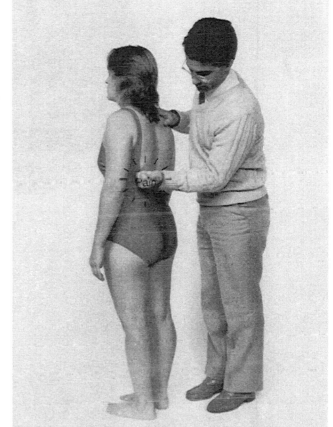

E

38 | *Nachlas Test*

Procedure: The patient is prone. Passively flex the knee of the patient bringing the heel to the ipsilateral buttock while pressing downward on the ipsilateral sacroiliac joint (Figs. A–C).

Rationale: This test causes a pulling first in the sacroiliac joint, then in the lumbosacral joint, and ultimately in the lumbar spine. It is important to do this test if a ligamentous sprain or discal lesion in the lumbar spine is suspected.

Classical Significance: Local lumbar, lumbosacral, or sacroiliac pain without radiation indicates strain or sprain injury (Fig. D).

Clinical Significance: An increase in radicular symptomatology indicates discal protrusion (Fig. E).

Follow-up: Perform the Valsalva maneuver, Dejerine's sign, or Lasegue's straight leg test.

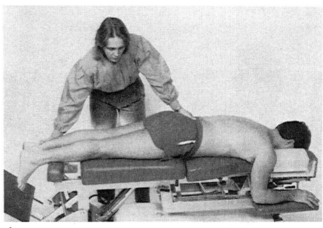

A

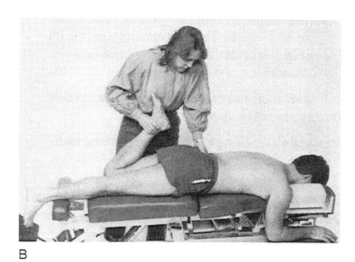

B

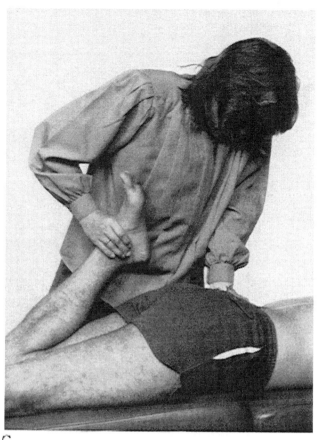

C

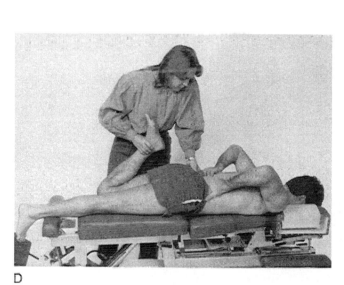

D

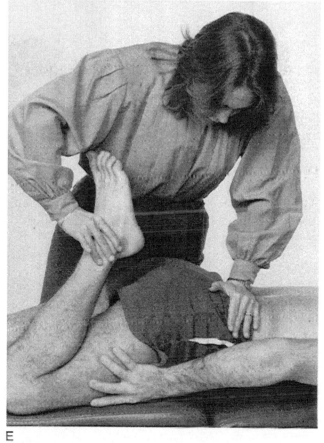

E

39 | *Naffziger's Test (Viet's Jugular Compression Test)*

Procedure: The patient is sitting. Place your hands around the patient's neck and manually compress the jugular veins for up to 45 seconds. This can also be performed using a blood pressure cuff inflated to 40 mmHg. Leave the blood pressure cuff in place for 10 to 15 seconds (this is Viet's jugular compression test) (Figs. A–E).

Rationale: Compression of the jugular veins increases intrathecal pressure, which will result in compromise of the cord by any space-occupying lesion.

Classical Significance: Radicular symptomatology along a specific dermatome indicates nerve root compression by a discal protrusion.

Clinical Significance: Perform this test with the patient supine if the patient has hypertension or is unable to sit. Check for flushing, which is a positive result. Then ask the patient to cough, which will increase or reproduce radicular pain.

Follow-up: Perform the Valsalva maneuver, Dejerine's sign, or Kemp's test.

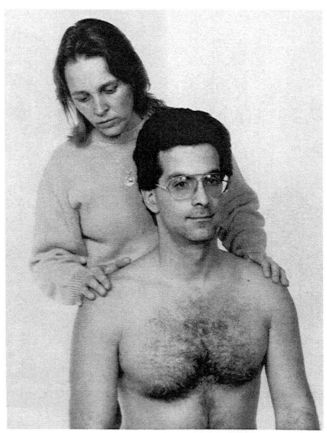

A

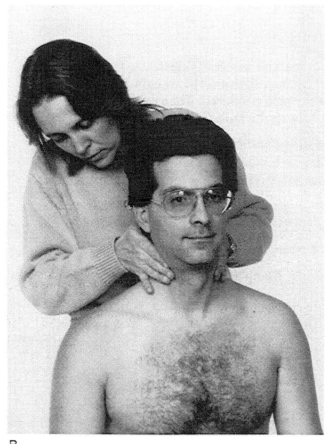

B

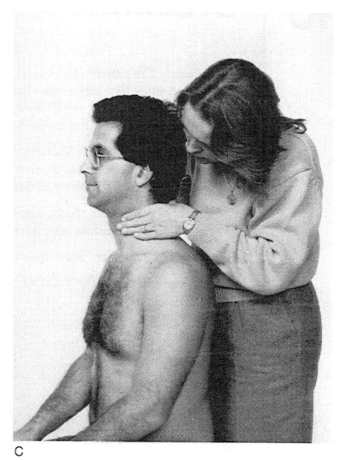

C

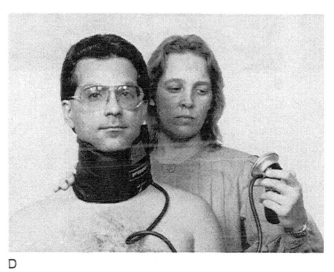

D

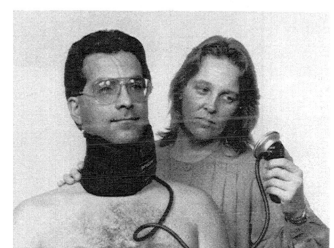

E

O'Connell Test

Procedure: The patient is supine. Perform the well leg raise (Fajersztajn's test), noting the site and angle that reproduces the pain (if any). Perform the straight leg test on the affected limb, noting the site and angle of the pain produced. Then raise both legs just short of the point of pain. Lower the well leg to the table (Figs. A–E).

Rationale: The separate lowering of the leg causes a pelvic shift, which alters the position of the discal lesion, causing pain. The lowering of the well leg is used as the indicator in this test; therefore, a positive response is suspicious for a medial disc lesion.

Classical Significance: An increase in pain when the well leg is lowered to the table indicates a positive finding only when the pain occurs in the leg of complaint (Fig. F).

Clinical Significance: See Classical Significance.

Follow-up: Perform the Valsalva maneuver, Kemp's test, or Dejerine's sign.

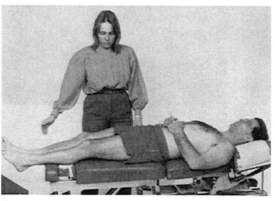

A

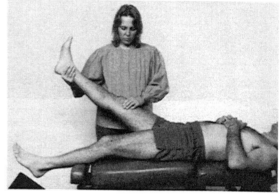

B

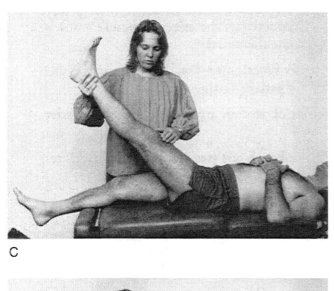

C

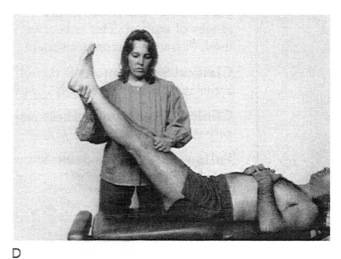

D

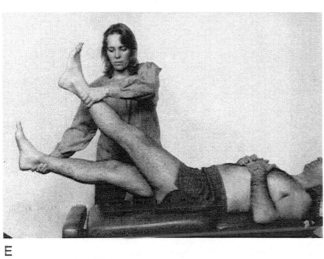

E

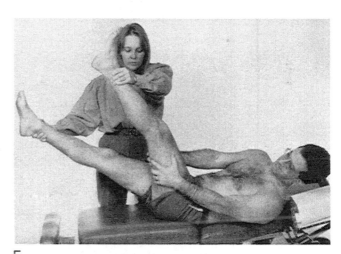

F

41 | O'Donoghues Maneuver

Procedure: The dorsolumbar spine is moved through its active and passive ranges of motion (Figs. A–F).

Rationale: The active ranges of motion are always less than or equal to the passive ranges of motion. This is because, to perform actively, the affected muscles must be used. Passive performance should not aggravate the muscles.

Classical Significance: If the active ranges of motion are less than the passive, then active muscle involvement is the cause of the patient's pain.

Clinical Significance: If the active ranges of motion are greater than the passive, suspect a malingerer.

Follow-up: Perform McBride's test, Burn's bench test (see Ch. 14) or Hoover's test (see Ch. 14).

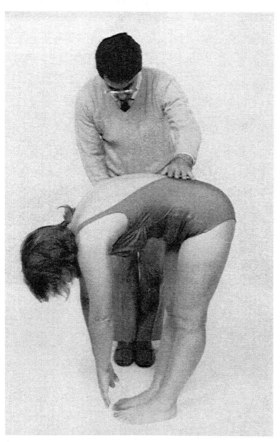

A

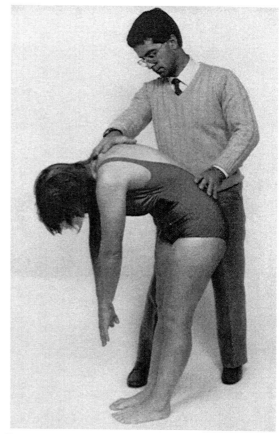

B

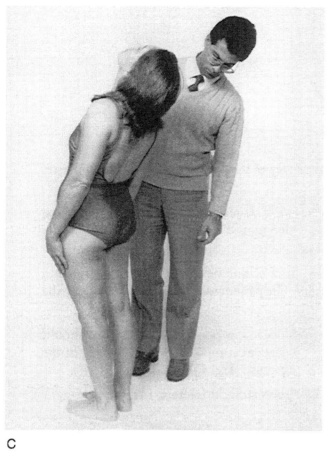

C

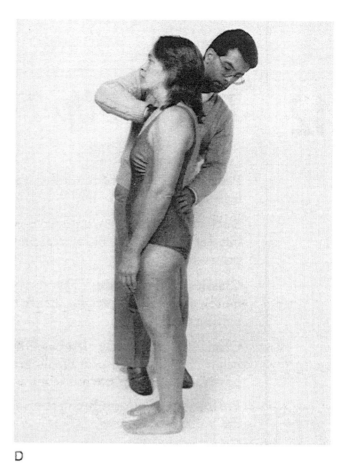

D

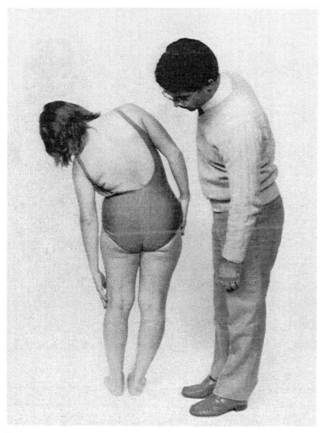

E

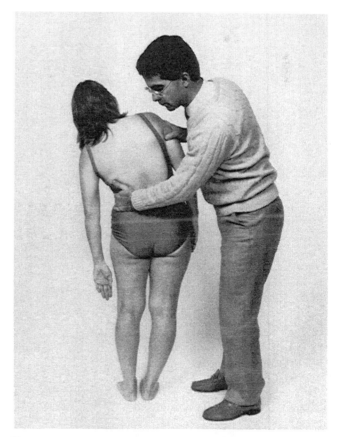

F

42 | *Petrin-Flip Test*

Procedure: The patient is seated. Extend one leg of the patient at a time and then both legs together (Figs. A–D).

Rationale: This test is a passive Bechterew's test. It places stress on the sciatic nerve but does not increase intrathecal pressure, which would increase the axial load on the protruding disc.

Classical Significance: This test will produce sciatic nerve radiculopathy when a muscle spasm is compressing the sciatic nerve. The patient will "flip" back to reduce the tension (Fig. E).

Clinical Significance: If a Lasegue's straight leg test is positive, this test also should be positive. If not, suspect a malingerer. If the patient complains of a stretching in the posterior thigh, hip extensor contracture is the cause (Fig. F).

Follow-up: Perform Bechterew's test, Lasegue's straight leg test, McBride's test, or the Valsalva maneuver.

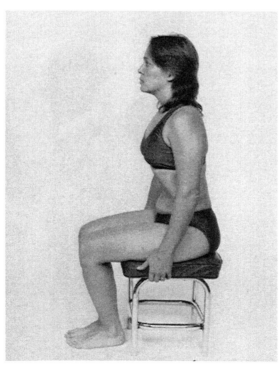

A

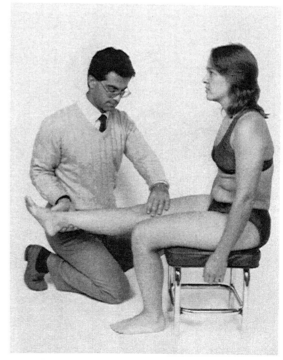

B

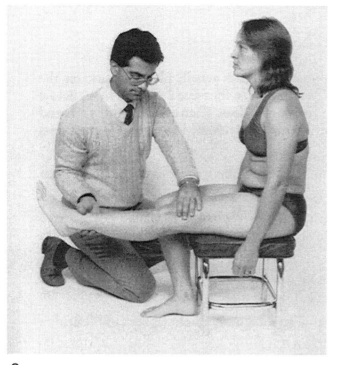

C

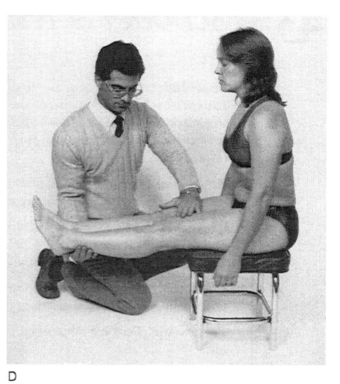

D

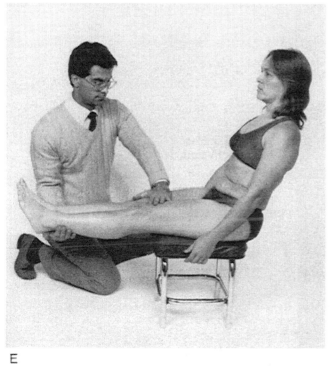

E

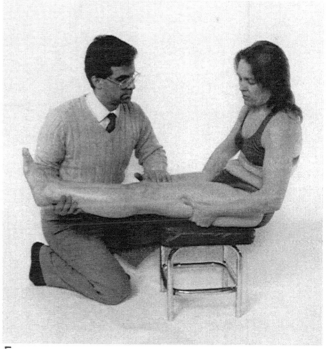

F

43 | *Schober's Test*

Procedure: The patient is standing. Using a grease pencil, place a mark on the patient's back midway between the dimples of Venus. Measure 2 inches (5 cm) below this mark and 4 inches (10 cm) above and place new dots. Then ask the patient to bend forward at the waist and remeasure the distance between the lowest and highest dots (Figs. A–D).

Rationale: In patients with normal lumbopelvic rhythm, the measurement between the two marks will increase more than 2 inches (5 cm).

Classical Significance: If, when the patient bends forward, the original distance of 6 inches (15 cm) is greater than 8 inches (20 cm) the patient has normal forward flexion and excursion of the lumbar spine (Fig. E).

Clinical Significance: In a suspected malingerer, although the patient may attempt to feign pain and lumbar restriction, there will be normal excursion.

Follow-up: Perform range of motion studies, Lasegue's straight leg test, or McBride's test.

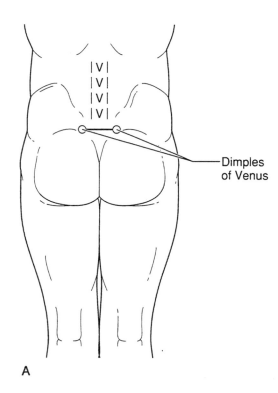

Dimples of Venus

A

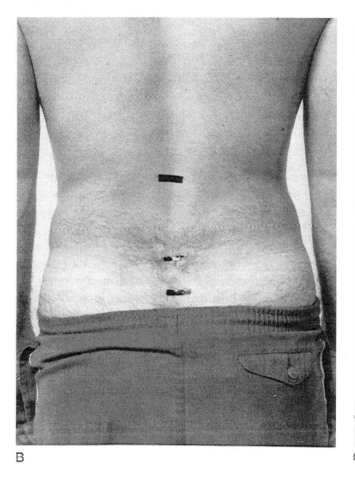

B

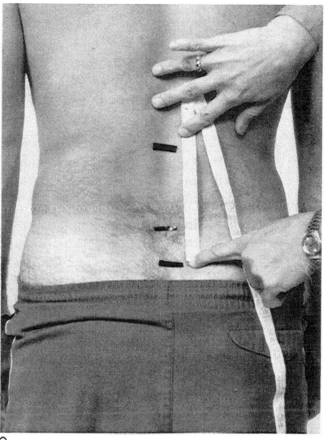

C

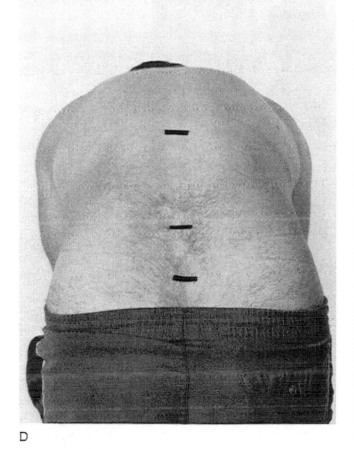

D

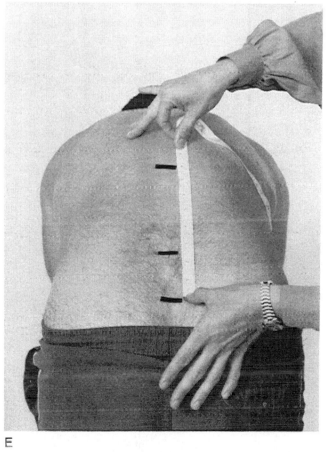

E

44 | *Seated Flexion Test*

Procedure: The patient is standing. Observe the patient performing active forward flexion. If the patient complains of pain while attempting to touch the toes ask the patient to be seated and to try and touch the toes (Figs. A–C).

Rationale: Lumbalgia that is produced on forward flexion can result from either a lumbar or pelvic lesion.

Classical Significance: The ability to perform the test better when seated than when standing is positive for a pelvic lesion and not for lumbar lesion. Being seated locks the pelvis out of forward flexion, which reduces the pain if a pelvic lesion is the problem (Fig. D).

Clinical Significance: If the patient has similar discomfort both seated and standing, the lesion is located within the lumbar spine (Fig. E).

Follow-up: Perform Beery's test, Burn's bench test (see Ch. 14), or Lasegue's straight leg test.

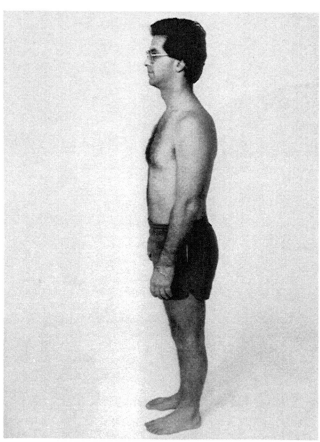

A

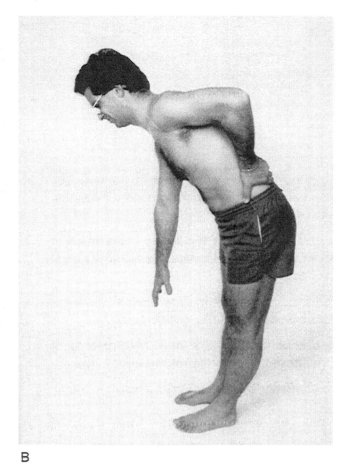

B

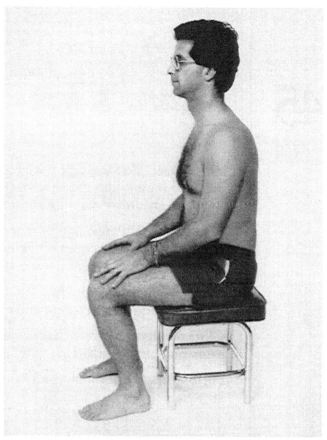

C

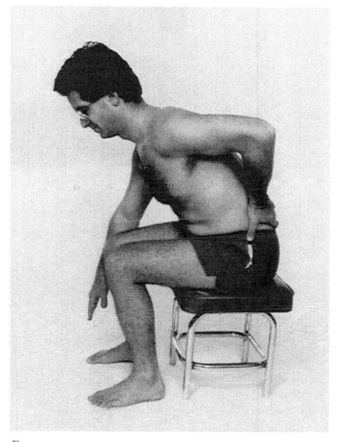

D

F

45 | *Sicard's Test*

Procedure: Perform this test only after a positive Lasegue's straight leg test. The patient is supine. Elevate one leg to the point of sciatic radiculopathy, lower it 5 degrees, and strongly dorsiflex the great toe (Figs. A–D).

Rationale: This test is similar to Braggard's test in that the sciatic nerve is being challenged and when stretched will produce symptoms. The dorsiflexion of the great toe exacerbates and confirms sciatic nerve root irritation.

Classical Significance: An increase in sciatic nerve root irritation when the leg is lowered 5 degrees and the great toe is dorsiflexed is a positive test (Fig. E).

Clinical Significance: Forced dorsiflexion of the great toe may exacerbate tight hamstrings, causing posterior thigh pain without radicular symptomatology (Fig. F).

Follow-up: Perform Braggard's test, the bowstring sign, or Turyn's test.

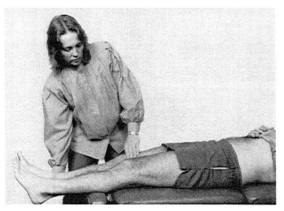

A

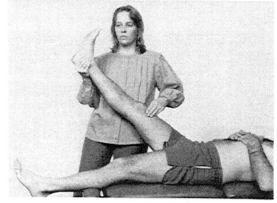

B

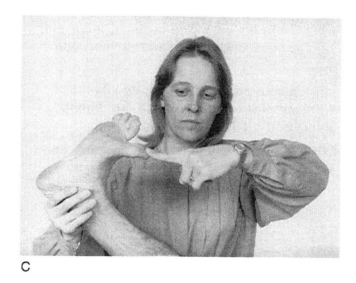

C

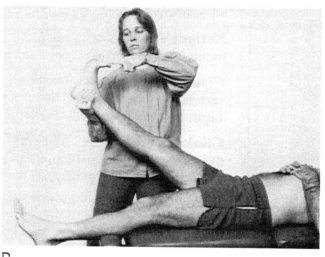

D

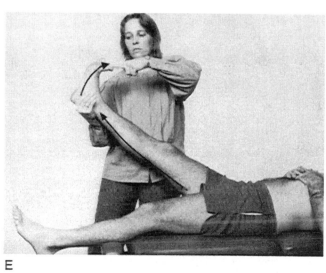

E

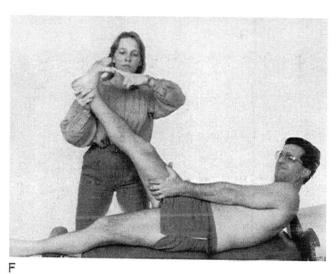

F

46 | *Spinous Percussion Test*

Procedure: The patient is seated. Instruct the patient to lean forward and support the forearms on the thighs. Using any neurologic hammer, strike the spinous processes of all lumbar vertebrae. Repeat by striking the paraspinal area (Figs. A–E).

Rationale: This test causes irritation to the spinous processes and surrounding ligamentous structures.

Classical Significance: Localized pain on a spinous process may indicate a fractured vertebral segment. An increase in radicular symptomatology indicates a discal lesion. Ligamentous sprains will also cause a nonradiating local pain.

Clinical Significance: When testing the paraspinal area, an increase in pain may be due to muscular strain. Also, the patient may have a low pain tolerance; be sure pain is not being caused by percussion alone.

Follow-up: Perform Lasegue's straight leg test, the hyperextension test, or the tuning fork test.

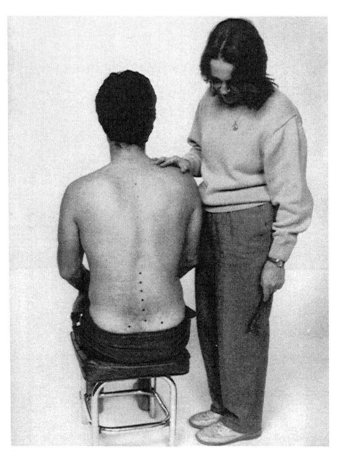

A

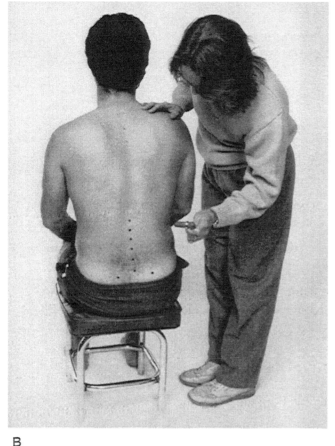

B

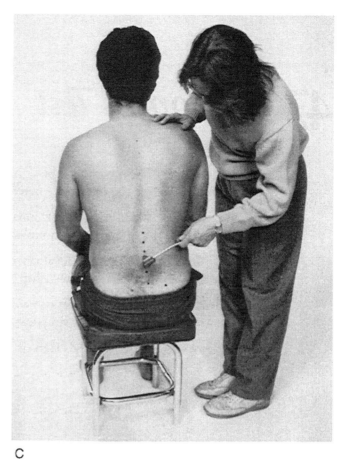

C

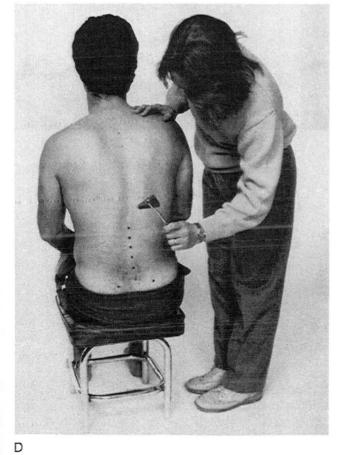

D

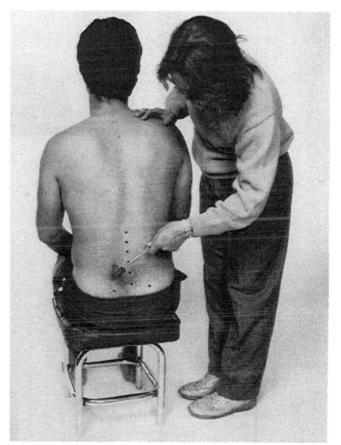

E

47 | *Thomas Test*

Procedure: The patient is supine. Instruct the patient to pull one knee to the chest and hold it. Observe the opposite knee for flexion (Figs. A–E).

Rationale: When the patient pulls the knee to the chest, a flattening of the lumbar lordosis occurs, putting additional stress on the iliopsoas musculature.

Classical Significance: Elevation of the leg or an increase in flexion of the knee on the side not being tested signifies a hip flexor contracture (Fig. F).

Clinical Significance: This test will be positive in rectus femoris contracture because the knee will flex to avoid stressing the rectus femoris musculature.

Follow-up: Perform Ely's sign or Ely's heel to buttock test.

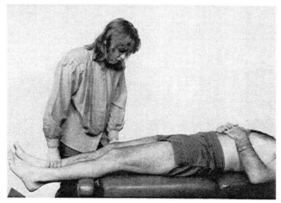

A

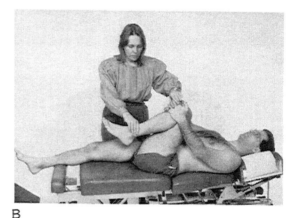

B

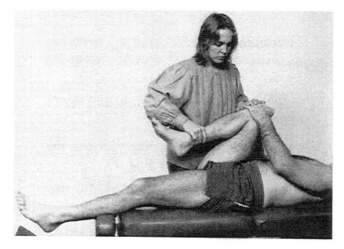

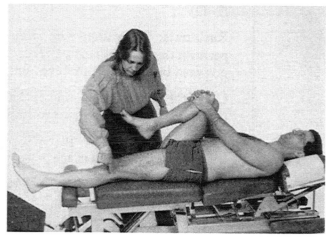

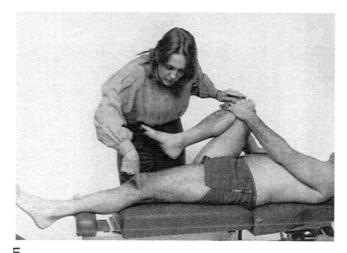

E

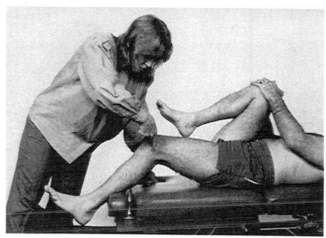

F

48 | *Toe Walk Test*

Procedure: The patient is standing. Ask the patient to walk on the toes forward and back for at least 10 steps. If it is possible that other muscles are being recruited when performing this test, ask the patient to walk on the toes while everting the feet (Figs. A–D).

Rationale: The patient with intact motor power from the S1 nerve root will be able to perform this test with ease. Eversion of the foot brings the peroneal muscles, which are powered by the S1 motor level, into use.

Classical Significance: The inability to perform this test indicates a lesion of the S1 nerve root, such as L5 disc protrusion or prolapse (Fig. E).

Clinical Significance: If the S2 nerve root level is spared due to innervation to the triceps surae, the patient will be able to toe walk but with less ease (Fig. F).

Follow-up: Perform Lasegue's straight leg test, Kemp's test, or the Valsalva maneuver.

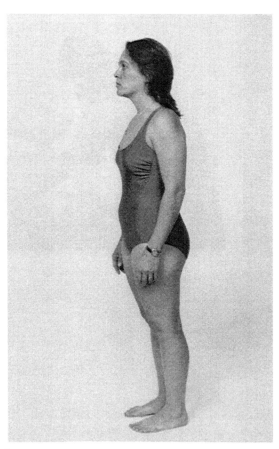

A

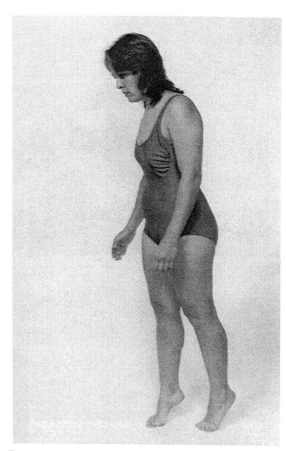

B

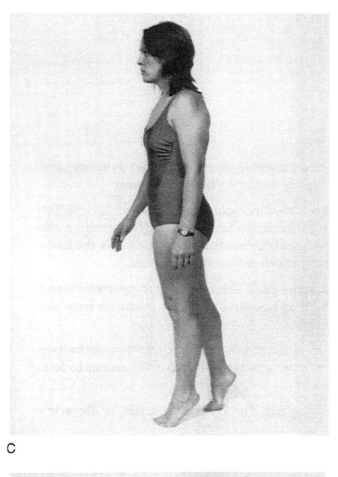

C

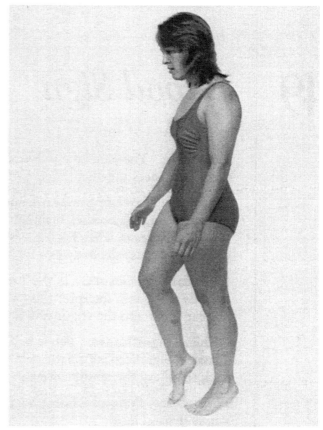

D

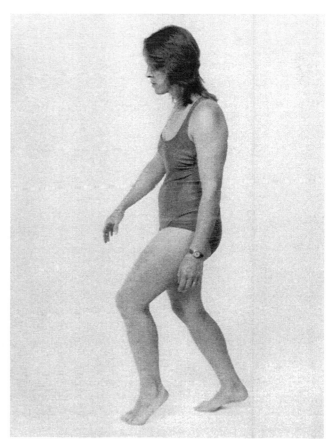

E

F

49 | *Tripod Sign*

Procedure: The patient is seated. Ask the patient to extend one knee at a time, and then both knees together (Figs. A–D). This is similar to Bechterew's test.

Rationale: Extending one knee puts strain on the hemipelvis on that side by a pull of the hamstring. The other hemipelvis will accommodate accordingly to relieve the tension. However, when both knees are extended, the extra strain caused by the hamstrings will cause the body as a whole to adapt to the postural stresses.

Classical Significance: If the patient leans back onto the upper extremities and extends the trunk, interpret this as hamstring tightness or spinal irritation from the lumbar spine into the sciatic notch (Fig. E).

Clinical Significance: Pelvic subluxation can cause the same effect as above (see Classical Significance). Sciatic nerve root irritation can also cause the patient to lean back to relieve the tension along its path.

Follow-up: Perform Lasegue's straight leg test, the advancement test, or Deyerle's sciatic tension test.

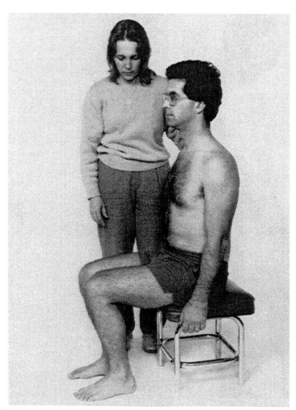

A

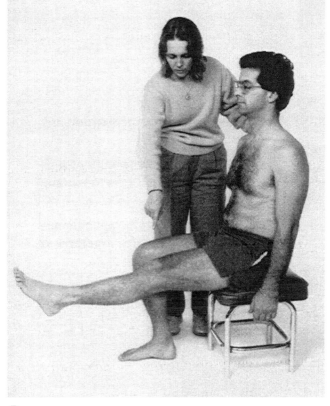

B

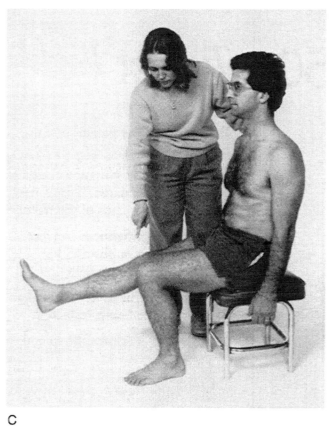

C

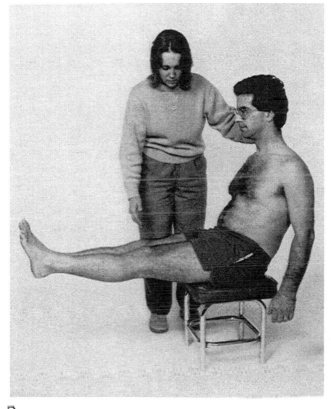

D

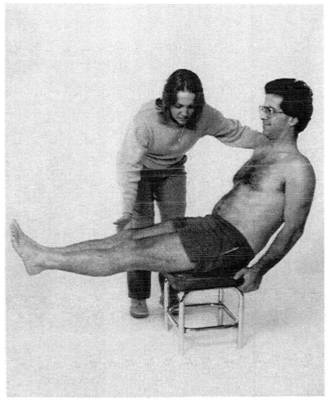

E

50 | *Tuning Fork Test*

Procedure: The patient is seated. Using a 128-cc tuning fork, place the stem on any bony prominence (Figs. A–D).

Rationale: The vibration caused by the tuning fork is transferred to the bony prominence being evaluated. If fracture is present, the underlying tissue will begin to vibrate, causing the two ends of the fracture to rub.

Classical Significance: An increase in sharp pain at the area of the bony prominence being tested is a positive test (Fig. E). This is a good way to test for fractures if radiography is unavailable.

Clinical Significance: Subtle hairline fractures may cause only a slight increase in pain at the site being evaluated.

Follow-up: Perform the spinous percussion test.

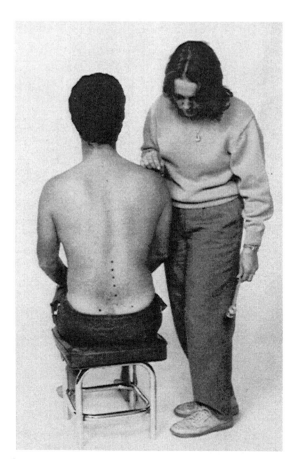

A

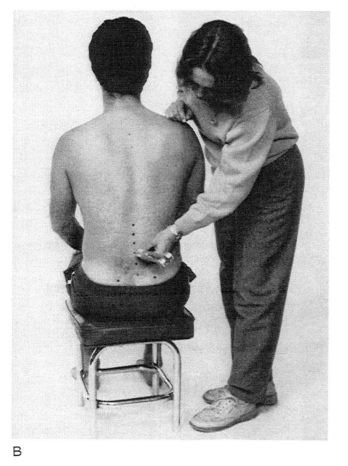

B

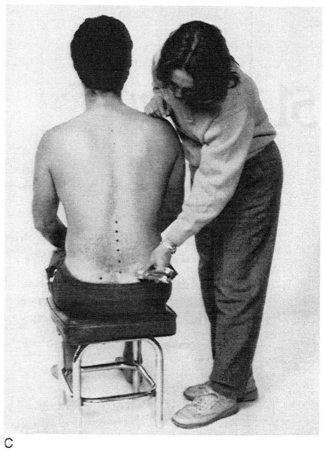

C

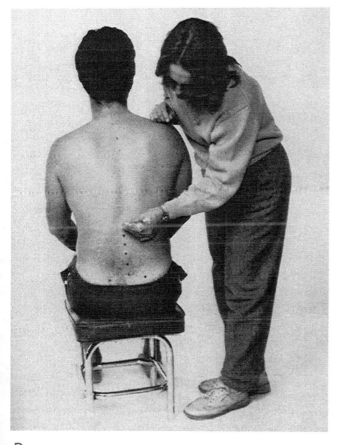

D

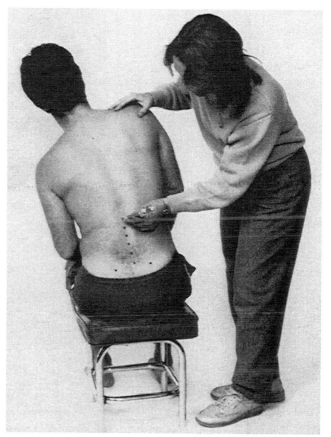

E

51 | *Turyn's Test*

Procedure: The patient is supine. Keeping both of the patient's legs on the examination table, forceably dorsiflex the patient's great toe (Figs. A–C).

Rationale: This test puts extra stress on the sciatic nerve by pulling on it.

Classical Significance: Reproduction of sciatic radiculopathy or pain, which may be limited to the gluteal region, is a positive test (Figs. D & E).

Clinical Significance: This test is less stressful than Sicard's test because the leg is flat on the table. If the sciatica is very slight, this test may not be positive, since reproduction of the complaint may not occur.

Follow-up: Perform Kemp's test, the Valsalva maneuver, or Sicard's test.

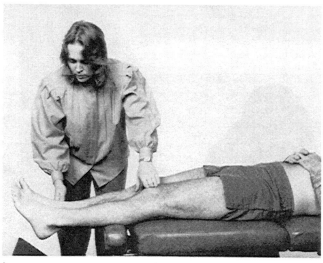

A

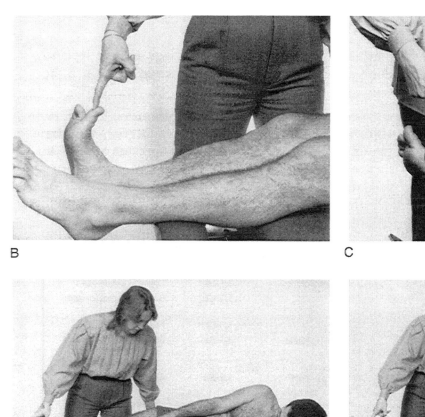

B

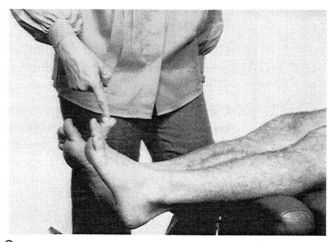

C

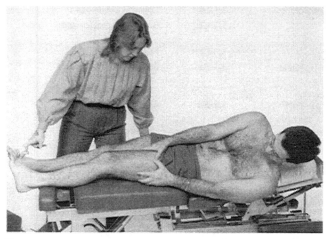

D

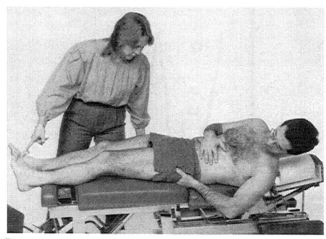

E

52 | *Valsalva Maneuver*

Procedure: The patient is seated. Ask the patient to breathe in deeply, hold it, and to bear down. If pain is produced, ask the patient to place the thumb in the mouth and try to puff the cheeks in an attempt to blow the thumb out of the mouth (Figs. C & D).

Rationale: This test causes an increase in intrathecal pressure.

Classical Significance: An increase in radicular symptomatology along a specific dermatome with both procedures indicates a space-occupying lesion (Figs. A, B, E, & F).

Clinical Significance: A space-occupying lesion can be a disc protrusion, tumor, or foraminal or lateral recess osteophytosis, or both. If the symptoms occur only with the first procedure and not with the second, suspect lumbar strain as the cause of the low back pain.

Follow-up: Perform Kemp's test, Lasegue's straight leg test, or the bowstring sign.

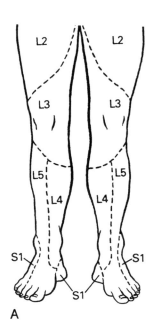

A

Nerve	Root Level	Muscle(s)
Branches of L2–L4	L2–L4	Iliopsoas; hip flexion
Femoral	L2–L4	Quadriceps; knee extension
Obturator	L2–L4	Adductors
Superior gluteal	L4–S1	Gluteus medius minimus & tensor fascia lata; abduction of the thigh
Inferior gluteal	L5–S2	Gluteus maximus; hip extension
Sciatic	L5–S2	Hamstrings; knee flexion
Deep peroneal	L4–L5	Tibialis anterior; dorsiflexion & inversion of the foot
Superficial peroneal	L5–S1	Peroneus longus & brevis; plantar flexion & eversion
Tibial	L5–S1	Tibialis posterior; plantar flexion
Deep peroneal	L4–S1	Extensor hallucis longus; extensor digitorum; dorsiflexion

When a disc lesion causes a nerve root problem, the disc level is located superior to the involved nerve root.

B

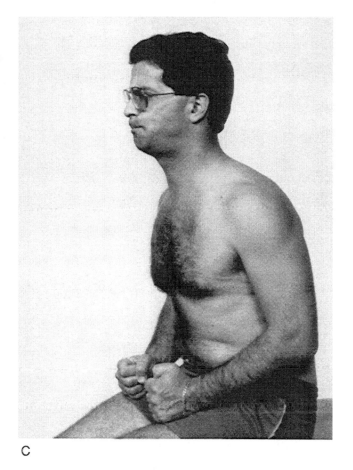

C

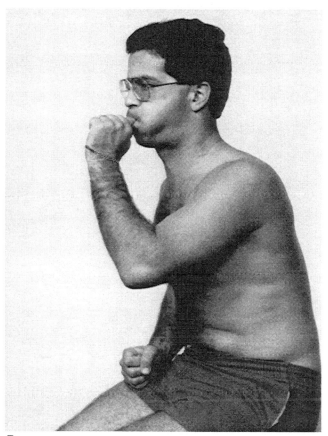

D

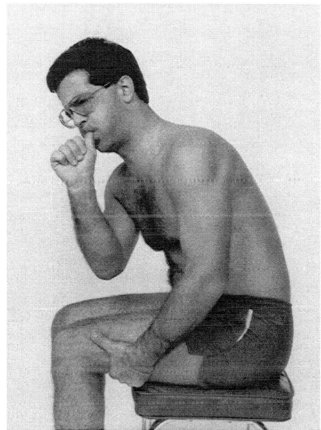

E

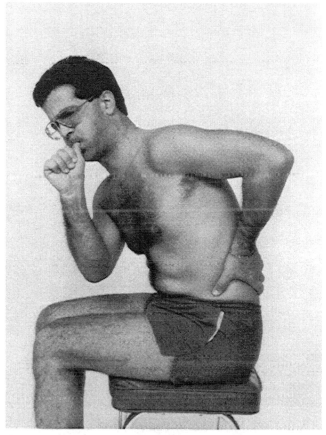

F

CHAPTER

9

Sacroiliac Testing

1. Belt Test
2. Erichsen's Test
3. Gaenslen's Test
4. Gillis' Test
5. Hibb's Test
6. Hip Abduction Stress Test
7. Hopping Test
8. Iliac Compression Test
9. Laguerre Test
10. Lewin's-Gaenslen's Test
11. Mennell's Test
12. Minor's Sign
13. Nachlas Test
14. Sacroiliac Stretch Test
15. Yeoman's Test

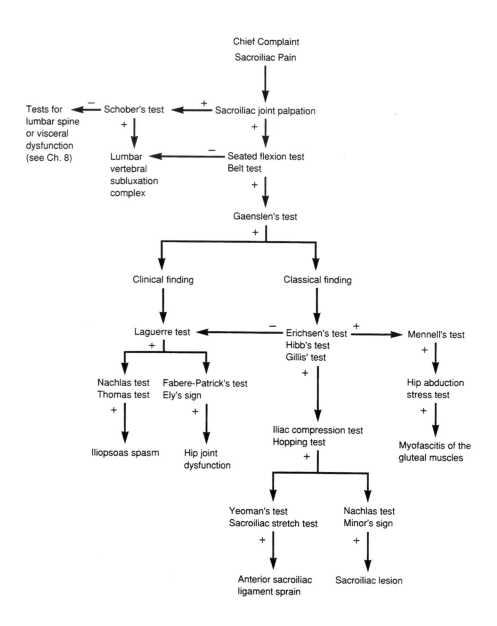

Procedures

1 | *Belt Test*

Procedure: Perform this test only on patients who present with some type of low back pain. The patient is standing. Stand behind the patient and ask the patient to bend forward to the level at which pain occurs. Then, support the patient's sacrum with your hip while the patient again bends forward (Figs. A–D).

Rationale: Forward flexion requires a properly functioning sacroiliac joint, lumbosacral joint, and individual lumbar vertebral movement. By comparing when the pain occurs with and without support, the level of dysfunction is determined.

Classical Significance: If pain occurs on forward flexion without support, but with support the pain is reduced, the problem occurs at the sacroiliac joint (Fig. E).

Clinical Significance: If pain occurs on forward flexion both with and without support, the problem occurs within the lumbar spine, including the lumbosacral junction (Fig. F).

Follow-up: Perform Mennell's test, Gaenslen's test, or the seated flexion test (see Ch. 8).

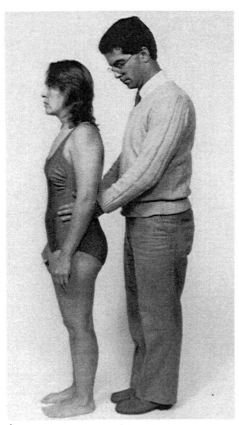

A

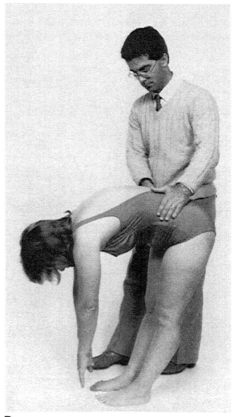

B

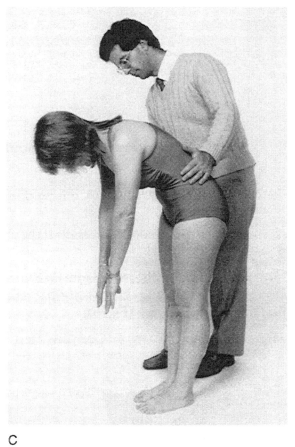

C

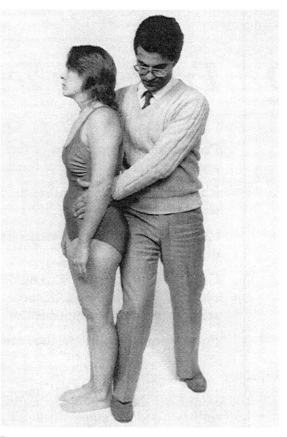

D

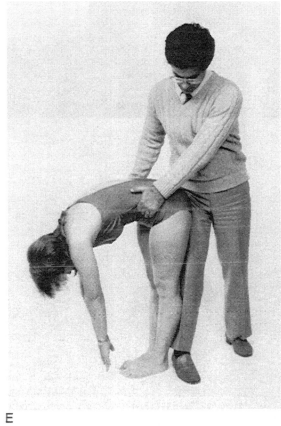

E

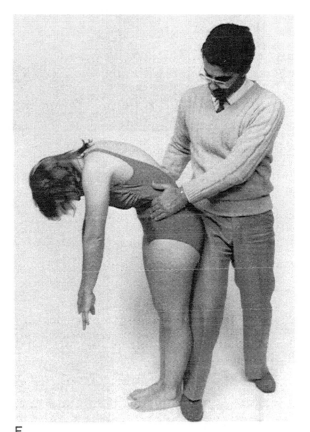

F

2 | *Erichsen's Test*

Procedure: The patient is prone. Place your hands over the dorsum of both ilia and give a sharp, forceful, lateral to medial thrust (Figs. A–D).

Rationale: This test compresses the sacroiliac joint and is similar to the iliac compression test.

Classical Significance: An increase in sacroiliac joint pain indicates a lesion at the site of pain (Fig. E).

Clinical Significance: This test helps to rule out hip joint disease because no contact occurs with the hip joint. If pain occurs in the buttocks and not in the sacroiliac joint, sciatic nerve entrapment or gluteal myofascitis may be present (Fig. F).

Follow-up: Perform the iliac compression test, Mennell's test, or Gaenslen's test.

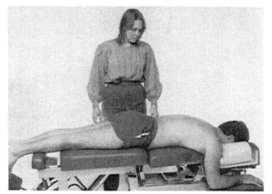

A

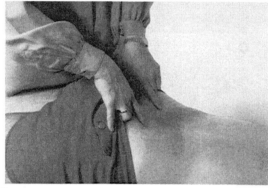

B

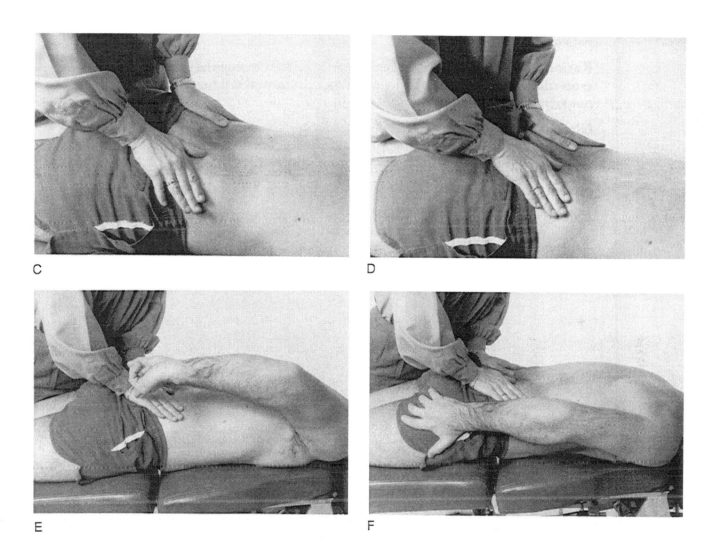

C

D

E

F

3 | ✳Gaenslen's Test

Procedure: The patient is supine. Ask the patient to grasp one knee and bring it to the chest. With the patient in this position, slide the extended leg off the side of the table. Then press downward on the extended leg while pushing the flexed knee onto the patient's chest (Figs. A–C).

Rationale: This test causes extreme rotational stress within the pelvis in general and especially within the sacroiliac joint. This is the classical test for confirming or ruling out sacroiliac joint lesion.

Classical Significance: Re-creation of pain in the sacroiliac joint on the side of the extended leg indicates a sacroiliac joint lesion (Fig. D).

Clinical Significance: This test can also re-create hip pain if hip joint lesion is present. Locating the area of pain will help determine where the lesion exists (Fig. E).

Follow-up: Perform Mennell's test, Gillis' test, or Yeoman's test.

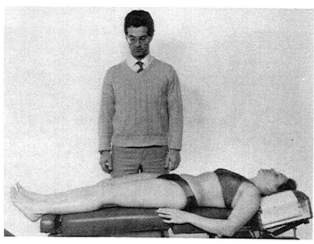

A

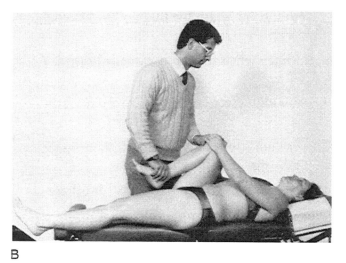

B

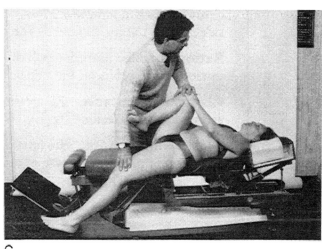

C

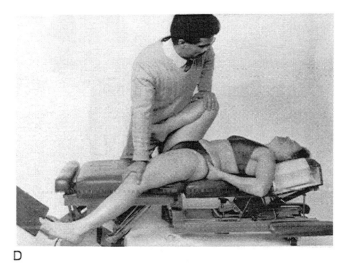

D

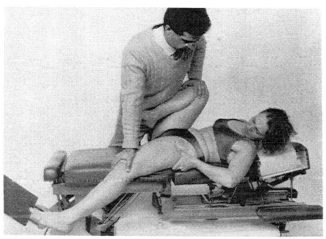

E

4 | *Gillis' Test*

Procedure: The patient is prone. Place the palm of your hand over the patient's sacroiliac joint on the unaffected side to stabilize the sacrum. The fingertips should fan over the affected sacroiliac joint. With the other hand, grasp the thigh of the affected side and lift the leg, extending the hip joint (Figs. A–D).

Rationale: The posterior pull of the hamstrings when the hip is extended causes a torsion of the pelvis on the side being tested.

Classical Significance: Re-creation of pain within the affected sacroiliac joint indicates a sacroiliac lesion (Fig. E).

Clinical Significance: Hip lesions such as malum coxae senilis can limit the amount of extension possible because of pain within the hip joint itself (Fig. F).

Follow-up: Perform the Nachlas test, Ely's heel to buttock test (see Ch. 8), or Fabere-Patrick's test (see Ch. 10).

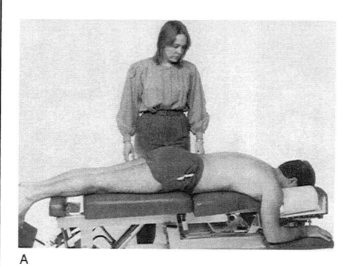

A

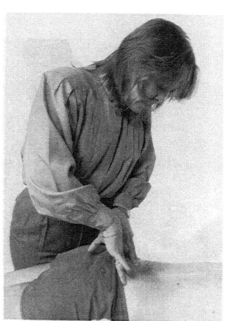

B

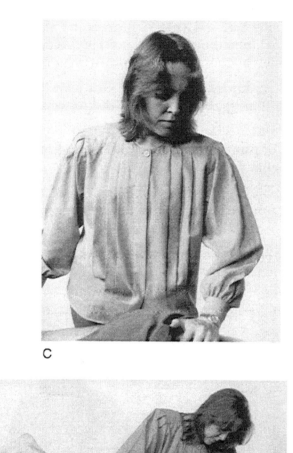

C

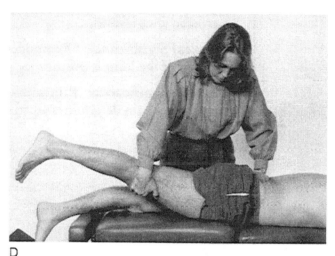

D

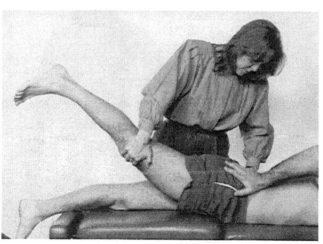

E

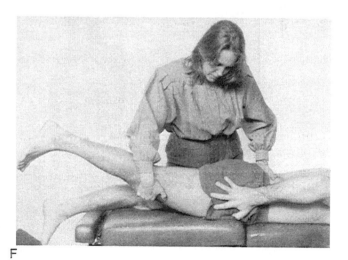

F

5 | *Hibb's Test*

Procedure: The patient is prone. Flex the heel and knee 90 degrees and rotate the femoral head internally by pushing the foot from the medial to lateral position. Repeat this test on the opposite side (Figs. A–D).

Rationale: Forces are transmitted from the hip joint into the sacroiliac joint. This test is primarily used to confirm hip joint pathology, but it is also useful for confirming sacroiliac joint lesions.

Classical Significance: Reproduction of pain within the sacroiliac joint from compression of the joint is positive for sacroiliac joint lesion (Fig. E).

Clinical Significance: Pain within the hip indicates hip joint lesion. The location of the patient's pain determines whether the problem is within the hip joint or sacroiliac joint (Fig. F).

Follow-up: Perform Gaenslen's test, Mennell's test, or Erichsen's test.

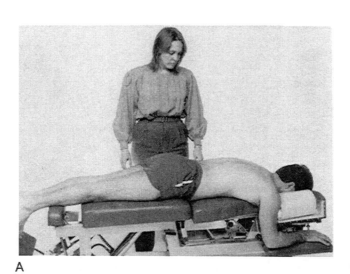

A

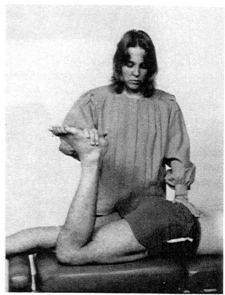

B

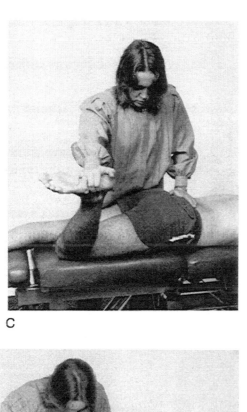

C

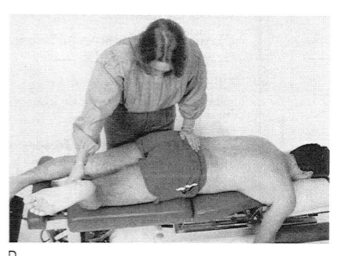

D

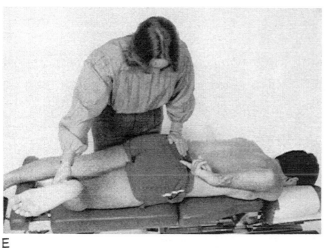

E

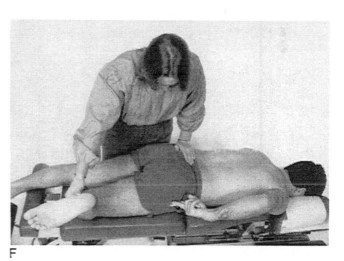

F

6 | *Hip Abduction Stress Test*

Procedure: The patient is lying on one side with the affected side up. Ask the patient to abduct the affected leg from the midline. Then, press downward against this leg as the patient resists the pressure (Figs. A–C).

Rationale: Testing the gluteus medius and gluteus minimus abductors with resistance stresses the ipsilateral sacroiliac joint.

Classical Significance: An increase in pain at the affected sacroiliac joint indicates a sacroiliac lesion (Fig. D).

Clinical Significance: A patient with hip joint pathology may have an increase of pain within the affected hip. The location of the pain helps pinpoint the type of lesion (Fig. E).

Follow-up: Perform the Trendelenburg test (see Ch. 8), Fabere-Patrick's test (see Ch. 10), or Erichsen's test.

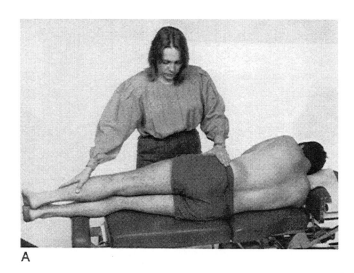

A

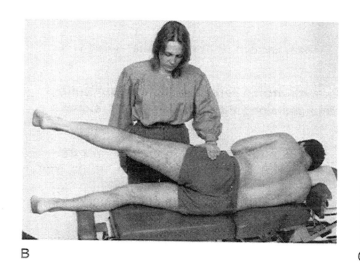

B

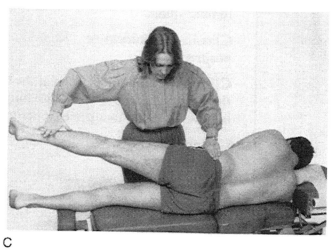

C

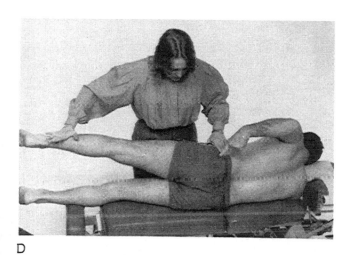

D

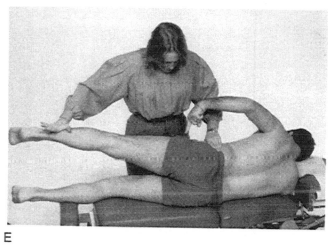

E

7 | *Hopping Test*

Procedure: The patient is standing. Ask the patient to hop first on one leg and then the other (Figs. A–E).

Rationale: Hopping produces a jarring force at the sacroiliac joint, hip joint, and lumbar spine.

Classical Significance: Reproduction of pain located at the sacroiliac joint is a positive test.

Clinical Significance: Pain at the hip may indicate hip pathology; diffuse pain along the posterior lumbar spine radiating around and along the flank can signify kidney involvement due to a stone or peritonitis.

Follow-up: Perform Fabere-Patrick's test (see Ch. 10), Kemp's test (see Ch. 8), or the Laguerre test.

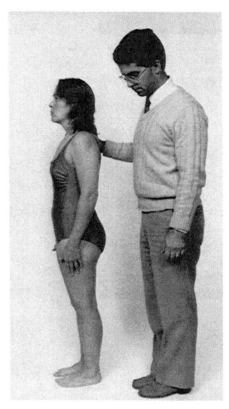

A

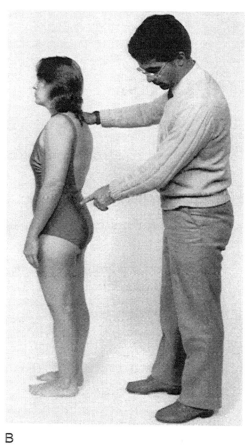

B

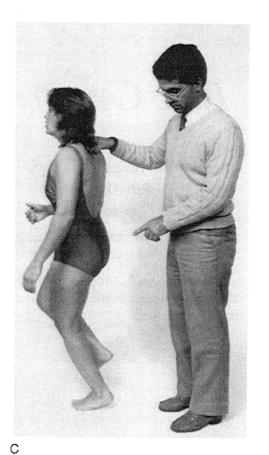

C

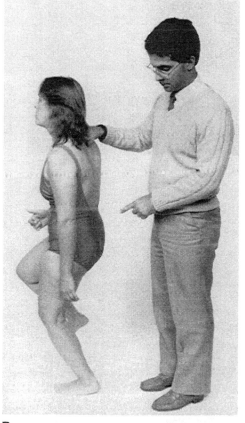

D

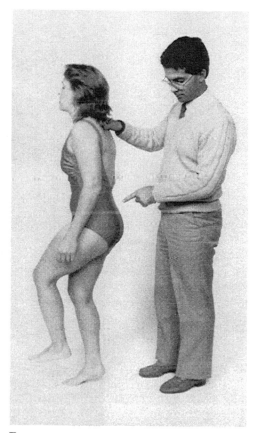

E

8 | *Iliac Compression Test*

Procedure: The patient is lying on one side. Place both hands on the innominate bone of the side facing up and press downward (Figs. A–C).

Rationale: The downward pressure compresses the sacroiliac joints.

Classical Significance: An increase in pain within the sacroiliac joint signifies a sacroiliac joint lesion in the affected side (Fig. D).

Clinical Significance: Pain at the site of pressure on the innominate bone can be a result of patient sensitivity and should be discounted (Fig. E).

Follow-up: Perform Erichsen's test or the sacroiliac stretch test.

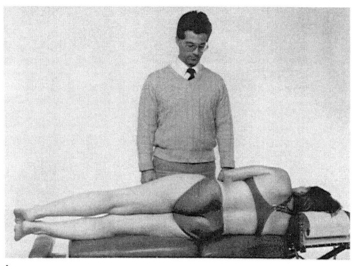

A

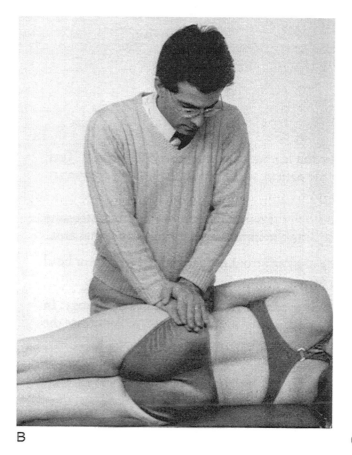

B

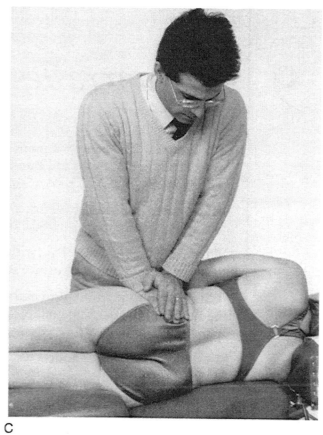

C

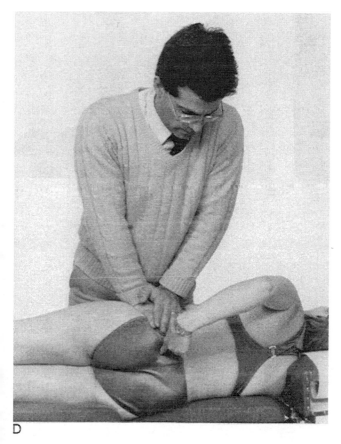

D

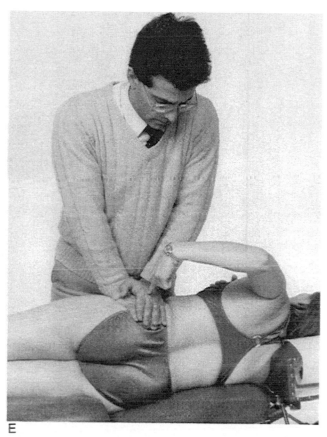

E

9 | *Laguerre Test*

Procedure: The patient is supine. Flex the leg and then the knee 90 degrees. Next, rotate the thigh outward and then force the patient's heel up while pressing downward on the knee (Figs. A–D).

Rationale: This maneuver forces the head of the femur into the acetabulum, stressing the anterior joint capsule, while not affecting the lumbosacral or lumbar spinal area.

Classical Significance: Pain within the hip joint from the pressure of the femur head into the acetabulum is a positive test (Fig. E).

Clinical Significance: Pain in the area of the sacroiliac joint indicates pathology. In addition, iliopsoas spasm on the ipsilateral side can be induced, which will increase the pain (Fig. F).

Follow-up: Perform Hibb's test, Gaenselen's test, or the sacroiliac stretch test.

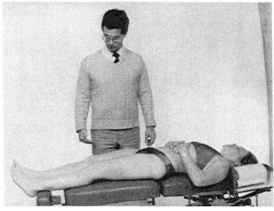

A

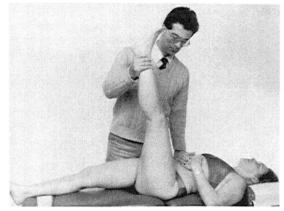

B

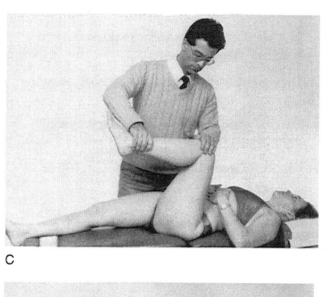

C

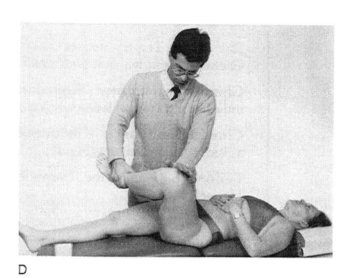

D

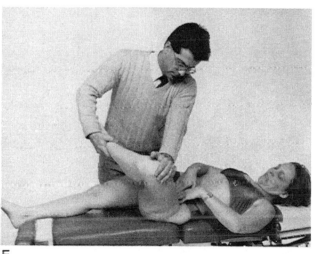

E

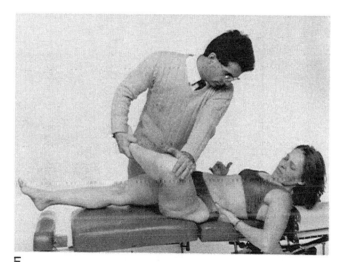

F

10 ✳*Lewin's-Gaenslen's Test*

Procedure: The patient is lying on the unaffected side. Ask the patient to grasp the knee of the unaffected side and pull it to the chest. Extend the affected thigh while pressing down on the flexed knee (Figs. A–C).

Rationale: This test stresses the extended sacroiliac joint. It is similar to the standard Gaenslen's test, which is performed with the patient supine.

Classical Significance: Reproduction of pain within the affected sacroiliac joint indicates a sacroiliac lesion on that side (Fig. D).

Clinical Significance: If the extension is limited, consider hip joint pathology, as well as iliopsoas contracture (Fig. E).

Follow-up: Perform the Thomas test (see Ch. 8), Fabere-Patrick's test (see Ch. 10), or Mennell's test.

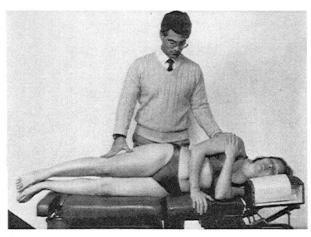

A

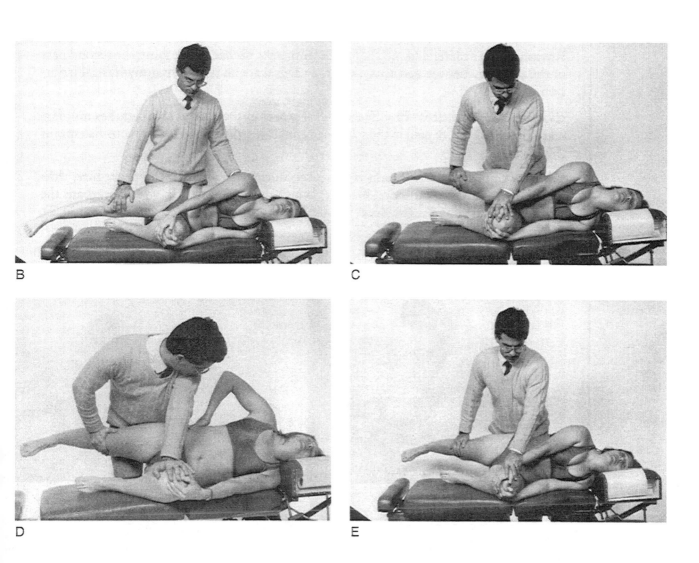

B

C

D

E

11 | *Mennell's Test*

Procedure: The patient is prone. First, palpate the posterior superior iliac spine (PSIS) bilaterally. Then apply a lateral to medial force against the PSIS. Finally, pull the soft tissue laterally until fully stretched (Figs. A–C).

Rationale: The lateral to medial force compresses the sacroiliac joint; the second part of the test stretches the soft tissue and may aggravate an underlying myofascial irritation.

Classical Significance: Pain in the lateral aspect of the gluteal area signifies myofascial irritation (Fig. D); pain in the sacroiliac joint can indicate a superior sacroiliac sprain (Fig. E).

Clinical Significance: If pain is increased during part one of the procedure, then grasping the anterior superior iliac spine and pulling posterior will exacerbate the problem, confirming the diagnosis of sacroiliac joint dysfunction due to sprain (Fig. F).

Follow-up: Perform Erichsen's test, Yeoman's test, Gaenslen's test, or Gillis' test.

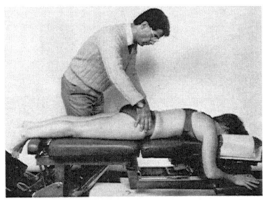

A

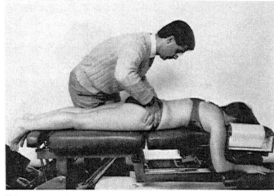

B

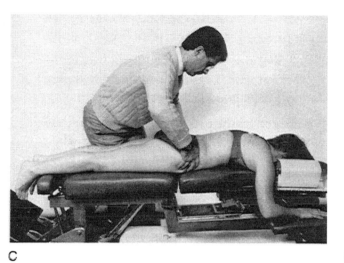

C

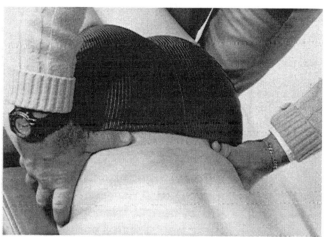

D

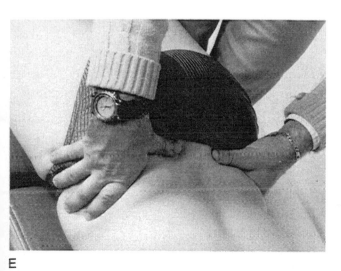

E

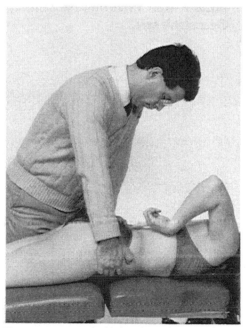

F

12 | *Minor's Sign*

Procedure: The patient is seated. Ask the patient to stand up and note the ease with which the patient is able to rise as well as the patient's facial expression (Figs. A & B).

Rationale: The patient with low back pain will not be able to stand up easily. In addition, the patient's face should indicate discomfort as a result of the increased pain caused by standing up. The normal patient will have good lumbopelvic rhythm.

Classical Significance: A positive test is indicated by the patient placing one hand on the thigh opposite the affected side, while putting the other hand on the pain when attempting to stand. The facial features will show a grimace (Figs. C–E).

Clinical Significance: Patients with ankylosing spondylitis will also have difficulty in rising from the seated position. This is due to stiffness in the spine, with subsequent loss of normal lumbopelvic rhythm. In addition, obese patients will have difficulty rising from a seated position because of weight imposed restrictions. However, this is not a significant finding.

Follow-up: Perform Kemp's test (see Ch. 8), Lasegue's straight leg test (see Ch. 8), or Gaenslen's test.

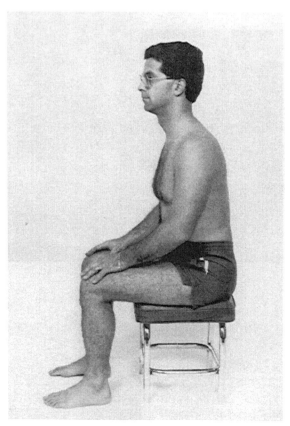

A

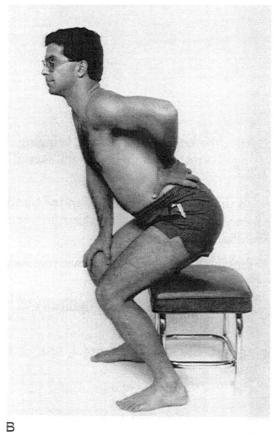

B

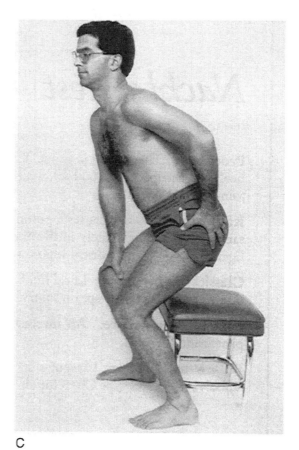

C

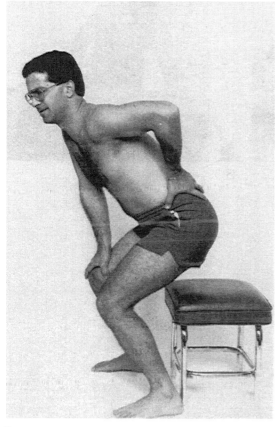

D

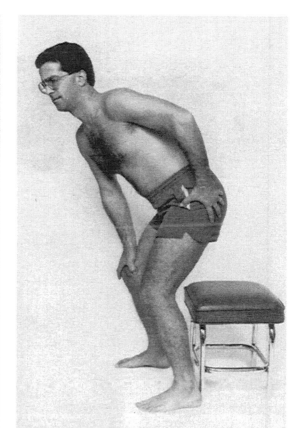

E

13 | *Nachlas Test*

Procedure: The patient is prone. Passively flex the knee of the patient, bringing the heel onto the ipsilateral buttock while pressing downward on the ipsilateral sacroiliac joint (Figs. A–D).

Rationale: This test causes a pulling first in the sacroiliac joint, then in the lumbosacral joint, and ultimately in the lumbar spine. It is important to perform this test if ligamentous sprain or discal lesion in the lumbar spine is suspected.

Classical Significance: Local lumbar, lumbosacral, or sacroiliac pain without radiation indicates strain or sprain injury (Fig. F).

Clinical Significance: An increase in radicular symptomatology indicates discal protrusion (Fig. E).

Follow-up: Perform Lasegue's straight leg test, Ely's heel to buttock test, or the Valsalva maneuver (see Ch. 8 for all three tests).

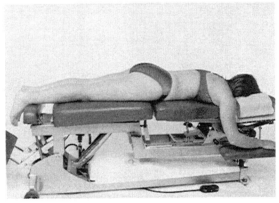

A

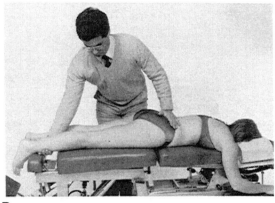

B

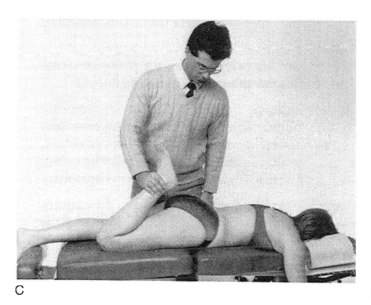

C

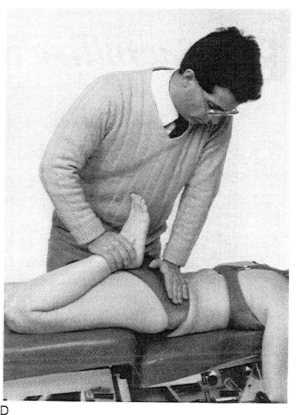

D

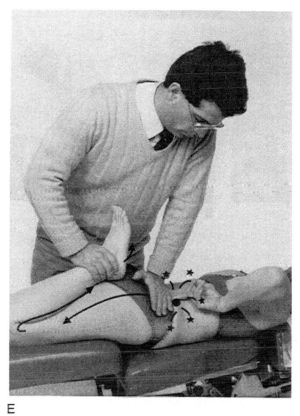

E

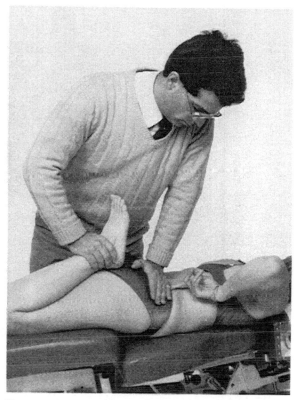

F

14 | *Sacroiliac Stretch Test*

Procedure: The patient is supine. Using crossed hands, press downward on the anterior superior iliac spines. The crossed-hands approach adds a lateral component to the downward pressure (Figs. A–D).

Rationale: The anterior to posterior force on the pelvis stresses the posterior sacroiliac joint while the lateral component stresses the anterior sacroiliac ligaments.

Classical Significance: Deep seated pain indicates a sprain of the anterior sacroiliac ligaments on the painful side (Fig. E: 1, iliolumbar ligament; 2, anterior superior iliac spine; 3, anterior inferior iliac spine; 4, lumbosacral ligament; 5, fifth lumbar vertebra; 6, anterior longitudinal ligament; 7, ventral sacroiliac ligament; 8, sacrospinous ligament; 9, ventral sacrococcygeal ligament; 10, sacrotuberous ligament; 11, pectineal ligament).

Clinical Significance: Pain in the posterior may be due to pressure from the examining table or from irritation of the posterior sacroiliac joint. The specific location of the pain will help determine which is the cause (Fig. F).

Follow-up: Perform Yeoman's test or Gaenslen's test.

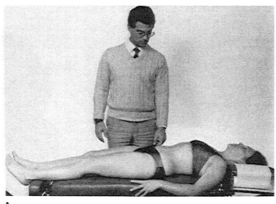

A

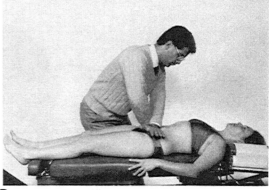

B

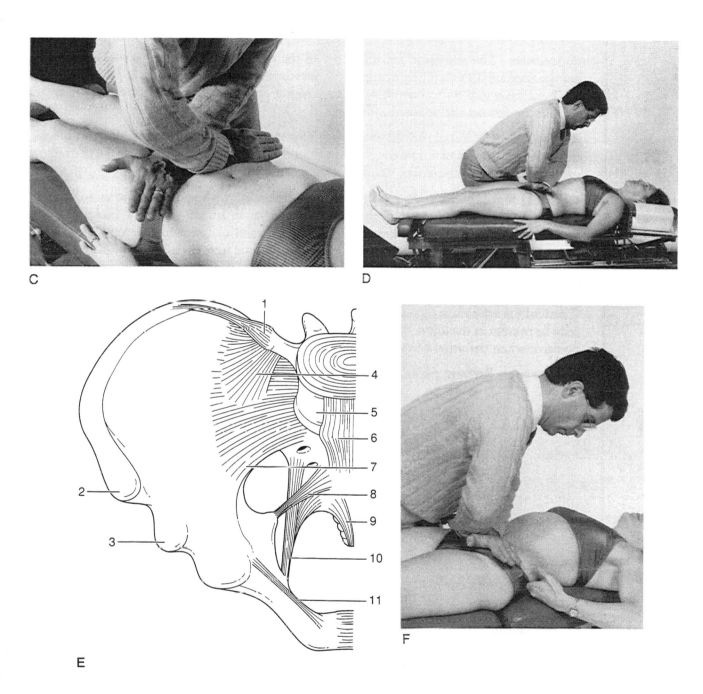

C

D

E

F

15 | *Yeoman's Test*

Procedure: The patient is prone. Stand on the opposite side of the sacroiliac joint being tested and flex the knee, bringing the heel onto the ipsilateral buttock. Then grasp the bent knee and extend the hip while pressing downward on the sacroiliac joint. Repeat the test on the opposite side (Figs. A–D).

Rationale: The initial part of the test slightly stresses the posterior sacroiliac structures. The addition of downward pressure will open up the anterior aspect of the sacroiliac joint and should stress the anterior sacroiliac ligaments.

Classical Significance: The test is positive, if pain is felt deep within the sacroiliac joint, which indicates a sprain of the anterior sacroiliac ligaments (Fig. E: 1, iliolumbar ligament; 2, anterior superior iliac spine; 3, anterior inferior iliac spine; 4, lumbosacral ligament; 5, fifth lumbar vertebra; 6, anterior longitudinal ligament; 7, ventral sacroiliac ligament; 8, sacrospinous ligament; 9, ventral sacrococcygeal ligament; 10, sacrotuberous ligament; 11, pectineal ligament).

Clinical Significance: Pain located within the posterior aspect of the sacroiliac joint may be present as the joint is stressed first. However, this test should only be considered positive when irritation at the anterior sacroiliac ligaments is increased (Fig. F).

Follow-up: Perform the sacroiliac stretch test or Ely's heel to buttock test (see Ch. 8).

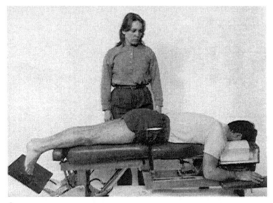

A

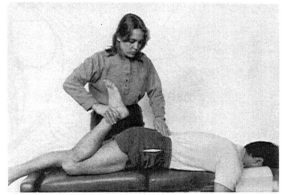

B

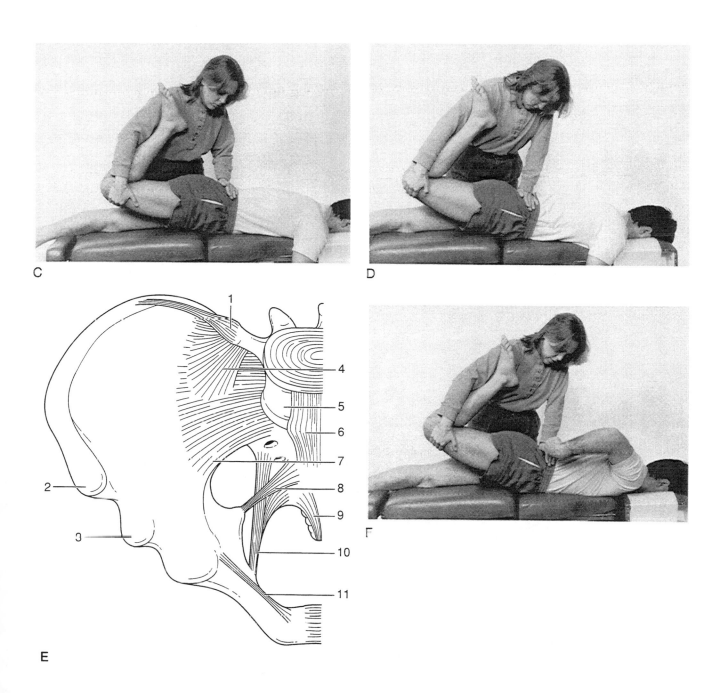

C

D

E

F

<table>
<tr><td>CHAPTER
10</td><td></td></tr>
</table>

Hip Testing

1. Range of Motion Studies
2. Actual Leg Length Test
3. Adduction/Abduction Contracture Tests
4. Allis Test
5. Anvil Test
6. Apparent Leg Length Test
7. Barlow's Test
8. Craig Test
9. Ely's Heel to Buttock Test
10. Ely's Sign
11. Fabere-Patrick's Test
12. Hamstring Contracture Test
13. Hibb's Test
14. Hopping Test
15. Hyperextension Hip Test
16. Laguerre Test
17. Nelaton's Line Test
18. Noble's Compression Test
19. Ober's Test
20. Ortolani's Test
21. Rectus Femoris Contracture Test
22. Telescoping Test
23. Thomas Test
24. Trendelenburg Test

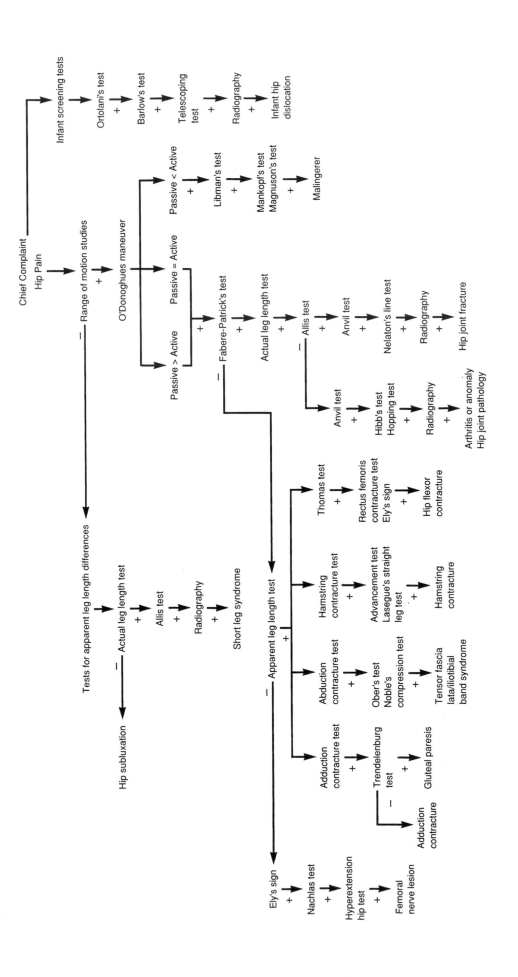

Range of Motion Studies

1

When performing range of motion studies, it is important to use either an arthrodial protractor or an inclinometer. The *American Medical Association Guides for Impairment Ratings* now recommend the use of the inclinometer exclusively. As a general rule, the active hip ranges of motion are performed by the patient without being measured to observe the degree of ease with which the patient performs them. However, with the inclinometer the active ranges of motion can be readily measured. Perform the passive ranges of motion after the active ones.

Flexion: The patient is supine with the knees fully extended. Place the inclinometer on the anterior thigh; record the number on the inclinometer (this is the zero position). Ask the patient to draw the knee into the chest. Record the new number; the difference between the zero position and the second number is the amount of flexion. Then, flex the patient's leg, bringing the knee to the chest. Normal flexion is 120 to 135 degrees.

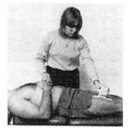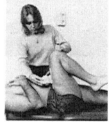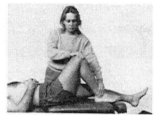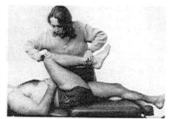

Extension: The patient is prone with the knees fully extended. Place the inclinometer on the posterior thigh (the zero position) and record the number. Ask the patient to flex the knee 90 degrees and to lift the thigh off the table as far as possible. Record this number; the difference between the two is the amount of extension. Stabilize the patient's hip, flex the patient's knee bringing the heel to the buttock, and lift the knee off the table. Normal extension is 20 to 30 degrees.

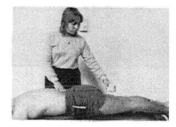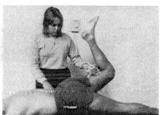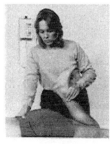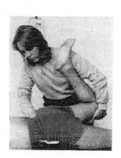

Abduction: The patient is lying on one side, with the top knee fully extended. Place the inclinometer on the lateral thigh; record the number. Ask the patient to abduct the leg as far as possible. Record this number; the difference between the two is the amount of abduction. With the patient supine and both legs together, separate one leg at a time, spreading the leg as wide as possible from the midline. Normal abduction is 45 to 50 degrees.

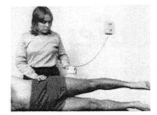 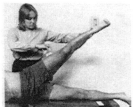 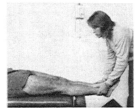 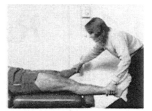

Adduction: The patient is lying on one side, with the top knee fully extended. Place the inclinometer on the lateral thigh; record the number. Ask the patient to adduct the leg off the table, pressing it to the floor as far as possible. Record this number; the difference between the two is the amount of adduction. With the patient supine and both legs together, lift one leg at a time and push it medially as far as possible. Normal adduction is 20 to 30 degrees.

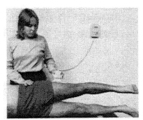 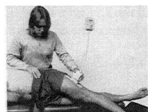 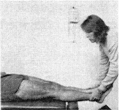 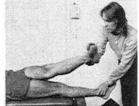

Internal Rotation: The patient is seated with the knees flexed 90 degrees. Place the inclinometer on the tibial tubercle; record this number (the zero position). Ask the patient to turn the foot in toward the midline; record this number. The difference is the amount of internal rotation. With the patient supine, grasp both heels and rotate the toes in toward each other. Normal internal rotation is 35 to 40 degrees.

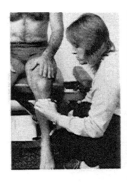 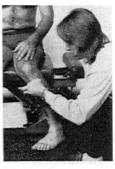 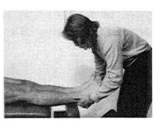 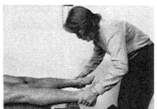

External Rotation: The patient is seated with the knees flexed 90 degrees. Place the inclinometer on the tibial tubercle; record this number. Ask the patient to turn the foot out away from the midline; record this number. The difference is the amount of external rotation. With the patient supine, grasp both heels and rotate the toes out away from each other. Normal external rotation is 40 to 45 degrees.

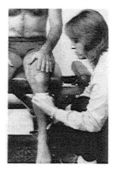 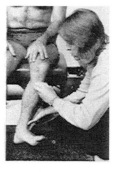 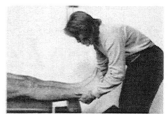 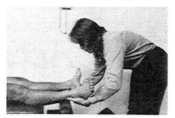

Quick Test: For a quick test of hip extension, ask the patient to stand from a seated position.

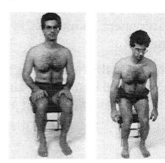

For abduction and then adduction, with the patient standing, ask the patient to spread the legs apart as far as possible and then to cross one leg in front of the other and walk this way (scissors position).

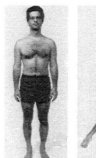 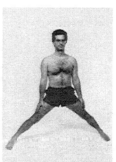 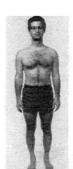 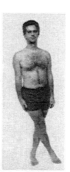

For internal rotation, with the patient seated, ask the patient to cross one thigh over the other. For external rotation, with the patient seated, ask the patient to place one heel on the contralateral knee.

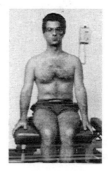 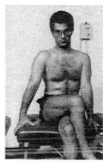 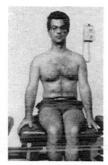 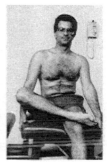

2 | *Actual Leg Length Test*

Procedure: The patient is supine. Mark the anterior superior iliac spine and the medial malleolus on each leg. Measure and record the distance of each leg. Compare the numbers (Figs. A–E). Should be equal

Rationale: This measurement is from one fixed point to another. Even in the presence of pelvic obliquity, muscle wasting, or obesity, this will indicate any congenital leg length or acquired leg length deficiency.

Classical Significance: Any difference in the measurement on one side as compared with the other indicates a true leg length discrepancy.

Clinical Significance: If the difference in length between the two legs is greater than one-quarter inch, it is considered a rateable impairment and is an important factor to consider in stabilization of the patient who presents with lower back and pelvic pain.

Follow-up: Refer the patient for radiography of the legs, or perform the Allis test or the apparent leg length test.

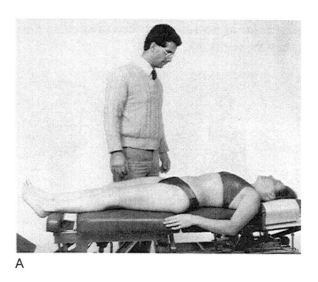

A

½ inch leg length discrepancy use heel lift. ⅛ inch at a time. > ½ inch. must get orthoses for outside of shoe.

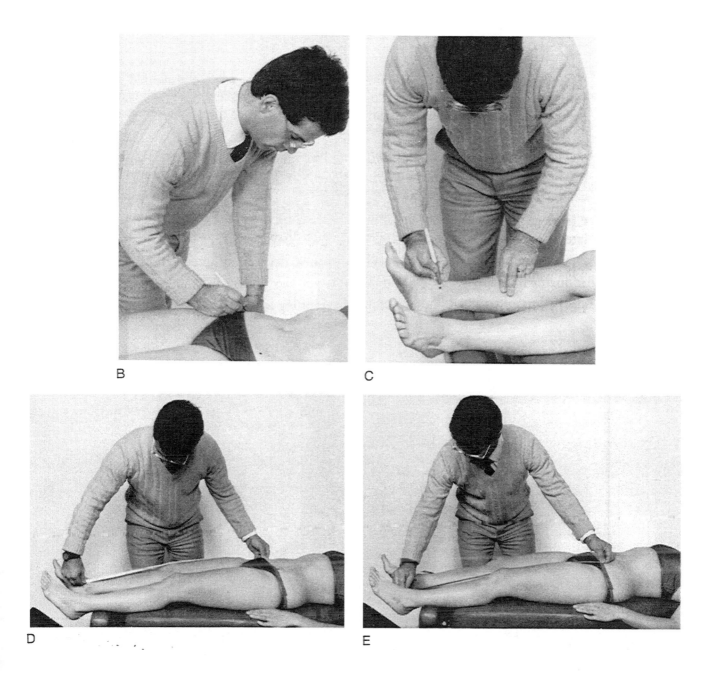

B

C

D

E

3 | *Adduction/Abduction Contracture Tests*

Procedure: This test is an observation of the patient when the patient is supine. Palpate the anterior superior iliac spines (ASISs) and align them with each other. In the normal pelvis, the angle the leg forms with the line between the ASISs is approximately 90 degrees (Figs. A–C).

Rationale: If the abductors and adductors are equally balanced, the ASISs are aligned. If any contracture is present, aligning the ASISs results in a shift in the pelvis and a change in the 90-degree angle.

Classical Significance: If the abductors are contracted, the leg will be pulled into a lateral position resulting in an angle of greater than 90 degrees (Fig. D).

Clinical Significance: An angle of less than 90 degrees indicates a contracture of the adductor musculature on that side (Fig. E).

Follow-up: Perform the actual and apparent leg length tests or Ober's test.

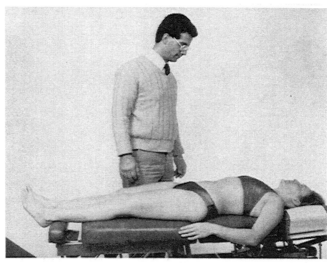

A

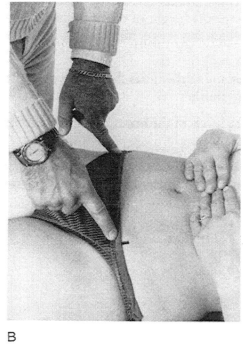

B

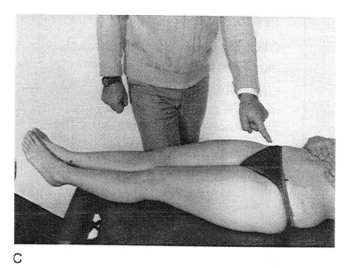

C

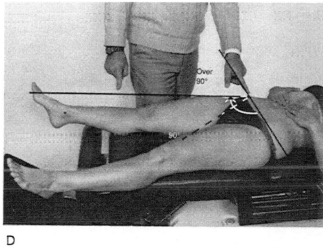

D

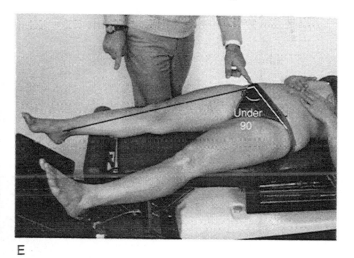

E

4 | *Allis Test*

Procedure: The patient is supine with the legs bent and the feet on the table, the heels are approximately parallel to each other. Observe the height of the femoral condyles (which one protrudes farther) and of tibias (which leg seems higher than the other) (Figs. A & B).

Rationale: The height of the femoral condyles and of the tibias should be equal if the feet are perfectly planted in relationship to one another.

Classical Significance: Any discrepancy in the levels of the knees, denoting shortening of the extremity, is a positive test (Figs. C & D).

Clinical Significance: The shortening may be a result of a posterior hip dislocation, in which case the femoral shaft on the involved side will be pulled backward creating the illusion of unequal femoral heights (Fig. E).

Follow-up: Perform the apparent and actual leg length tests or refer the patient for radiography.

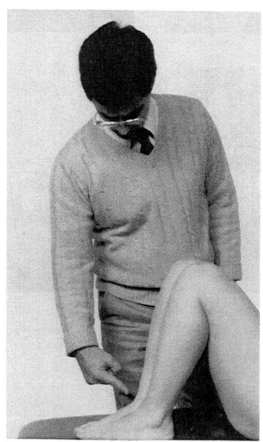

A

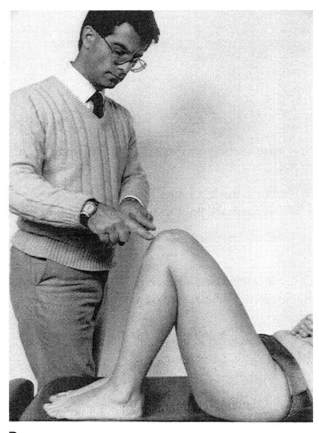

B

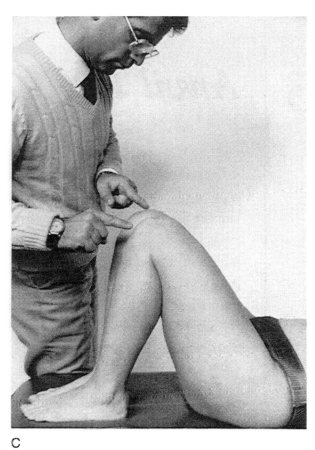

C

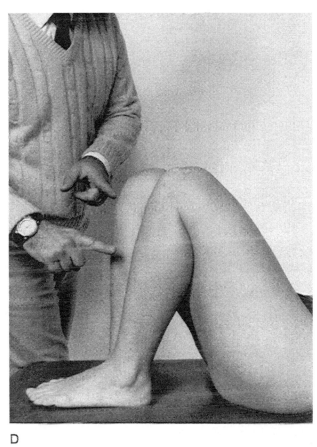

D

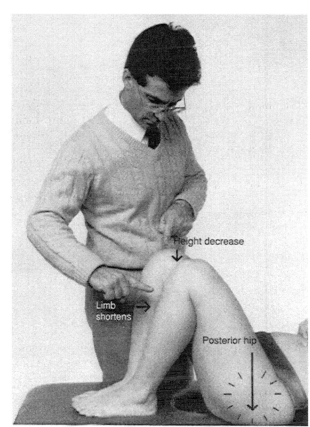

E

5 | *Anvil Test*

Procedure: The patient is supine. Slightly raise the leg on the side being tested and deliver a forceful blow to the heel (Figs. A–C).

Rationale: The force of the blow is delivered into the hip joint. This is an attempt to jam the femur head into the joint, which will exacerbate pain in a hip with a lesion.

Classical Significance: Reproduction of pain within the hip joint is positive for hip joint lesion (Fig. D).

Clinical Significance: If a patient's range of motion is limited, perform this test with the patient's leg lying neutral and flat on the table (Fig. E). The degree of increase in symptomatology within the hip is significant.

Follow-up: Perform the Allis test, the Thomas test, Ely's heel to buttock test, or Ober's test.

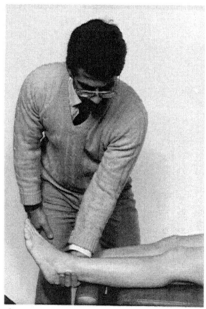

A

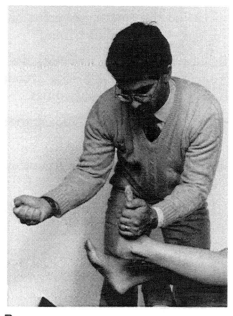

B

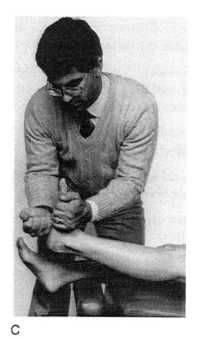

C

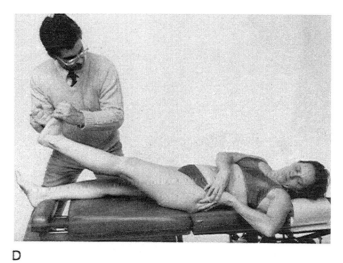

D

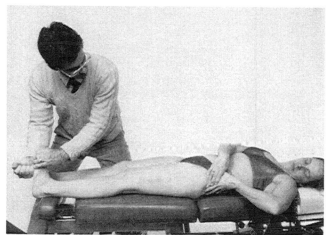

E

6 | *Apparent Leg Length Test*

Procedure: The patient is supine. Mark the umbilicus and the medial malleoli. Measure the distance between the umbilicus and the medial malleolus of each leg and compare the measurements (Figs. A–E).

Rationale: A soft tissue (nonfixed) and a bony (fixed) landmark are used because many variables affect leg length. This measurement takes into account soft tissue contracture, which can affect the pelvis, as well as pelvic obliquities.

Classical Significance: Any discrepancy in leg length is significant; the shorter side is the affected one.

Clinical Significance: Many variables can account for the discrepancies in results and further investigation is necessary.

Follow-up: Perform the actual leg length test or the contracture tests.

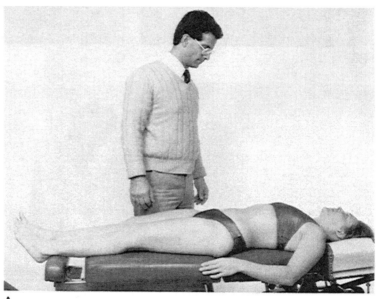

A

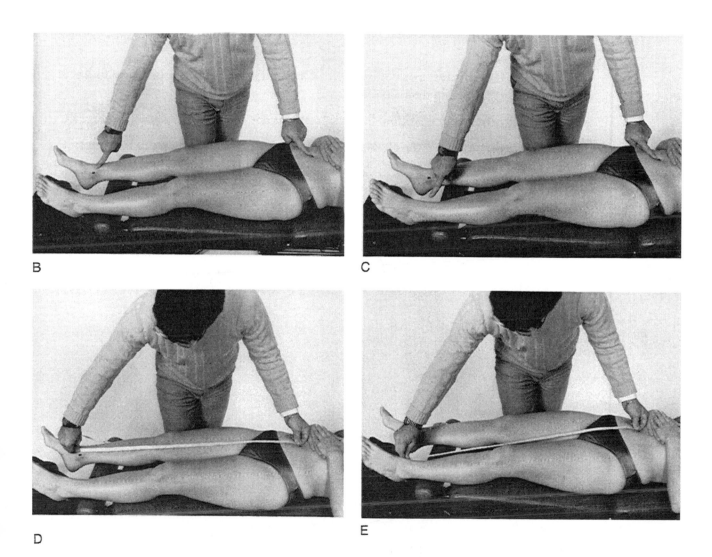

B

C

D

E

7 | *Barlow's Test*

Procedure: This test is used on infants up to 6 months of age. The infant is supine. Position your hands so that the thumb lies along the patient's inner thigh and the index and middle fingers lie on the outer thigh. Apply pressure along the posterior to anterior plane to produce a palpable click. Repeat this in the anterior to posterior plane (Figs. A–D).

Rationale: Use this test as a follow up to Ortolani's test with the infant who has a history of congenital hip dislocation.

Classical Significance: A palpable click confirms the dislocation of the hip (Fig. E).

Clinical Significance: If the click occurs when pressure is applied from the anterior to posterior plane, the infant has "unstable" congenital hip dislocation.

Follow-up: Perform the telescoping test.

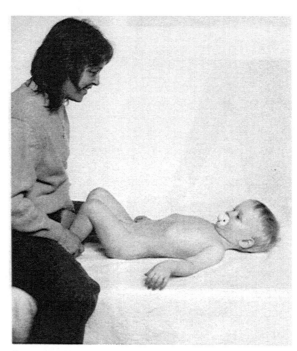

A

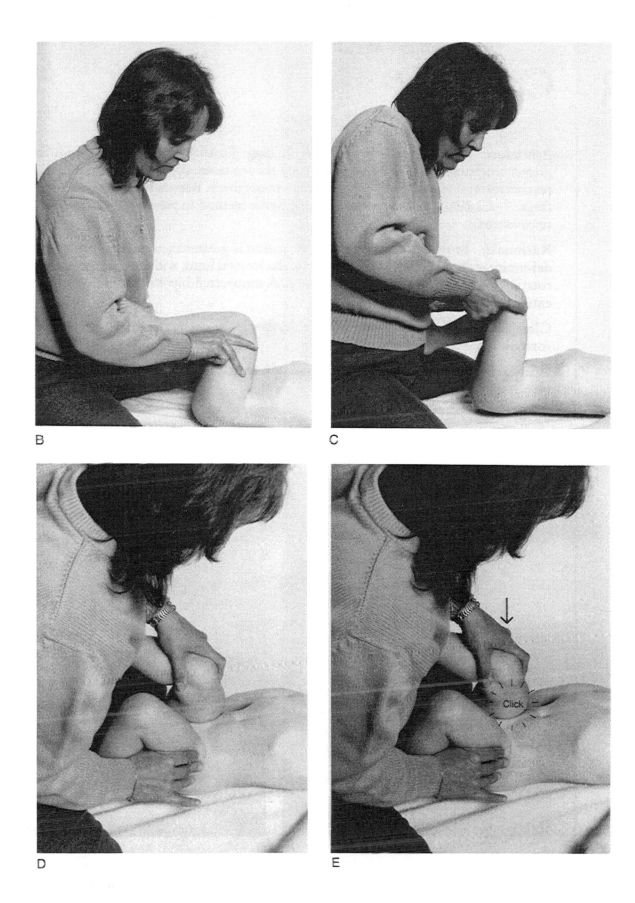

B

C

D

E

8 | *Craig Test*

Procedure: The patient is prone with the knee flexed 90 degrees. Palpate for the greater trochanter and then passively rotate the leg internally and externally until it reaches its most medial and lateral positions, respectively. Record the degree of motion (Figs. A–C). (This test is also known as the Ryder method to measure anteversion and retroversion.)

Rationale: In the normal hip, external rotation is greater than internal rotation. A deformity of the hip, such as anteversion of the femoral head, will result in the internal rotation far exceeding the external rotation. A retroverted hip will result in excessive external rotation.

Classical Significance: External rotation should be slightly greater than internal rotation if the test is normal (Figs. D–F).

Clinical Significance: Internal rotation that is greater than external indicates a possible deformity of the angle of the femoral head.

Follow-up: Perform Nelaton's line test or Hibb's test.

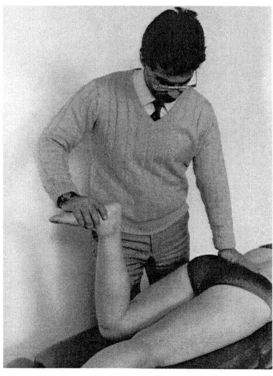

A

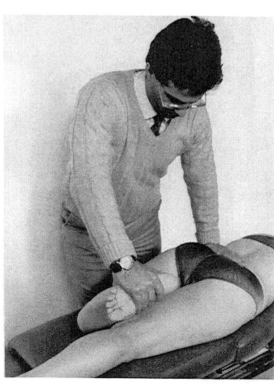

B

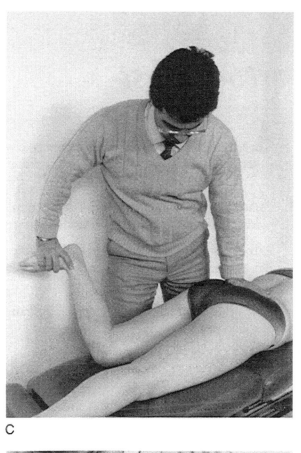

C

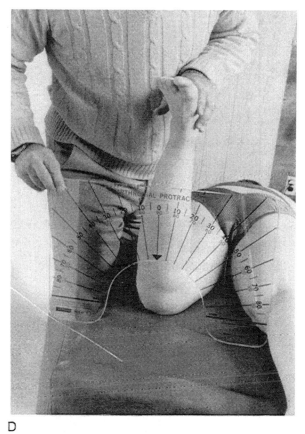

D

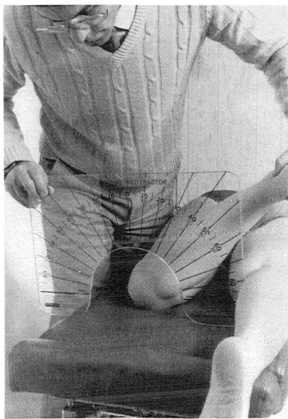

E

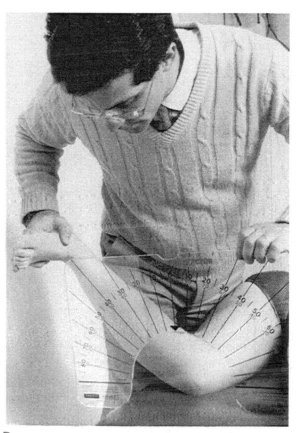

F

9 | *Ely's Heel to Buttock Test*

Procedure: The patient is prone. Flex the knee, bringing the heel onto the contralateral buttock. If this is possible, then lift the flexed knee off the table to hyperextend the hip (Figs. A–D).

Rationale: Bringing the heel to the contralateral hip causes a torsional stress that occurs first in the hip. The hyperextension adds a pull in the iliopsoas muscle.

Classical Significance: The inability to perform the above procedures can indicate aggravation of the lumbar nerve roots, lumbar adhesions, psoas irritation, or hip dysfunction (Fig. E).

Clinical Significance: Hyperextension of the hip extends the lumbar spine and can aggravate a facet irritation, resulting in scleratogenous pain.

Follow-up: Perform Fabere-Patrick's test, the Laguerre test, or Ely's sign.

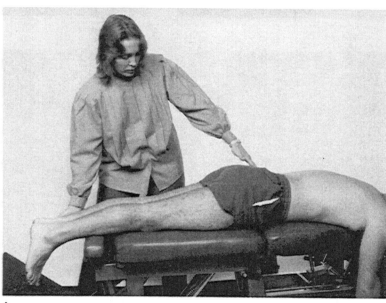

A

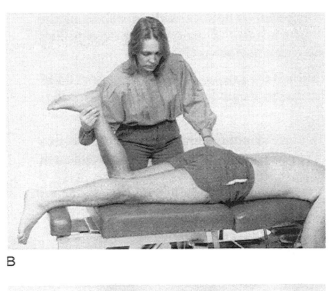

B

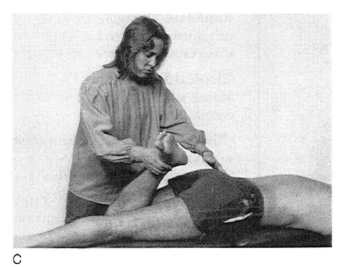

C

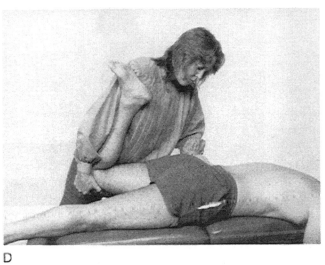

D

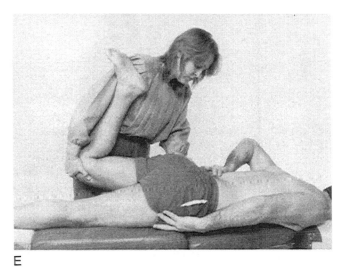

E

10 | *Ely's Sign*

Procedure: The patient is prone. Flex the knee, bringing the heel of the patient onto the ipsilateral buttock. Do not stabilize the pelvis (Figs. A–D).

Rationale: Bringing the lower leg to the ipsilateral buttock without stabilizing the pelvis stresses the rectus femoris muscle, which is part of the quadriceps group. This stress causes an anterior rotational torque within the pelvis (Fig. E).

Classical Significance: Ely's sign is positive if the pelvis on the side being tested lifts off the table. The thigh will also abduct due to rectus femoris or tensor fascia lata contracture (Fig. F).

Clinical Significance: Hip pathology or range of motion limitations in the hip due to subluxation can cause a false-positive test. It is important to test the ease of movement in the hip ranges of motion before performing this test.

Follow-up: Perform Fabere-Patrick's test, the Laguerre test, Ober's test, the Thomas test, or the rectus femoris contracture test.

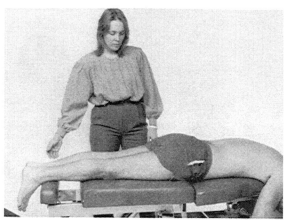

A

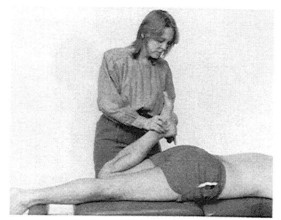

B

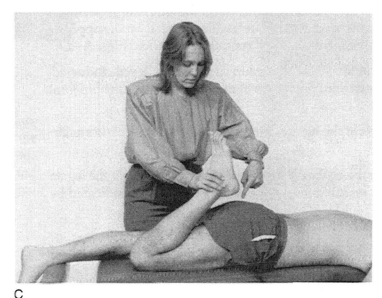

C

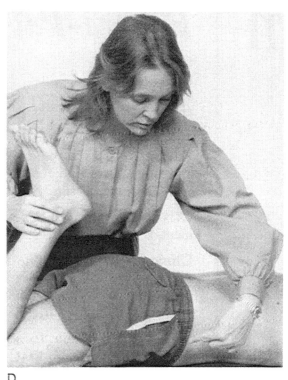

D

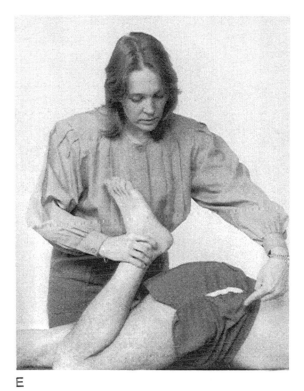

E

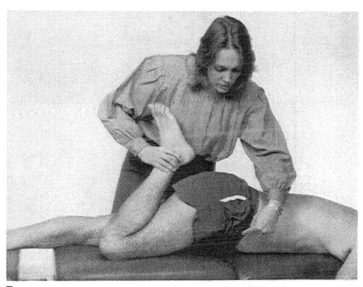

F

11 | *Fabere-Patrick's Test*

Procedure: The patient is supine. Flex the patient's knee on the side being tested and abduct and externally rotate the femur so that that outer malleolus rests on the opposite knee. Stress this side further by pressing downward on the flexed knee (Figs. A–D).

Rationale: This test places maximum stress on the hip because it is flexed, abducted, and externally rotated. Adding downward pressure will exacerbate pain in the hip joint with a suspected lesion.

Classical Significance: Pain within the hip joint, especially at the hip flexor attachment, is a positive test (Fig. E).

Clinical Significance: Iliopsoas spasm may result in the inability to abduct the leg on the side being tested. A sacroiliac joint lesion (not hip joint pathology) is indicated by pain within the sacroiliac joint (Fig. F).

Follow-up: Perform Ober's test, the anvil test, the Allis test, the Laguerre test, or sacroiliac tests (see Ch. 9).

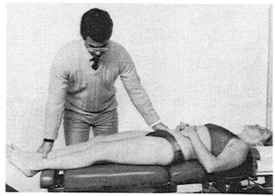

A

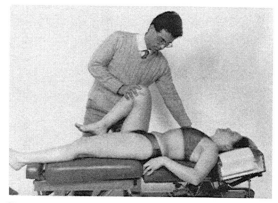

B

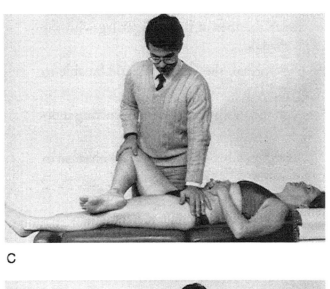

C

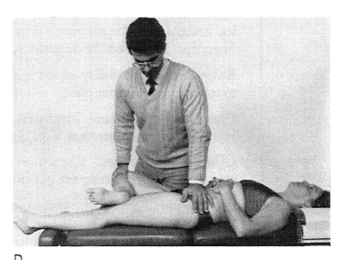

D

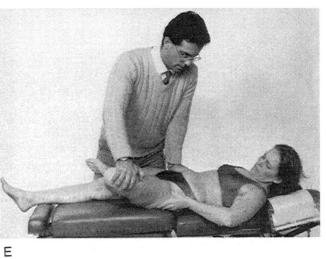

E

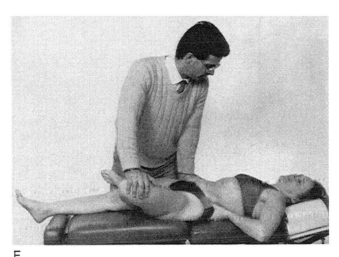

F

12 | *Hamstring Contracture Test*

Procedure: Instruct the patient to sit with one knee flexed to the chest and the other leg straight. Ask the patient to attempt to touch the toes of the straight leg with the fingertips. Repeat on the opposite side (Figs. A–C).

Rationale: If flexibility of the hamstrings is normal, the patient should be able to touch the toes without pain.

Classical Significance: The inability to touch the toes without pain occurring indicates hamstring contracture (Fig. D).

Clinical Significance: Certain nerve root compressions will result in an increase in pain into the leg, causing the patient to limit forward flexion (Fig. E).

Follow-up: Perform the straight leg test or the advancement test (see Ch. 8).

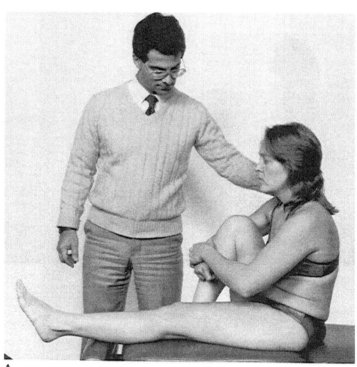

A

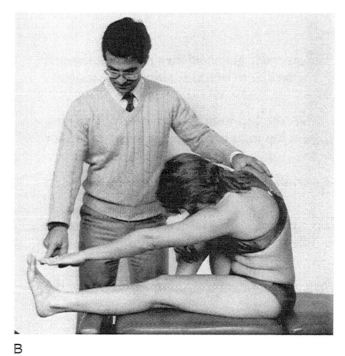

B

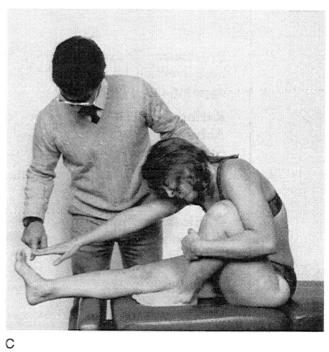

C

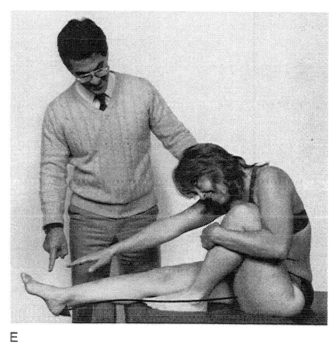

D

E

13 | *Hibb's Test*

Procedure: The patient is prone. Flex the knee 90 degrees and then rotate the femoral head internally by pushing the foot from the medial to lateral position. Repeat on the opposite side (Figs. A–D).

Rationale: This test transmits forces from the hip joint into the sacroiliac joint. Although the test is normally used to confirm hip joint pathology, it is also useful for confirming a sacroiliac joint lesion.

Classical Significance: Pain within the sacroiliac joint from compression is a positive test (Fig. E).

Clinical Significance: Pain within the hip indicates a hip joint lesion. The diagnosis of hip joint or sacroiliac joint pathology is determined by the location of the patient's pain (Fig. F).

Follow-up: Perform Fabere-Patrick's test, the Laguerre test, the Thomas test, or the sacroiliac tests (see Ch. 9).

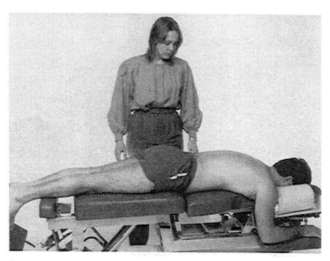

A

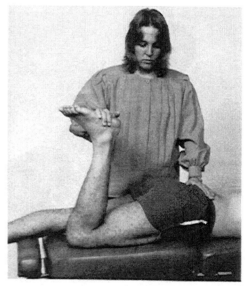

B

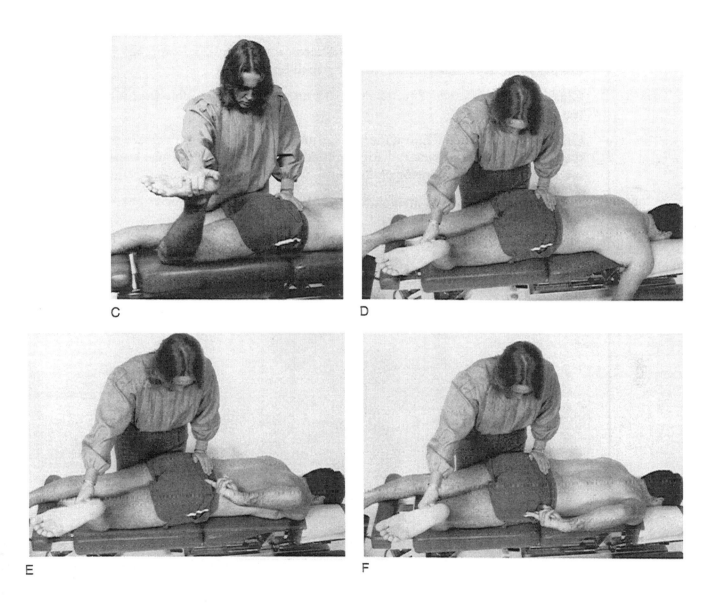

C

D

E

F

14 | *Hopping Test*

Procedure: The patient is standing. Ask the patient to hop first on one leg and then on the other (Figs. A–E).

Rationale: This test produces a jarring force at the sacroiliac joint, hip joint, and lumbar spine. It is similar to the standing anvil test.

Classical Significance: Reproduction of pain within the sacroiliac joint is a positive test.

Clinical Significance: Pain at the hip may indicate hip pathology; a diffuse pain along the posterior lumbar spine radiating around and along the flank can mean kidney involvement due to a stone or peritonitis.

Follow-up: Perform the anvil test, Fabere-Patrick's test, the Laguerre test, or the toe and heel walk tests (see Ch. 8).

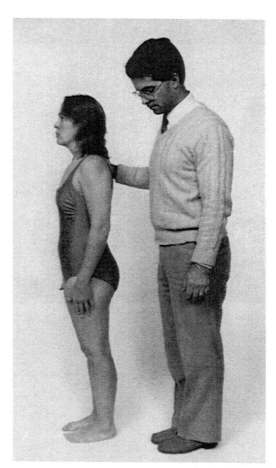

A

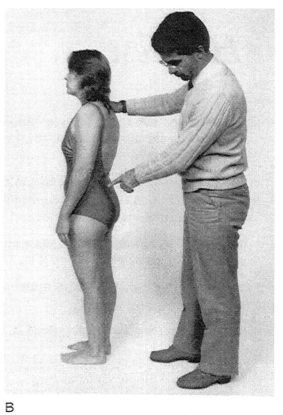

B

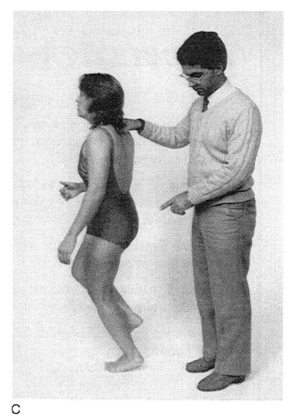

C

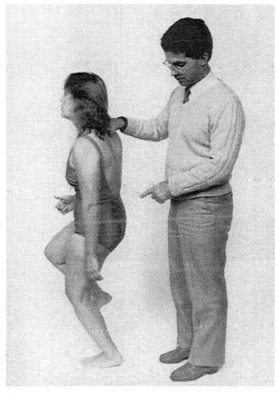

D

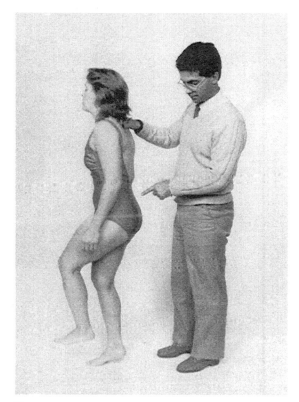

E

15 | *Hyperextension Hip Test*

Procedure: The patient is prone. Stand on the unaffected side and place your hand on the dorsum of the ilia being tested while slowly extending the hip on that side (the knee is slightly flexed) (Figs. A–C).

Rationale: This test produces hyperextension forces in the lumbar spine by passive hyperextension of the hip. Hip pathology will cause restriction and pain, felt when the joint is moved. If the hip is normal, the forces move up into the lumbar spine.

Classical Significance: Pain within the hip at the inception of this test, with a resultant loss of normal joint mechanics, is positive for hip joint pathology (Fig. D).

Clinical Significance: A burning pain in the anterior thigh may be due to stretching of the femoral nerve caused by tractioning of the nerve roots (Fig. E).

Follow-up: Perform Ely's sign, Ely's heel to buttock test, the Nachlas test (see Ch. 9), or the Thomas test.

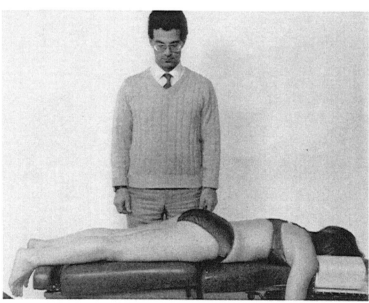

A

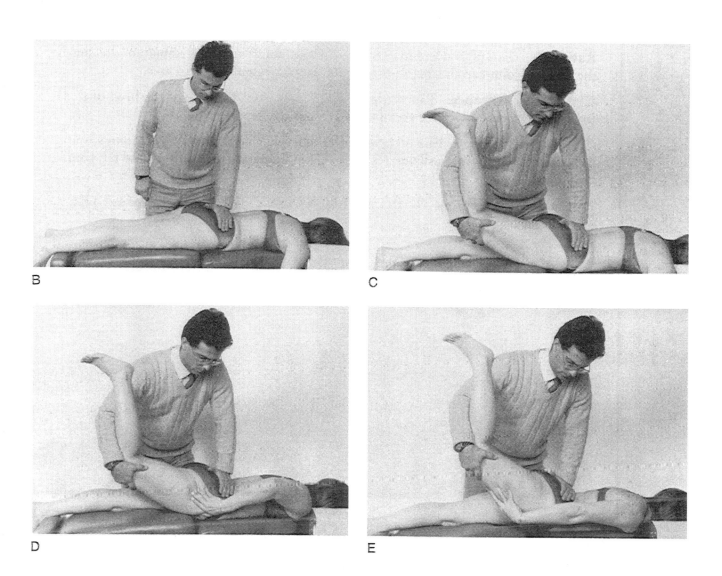

B

C

D

E

16 | *Laguerre Test*

Procedure: The patient is supine. First, flex the hip 90 degrees and then flex the knee 90 degrees. Next, rotate the thigh outward and force the patient's heel up while pressing downward on the knee (Figs. A–D).

Rationale: This maneuver forces the head of the femur into the acetabulum, stressing the anterior joint capsule, but not the lumbosacral or lumbar spinal area.

Classical Significance: Pain within the hip joint from pressure of the head of the femur being pushed into the acetabulum is a positive test (Fig. E).

Clinical Significance: Pain in the area of the sacroiliac joint indicates pathology, and iliopsoas spasm on the ipsilateral side can be induced, which will increase the pain (Fig. F).

Follow-up: Perform the Thomas test, Fabere-Patrick's test, Hibb's test, or sacroiliac tests (see Ch. 9).

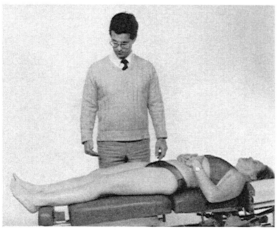

A

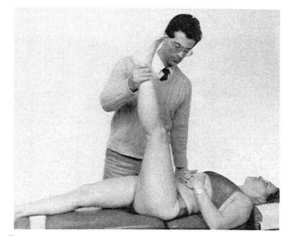

B

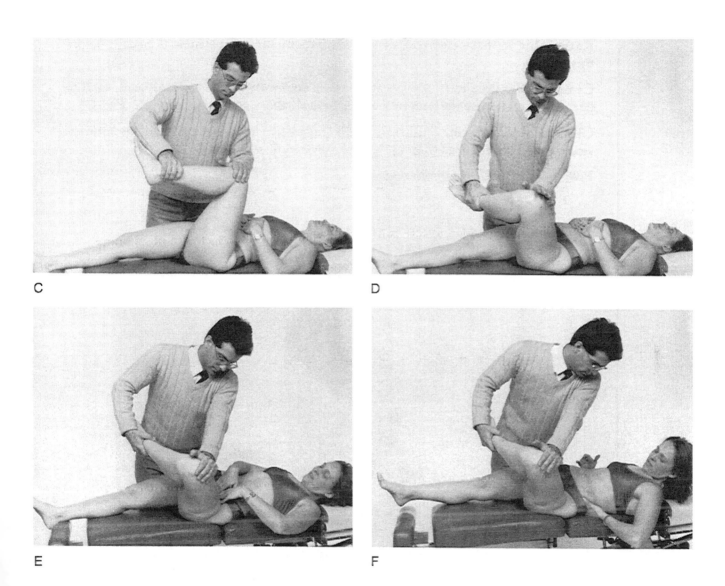

C

D

E

F

17 | *Nelaton's Line Test*

Procedure: The patient is supine. Visualize an imaginary line that transects the anterior superior iliac spine and the ischial tuberosity on the same side (Figs. A–C).

Rationale: In the normal pelvis, the greater trochanter will just meet or be right below this line.

Classical Significance: A dislocated hip or deformity of the femoral head, such as coxa vara, will cause the femoral head to be well above the imaginary line (Fig. D).

Clinical Significance: This test will also be positive in the patient who has anteversion of the femoral head (Fig. E).

Follow-up: Perform the Craig test.

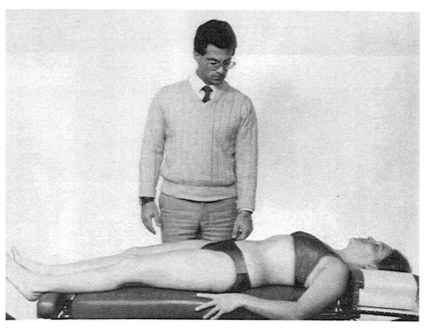

A

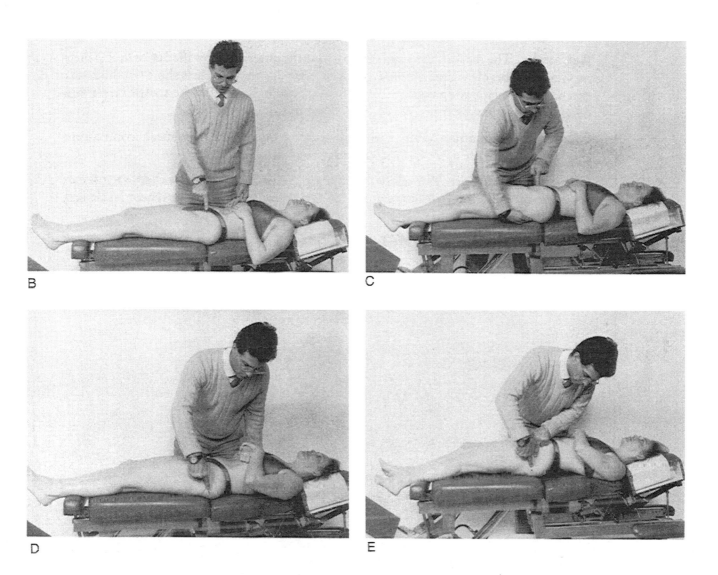

B

C

D

E

18 | *Noble's Compression Test*

Procedure: The patient is supine with the knees flexed 90 degrees and the hips flexed slightly. Apply pressure at the lateral femoral condyle, extend the knee 60 degrees, and ask the patient to slowly extend the leg from 30 degrees to zero (Figs. A–C).

Rationale: The tensor fascia lata originates at the anterior outer iliac crest and inserts on Gerdy's tubercle via the iliotibial band. The belly of the muscle is short but the fascia extends to the lateral epicondyle. Maximum stress is placed on the tensor fascia lata when the knee moves from 30 degrees flexion to full extension.

Classical Significance: Pain within the tensor fascia lata may mean contracture (Fig. D).

Clinical Significance: Pain elicited from the posterior thigh when the leg extends can result from hamstring tightness and should not be confused with the tensor fascia lata contracture (Fig. E).

Follow-up: Perform Ober's test.

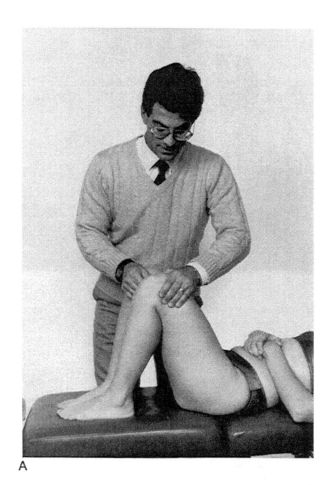

A

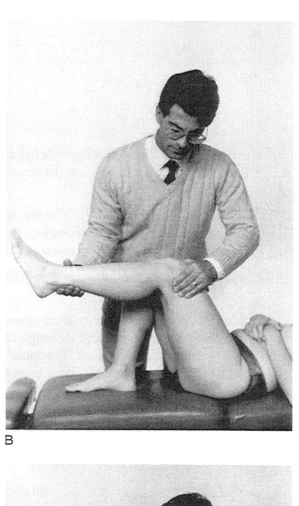

B

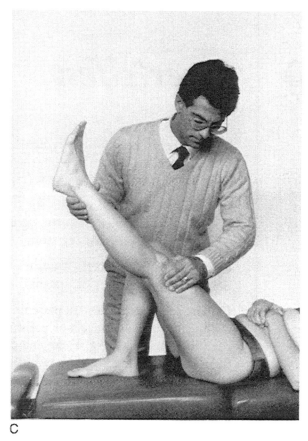

C

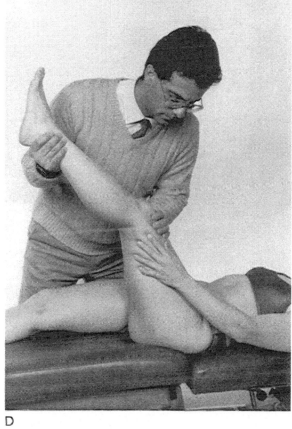

D

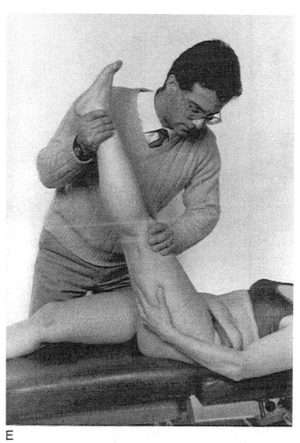

E

19 | *Ober's Test*

Procedure: The patient is lying on the side not being tested. The lower leg is flexed at the knee for stability. The upper leg is straight and parallel with the line of the torso. Raise the leg and then release it (Figs. A–D).

Rationale: This test stresses the tensor fascia lata (TFL) of the upper leg. The test as described by Ober is as above, except that the upper leg is also flexed. However, we believe that keeping the leg straight stresses the TFL more than if the leg is bent.

Classical Significance: Failure of the limb to fall back to the table or if it falls posteriorly indicates TFL spasm (Fig. E).

Clinical Significance: In patients with disease of the hip joint, such as malum coxae senilis, it may be difficult or painful to complete this test solely because of range of motion restriction (Fig. F: degenerative joint disease; main characteristics: 1, nonuniform joint spacing; 2, subchondral sclerosis; 3, cysts [geodes]; 4, osteophytosis; minor characteristics: 5, weightbearing trabecular thickening; 6, superior and lateral translation of femur).

Follow-up: Perform Noble's compression test.

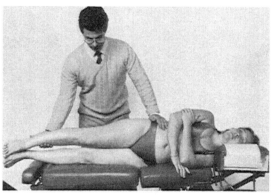

A

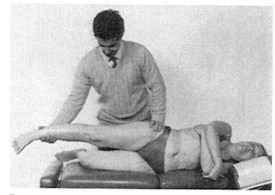

B

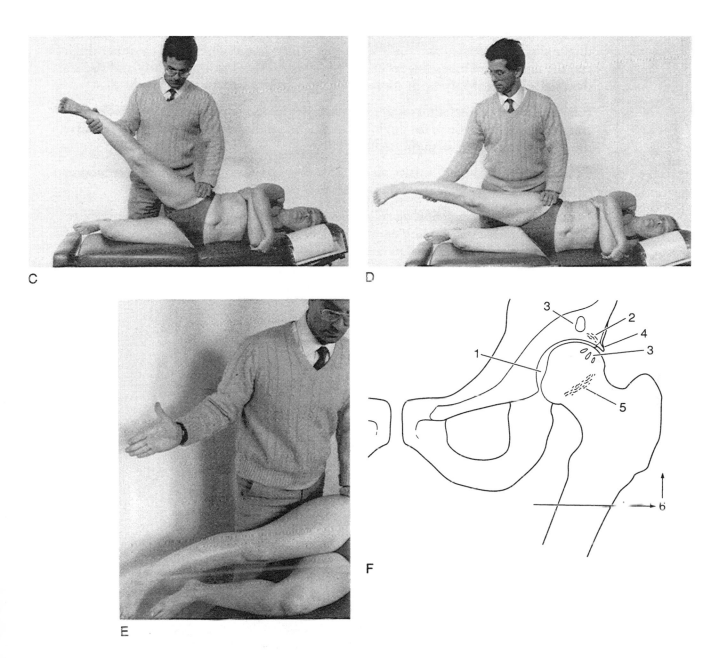

C

D

E

F

20 | *Ortolani's Test*

Procedure: This test is performed only on infants. The patient is supine with the thighs slightly abducted and the knees flexed. Place your thumb along the inner thigh and the middle and index fingers on the outer thigh. Flex the hips slightly and abduct the thighs in turn applying pressure against the greater trochanter (Figs. A–E).

Rationale: In infants up to 8 weeks of age, the force against the greater trochanter, coupled with abduction of the thigh, causes the dislocated hip to slip over the acetabular rim and relocate with an audible click.

Classical Significance: A palpable or audible click, or both, demonstrates a reduction of a congenital hip dislocation (Fig. F: arrows, false acetabula).

Clinical Significance: Soft clicks may occur without dislocation and are thought to be associated with the slipping of the iliofemoral ligament over the anterior surface of the femoral head as it moves laterally.

Follow-up: Perform the Allis test, Barlow's test, or the telescoping test.

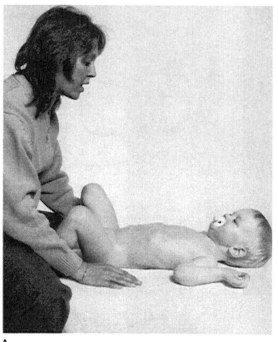

A

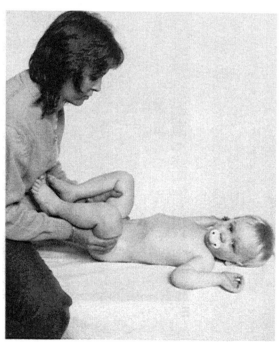

B

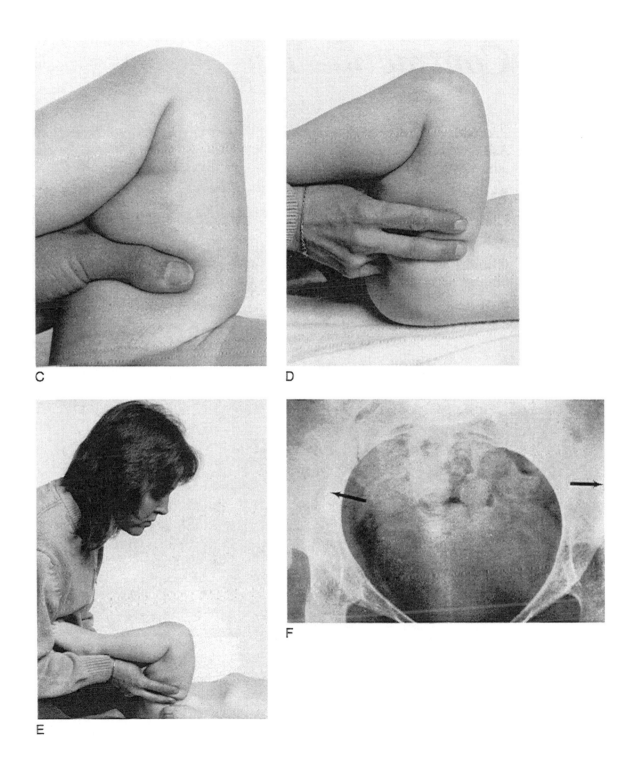

C

D

E

F

21 | *Rectus Femoris Contracture Test*

Procedure: The patient is supine with the lower legs draped over the edge of the table. Ask the patient to grasp one knee and bring it to the chest. Observe the angle maintained by the dangling leg. Repeat this test on the other side (Figs. A–C).

Rationale: If rectus femoris contracture is not present, the dangling leg will not move.

Classical Significance: Rectus femoris contracture will cause the dangling leg to slightly extend (Fig. D).

Clinical Significance: Iliopsoas spasm may cause a response similar to the classical finding; perform the Thomas test to rule out iliopsoas spasm (Fig. E).

Follow-up: Perform the Thomas test or Ely's heel to buttock test.

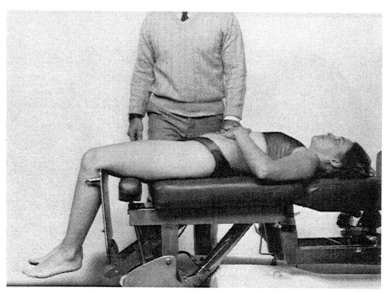

A

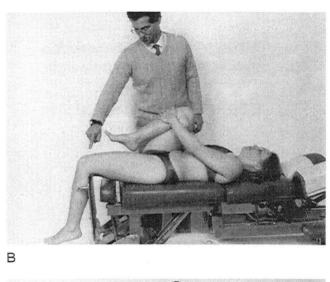

B

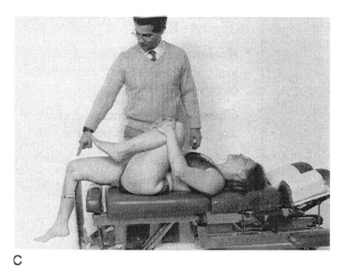

C

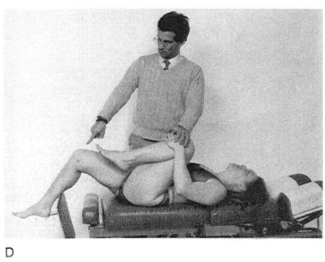

D

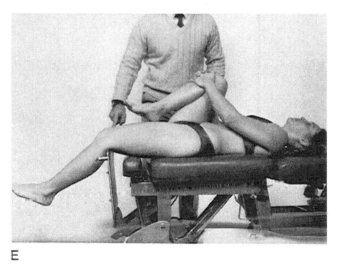

E

22 | *Telescoping Test*

Procedure: The infant is supine with the knees and hips flexed. Apply pressure downward against the knee toward or into the examining table. Then, keeping the knee flexed, pull the thigh upwards. Compare the results with those of the opposite side (Figs. A–E).

Rationale: In the normal child, this movement will result in little motion in the hip joint. In the child with a congenital hip problem, excessive movement occurs throughout this maneuver.

Classical Significance: Excessive joint play (called telescoping or pistoning) in the hip being tested is a positive test.

Clinical Significance: A positive test indicates congenital hip dysplasia.

Follow-up: Perform Ortolani's test or Barlow's test.

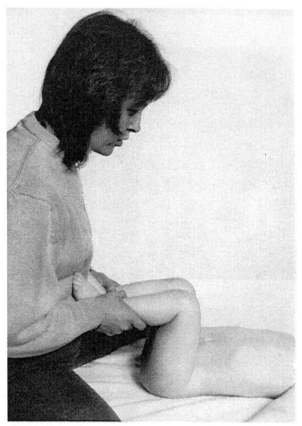

A

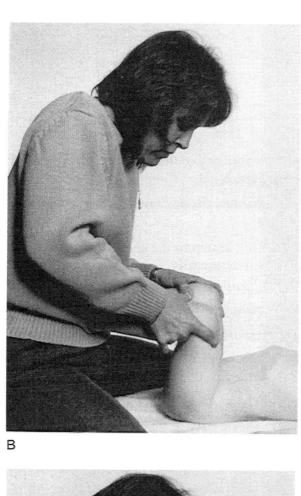

B

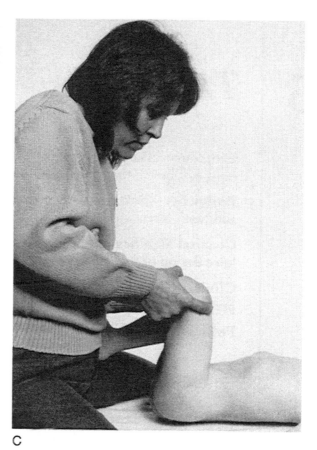

C

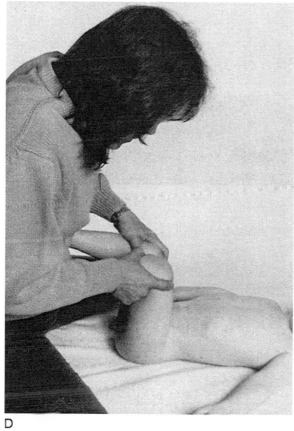

D

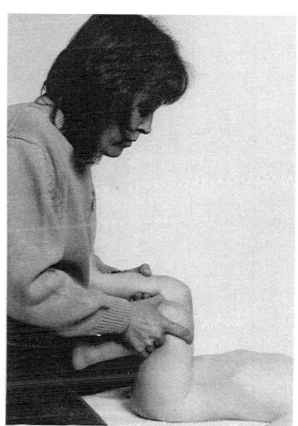

E

23 | *Thomas Test*

Procedure: The patient is supine. Instruct the patient to pull one knee to the chest and hold it. Observe the other knee for flexion (Figs. A–D).

Rationale: Drawing the knee to the chest flattens the lumbar lordosis, which puts additional stress on the iliopsoas musculature.

Classical Significance: Elevation of the leg not drawn to the chest or an increase in knee flexion of that leg signifies hip flexor contracture (Fig. E).

Clinical Significance: This test will be positive if rectus femoris contracture is present because the knee will flex to avoid stressing the rectus femoris musculature.

Follow-up: Perform Ely's heel to buttock test or the rectus femoris contracture test.

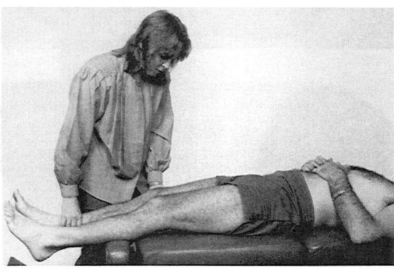

A

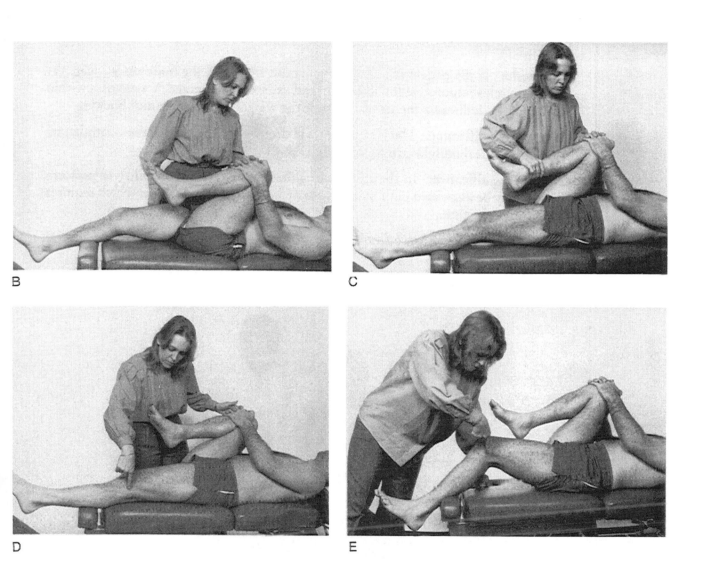

B

C

D

E

24 | *Trendelenburg Test*

Procedure: The patient is standing. Ask the patient to raise one knee toward the chest, balancing on the supporting limb. The patient should be supported by a table or a nearby wall if unable to balance on one leg. Observe the gluteal fold of the supporting leg (Figs. A–C).

Rationale: If the patient is able to support the weight of the body on one leg, the gluteal muscles responsible for abduction and extension are intact. A weakness within these muscles will cause the patient to shift the weight as the extremity buckles.

Classical Significance: The gluteal fold will drop below the level of the contralateral side if the gluteal muscles are weak (Figs. D & E).

Clinical Significance: In the absence of gluteal weakness, the inability to perform this test may be associated with an unrelated dysequilibrium syndrome, which requires further investigation.

Follow-up: Perform cerebellar testing (see Ch. 1) or muscle testing of the gluteal musculature.

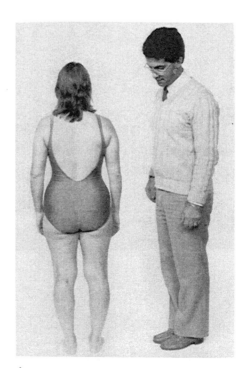

A

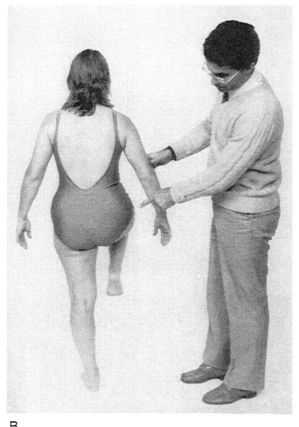

B

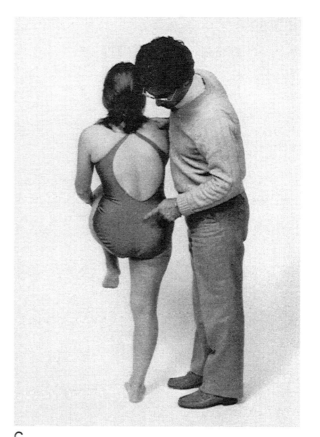

C

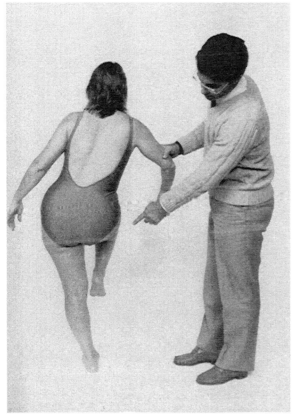

D

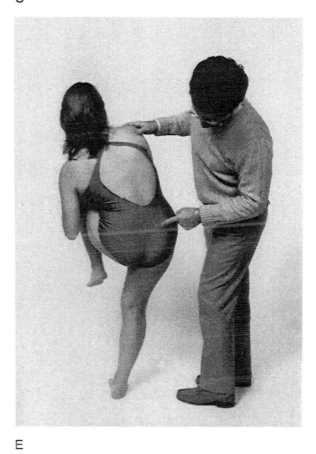

E

Knee Testing

1. Range of Motion Studies
2. Anterior to Posterior and Posterior to Anterior Drawer Tests
3. Apley's Compression Test
4. Apley's Distraction Test
5. Ballotment Test
6. Bounce Home Test
7. Brush Stroke Test
8. Childress Duck Waddle Test
9. Clark's Sign
10. Crossover Test
11. Dreyer's Test
12. Extension Lag Test
13. External Rotation Recurvatum Test
14. Fluctuation Test
15. Fouchet's Sign
16. Genu Valgum Test
17. Genu Varum Test
18. Godfrey's Test
19. Helfet Pivot Shift Test
20. Hyperextension Test
21. Hyperflexion Meniscus Test
22. Jakob's Test
23. Jerk Test of Hughston
24. Knee Drop Test
25. Knee Flexion Stress Test
26. Lachman's Test
27. Losee's Test
28. Macintosh Test
29. McMurray's Test
30. Mediopatella Plica Test
31. Noble's Compression Test
32. O'Donoghues Maneuver
33. Patella Apprehension Test
34. Patella Grind Test
35. Patella Inhibition Test
36. Patella Tap
37. Payr's Sign
38. Plica Stutter Test
39. Posterior Sag Sign
40. Q-Angle Test
41. Screw Home Test
42. Slocum Test
43. Steinmann's Tenderness Displacement Sign
44. Valgus Stress Test
45. Varus Stress Test
46. Waldron Test
47. Wilson's Test

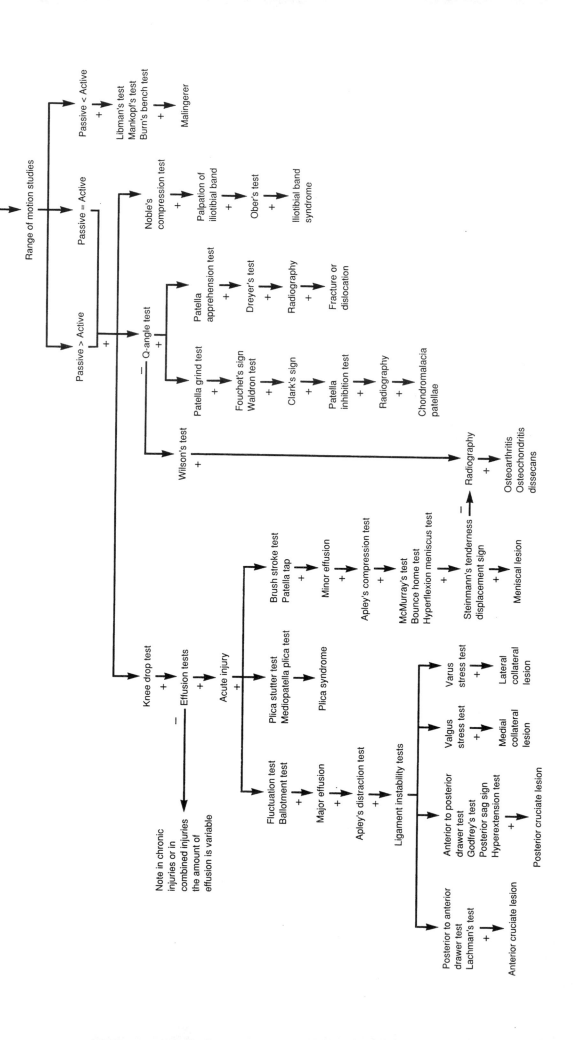

1 | *Range of Motion Studies*

When performing range of motion studies, it is important to use either an arthrodial protractor or an inclinometer. The *American Medical Association Guides for Impairment Ratings* now recommend the use of the inclinometer exclusively

Flexion: The patient is prone with the legs fully extended. Ask the patient to flex one knee and bring the heel as close to the buttock as possible. Next, with the patient supine and the legs fully extended, raise the leg 60 degrees. Place the inclinometer on the anterior shin (this is the zero position); flex the knee bringing the heel to the buttock and record this measurement with the inclinometer. The difference between the two measurements is the patient's degree of flexion at the knee. Normal flexion is 135 degrees.

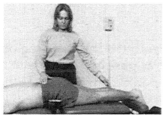 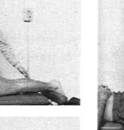 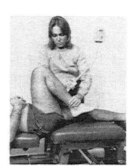

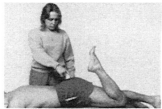

Extension: The patient is supine with the legs straight (this is the zero position). Normally, no extension occurs in the knee beyond this point. However, women may have a slight recurvatum; in women up to 15 degrees of hyperextension is considered normal. To quickly assess knee extension, ask the patient to perform a deep knee bend and rise from that position. Observe the knees for fluidity of motion and that the knees are straight when the patient has finished standing up. Normal extension is 0 to 15 degrees.

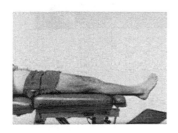 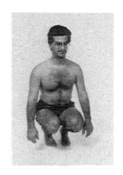 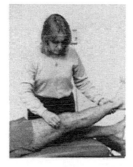 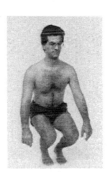

Medial Tibial Rotation: The patient is seated with the legs dangling off the table. Ask the patient to rotate the ankle medially as far as possible. Then, with the patient supine and the legs straight, place the inclinometer on the tibial tubercle (this is zero). Ask the patient to rotate the leg medially as far as possible. Record this measurement; the difference between the two is the patient's degree of medial tibial rotation. Normal medial tibial rotation is 20 to 30 degrees.

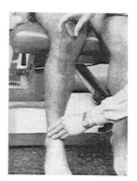 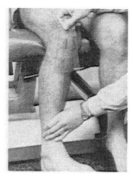 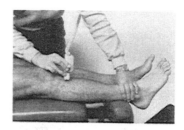

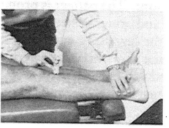

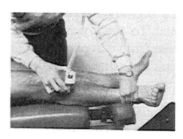

Lateral Tibial Rotation: The patient is seated with the legs dangling off the table. Ask the patient to rotate the ankle laterally as far as possible. Next, with the patient supine and the legs straight, place the inclinometer on the tibial tubercle (this is zero). Ask the patient to rotate the leg laterally as far as possible. Record this measurement; the difference between the two is the patient's degree of lateral tibial rotation. Normal lateral tibial rotation is 30 to 40 degrees.

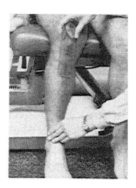 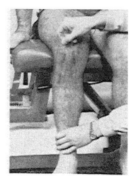 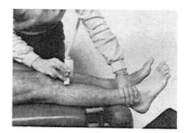

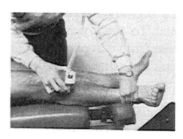

Quick Test: Proper functioning of the knee can be quickly tested by having the patient squat into a deep knee bend and stand up again, or by having the patient rise from a seated position. In the normal patient, the weight will be equally distributed and the knees will be fully extended at the end of the movement. Finally, ask the patient to rotate each ankle medially and laterally.

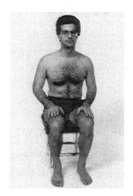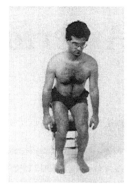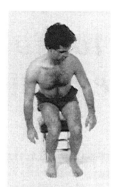

Note: Most authors believe it is only necessary to assess flexion and extension, as the true ranges of motion of the knee. It is our opinion that the rotary component that occurs at the tibial femoral junction also should be assessed.

2 | Anterior to Posterior and Posterior to Anterior Drawer Tests

Procedure: The patient is supine with the knees flexed and the heels flat on the table. Grasp the proximal tibia with two hands and force the tibia forward and then backward at the same time keeping the feet on the table (Figs. A–D).

Rationale: This test evaluates the integrity of the anterior and the posterior cruciate ligaments. Normally, no anterior or posterior displacement will occur (Figs. E & F).

Classical Significance: Anterior displacement may result from damage to the anterior cruciate ligament; posterior displacement from damage to the posterior cruciate ligament.

Clinical Significance: In patients with degenerative joint disease of the knee, the supporting ligaments may be lax, which will allow some displacement. Before testing, be sure posterior lag is not present.

Follow-up: Perform Lachman's test, the Macintosh test, or the Slocum test.

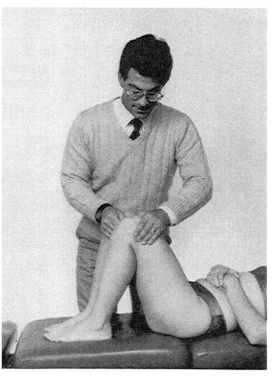

A

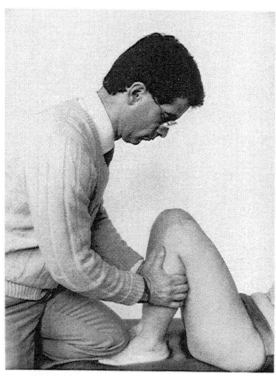

B

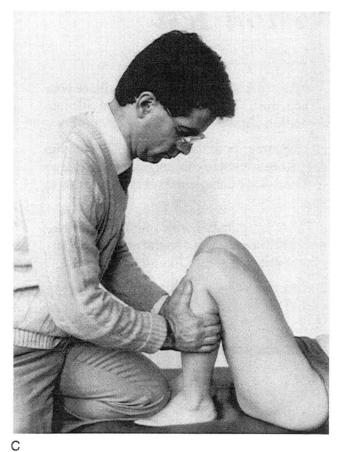

C

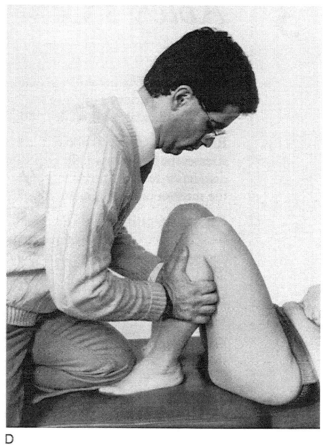

D

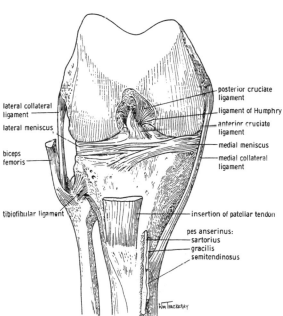

E

lateral collateral ligament
lateral meniscus
biceps femoris
tibiofibular ligament

posterior cruciate ligament
ligament of Humphry
anterior cruciate ligament
medial meniscus
medial collateral ligament

insertion of patellar tendon

pes anserinus:
sartorius
gracilis
semitendinosus

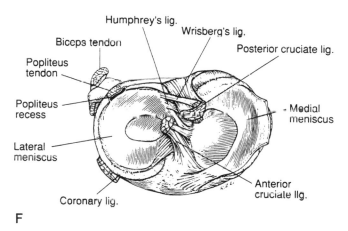

F

Biceps tendon
Popliteus tendon
Popliteus recess
Lateral meniscus
Coronary lig.

Humphrey's lig.
Wrisberg's lig.
Posterior cruciate lig.
Medial meniscus
Anterior cruciate llg.

3 | *Apley's Compression Test*

Procedure: The patient is prone with the affected knee flexed 90 degrees. Place your knee on the patient's thigh to stabilize it. Then, push the ankle of the affected side into the table. Repeat with medial and lateral rotation (Apley's grind test) (Figs. A–D).

Rationale: Compression of the knee tests the integrity of the meniscus. The rotation stresses the meniscus on the opposite side. This test is used in combination with Apley's distraction test to determine whether the patient's knee complaint is caused by injury to the menisci or to the ligaments.

Classical Significance: Pain within the knee that increases with compression signifies a meniscus injury. Pain felt with medial rotation indicates a lateral meniscus injury and with lateral rotation, a medial meniscus injury (Figs. E & F).

Clinical Significance: An inflammatory process present within the knee, such as Baker's cyst or rheumatoid arthritis, may produce a false-positive test, since compression of the inflamed joint may cause pain.

Follow-up: Perform McMurray's test, Steinmann's tenderness displacement sign, or the O'Donoghues maneuver.

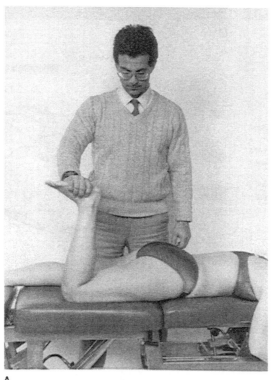

A

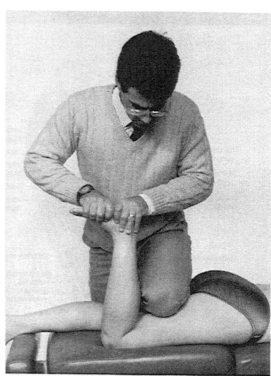

B

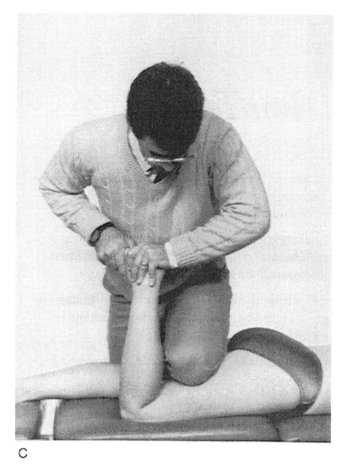

C

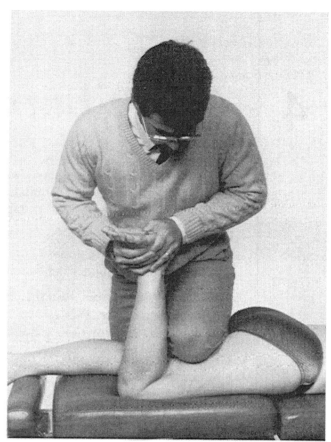

D

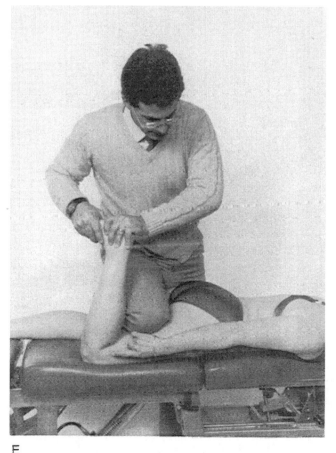

E

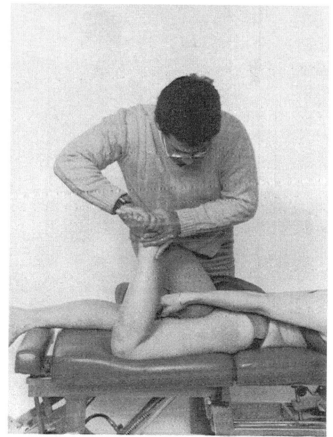

F

4 | *Apley's Distraction Test*

Procedure: The patient is prone with the affected knee flexed 90 degrees. Place your knee on the patient's thigh to stabilize it. Then grasp the ankle of the affected leg and apply a distractive force. Repeat with medial and lateral rotation (Figs. A–D).

Rationale: Distraction of the knee tests the integrity of the ligaments. The medial and lateral rotation tests the opposite ligaments. This test is used with Apley's compression test to determine whether the ligaments or menisci are injured.

Classical Significance: Pain that increases within the knee with distraction indicates a ligamentous injury. Pain felt with medial rotation indicates a lateral ligamentous injury; with lateral rotation, a medial ligamentous injury (Figs. E & F).

Clinical Significance: Distraction of the joint may alleviate the patient's symptoms if a minor meniscal tear is present.

Follow-up: Perform the valgus and varus stress tests or the crossover test.

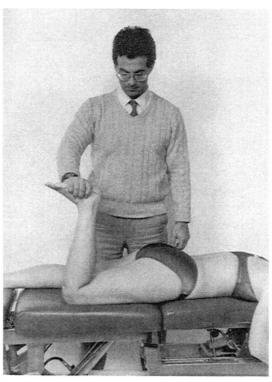

A

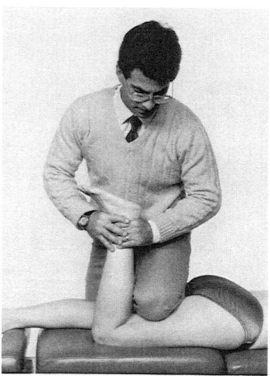

B

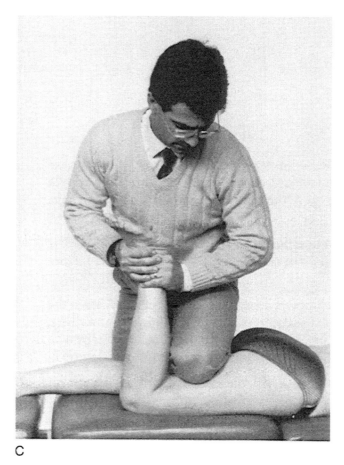

C

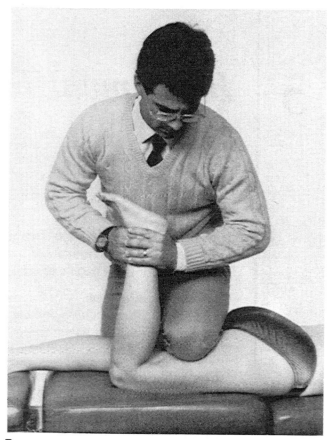

D

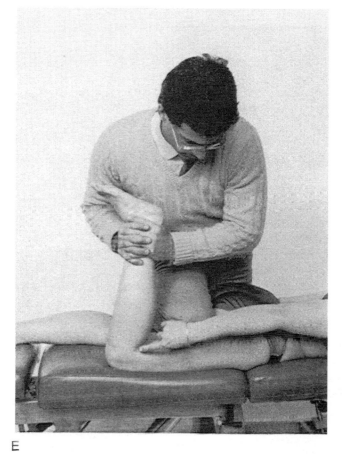

E

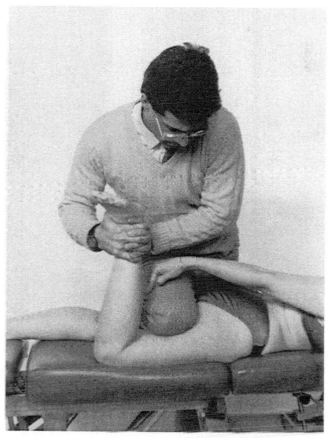

F

5 | *Ballotment Test*

Procedure: The patient is supine with the joint with visible effusion carefully extended fully. Ask the patient to relax the quadriceps muscles. Then, force the patella into the patellar groove and quickly release it. Observe the patella for rebound (Figs. A–D).

Rationale: In the joint with large amounts of fluid, forcing the patella into the patellar groove displaces the fluid laterally. On the release, the fluid flows back to its former position, forcing the patella to rebound.

Classical Significance: This test will be positive if large amounts of effusion are in the joint (Fig. E). Fluid accumulation changes the contour of the knee joint. The swelling, however, is diffuse and encompasses the entire synovial cavity and suprapatellar pouch. This creates the periarticular edema shown in the anteroposterior (AP) view of Figure E.

Clinical Significance: Do not confuse this test with the patella tap, which is a test for minor effusion. If bursal swelling is the cause of the effusion, this test will be negative because the bursal sac contains the fluid even against compression.

Follow-up: Perform the fluctuation test or the bounce home test.

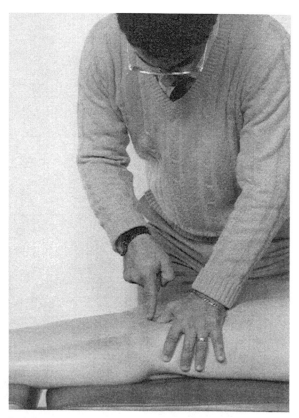

A

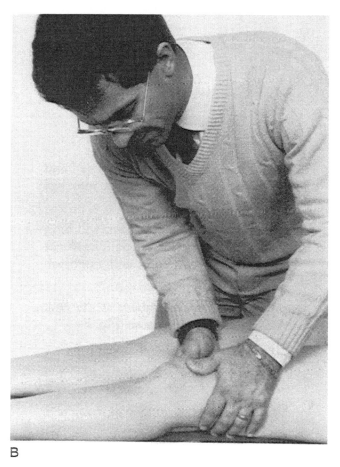

B

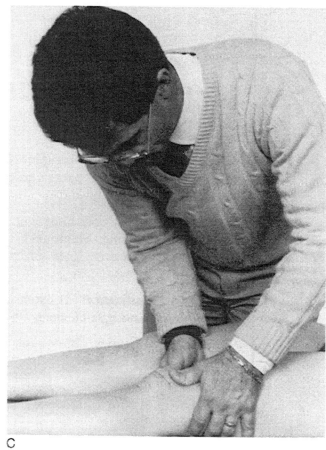

C

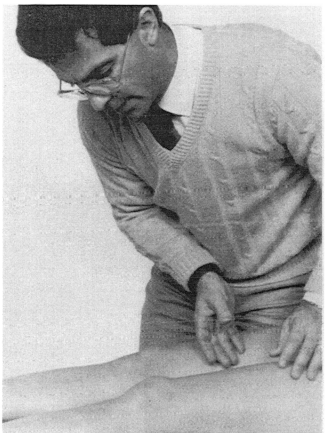

D

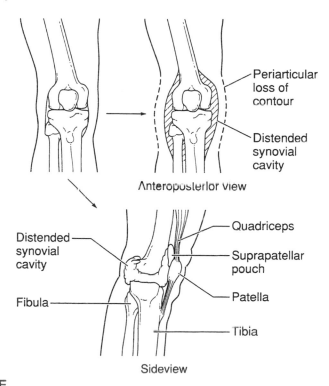

Periarticular
loss of
contour

Distended
synovial
cavity

Anteroposterior view

Distended
synovial
cavity

Quadriceps

Suprapatellar
pouch

Fibula

Patella

Tibia

Sideview

E

6 | *Bounce Home Test*

Procedure: The patient is supine. Cup the patient's heel on the side being tested and flex the knee. Ask the patient to relax and allow the knee to drop back into full extension (Figs. A–C).

Rationale: In the normal patient, the knee dropping back into extension will have a good, crisp feeling. The knee may hyperextend if the posterior cruciate ligament is damaged. However, knee inflammation will restrict both flexion and extension (Fig. D).

Classical Significance: If extension is restricted or if it feels rubbery at the end, something is causing a blockage. A torn meniscus is the probable cause (Fig. E).

Clinical Significance: If the patient is not fully relaxed, the guarding mechanism may keep the knee from locking into extension normally. Repeat the test on the opposite side for comparison.

Follow-up: Perform McMurray's test, Apley's compression test, or the O'Donoghues maneuver.

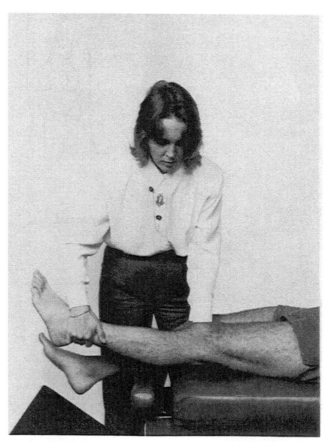

A

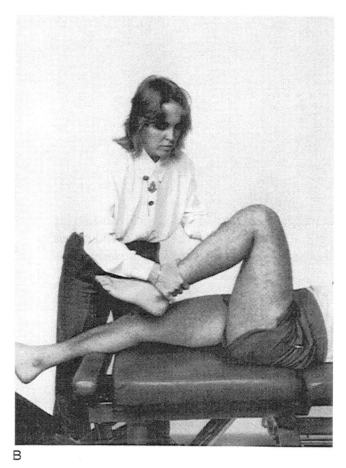

B

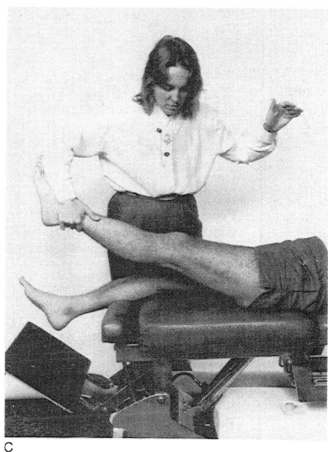

C

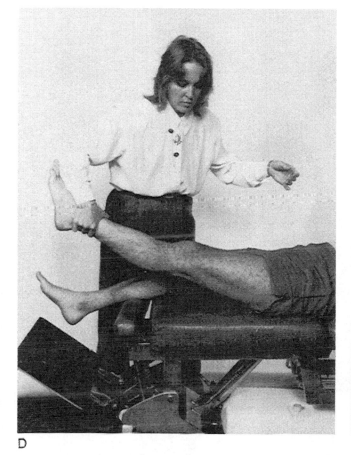

D

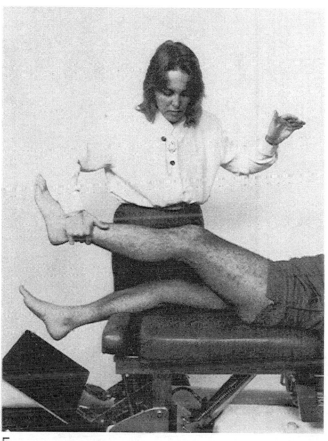

E

7 | *Brush Stroke Test (Wipe Test)*

Procedure: The patient is supine with both knees fully extended. Using brush-like (or wiping) strokes with the fingers, start at the medial side of the patella and brush cephalad while the opposite hand starts on the lateral side and strokes caudally (Figs. A–C).

Rationale: This test will milk any small amount of effusion from the medial to the lateral side, with a fluid wave then observed going back laterally to medially.

Classical Significance: Bulging at the medial inferior aspect of the patella signifies joint effusion (Fig. D).

Clinical Significance: This test is useful when small amounts of effusion are suspected. As little as 4 to 8 ml of extra fluid will cause a positive finding (Fig. E).

Follow-up: Perform the patella tap or the fluctuation test.

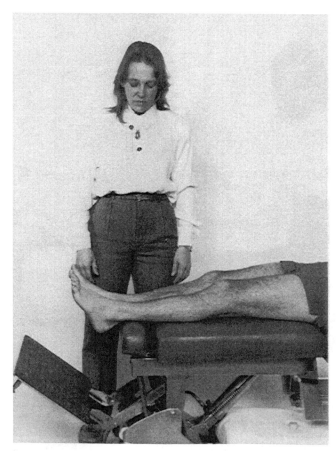

A

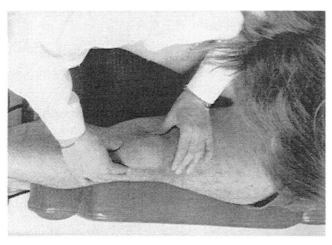

B

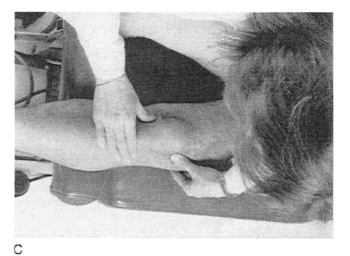

C

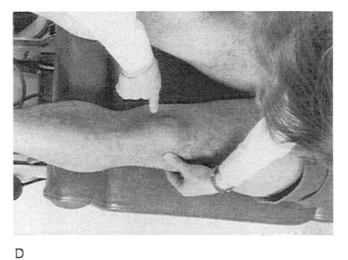

D

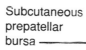

Suprapatellar
bursa

Subcutaneous
prepatellar
bursa

Patellar
ligament

Deep infrapatellar
bursa

E

8 | *Childress Duck Waddle Test*

Procedure: The patient is standing with the feet shoulder width apart. Ask the patient to rotate the legs internally as much as possible and then to squat fully. Ask the patient to repeat the maneuver with the legs fully rotated externally. (Figs. A–F).

Rationale: The internal rotation stresses the lateral meniscus and medial collateral ligament; the external rotation stresses the medial meniscus and lateral collateral ligament.

Classical Significance: If the patient experiences pain in the knee joint, cannot fully flex the leg when performing the squat, or a clicking sound occurs in the knee joint, a meniscal tear may be present.

Clinical Significance: See Classical Significance.

Follow-up: Perform McMurray's test, Apley's compression test, or the bounce home test.

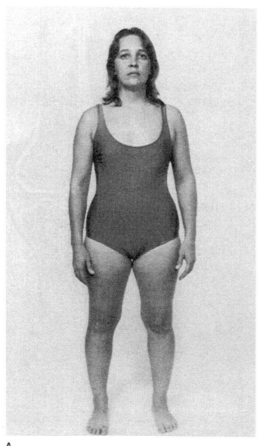 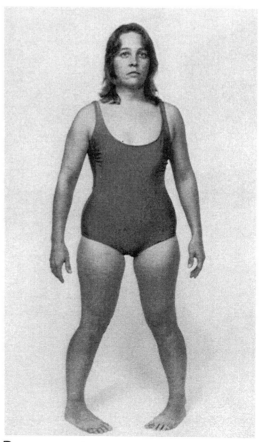

A   B

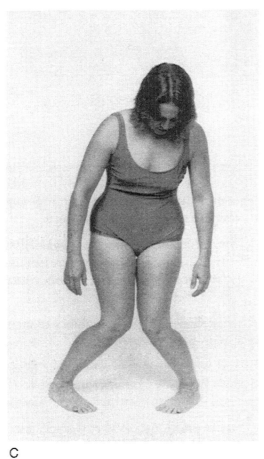

C

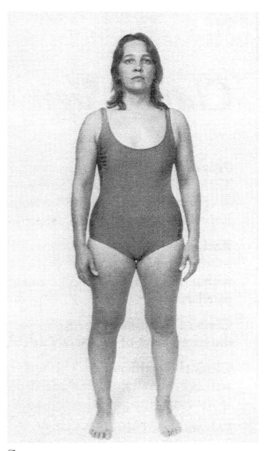

D

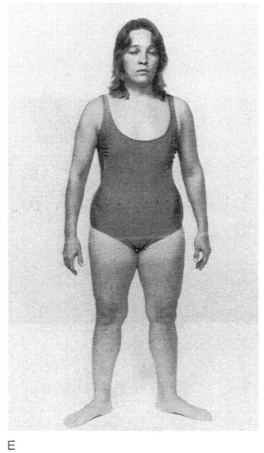

E

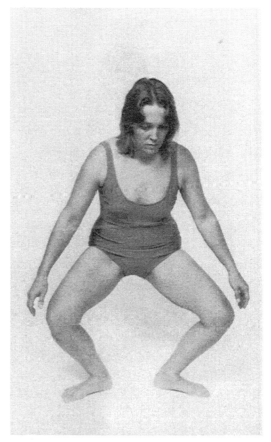

F

9 | *Clark's Sign*

Procedure: The patient is supine. Press downward at the superior pole of the patella. Then ask the patient to contract the quadriceps of the leg being tested and to hold them in contraction. Repeat the test with the patient's knee flexed 30, 60, and 90 degrees. Repeat the above on the opposite leg and compare the results (Figs. A–F).

Rationale: This procedure tests for chondromalacia patellae. The downward pressure restricts upward movement of the patella. Contracting the quadriceps increases tension within the retropatellar space and aggravates the knee suffering from chondromalacia patellae.

Classical Significance: An increase in retropatellar pain or the inability to maintain the contraction of the quadriceps because of pain is a positive test.

Clinical Significance: This test is performed at different degrees of knee flexion as well as bilaterally to avoid a false-positive result from the examiner pressing too hard. Individuals with patella tendinitis will have pain just from contracting the quadriceps.

Follow-up: Perform Fouchet's sign, the patella grind test, or the Q-angle test.

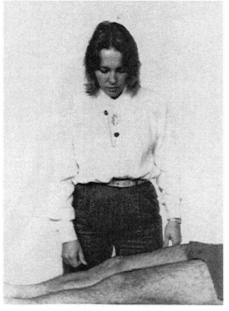

A

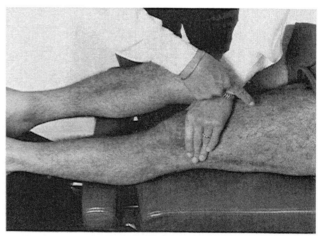

B

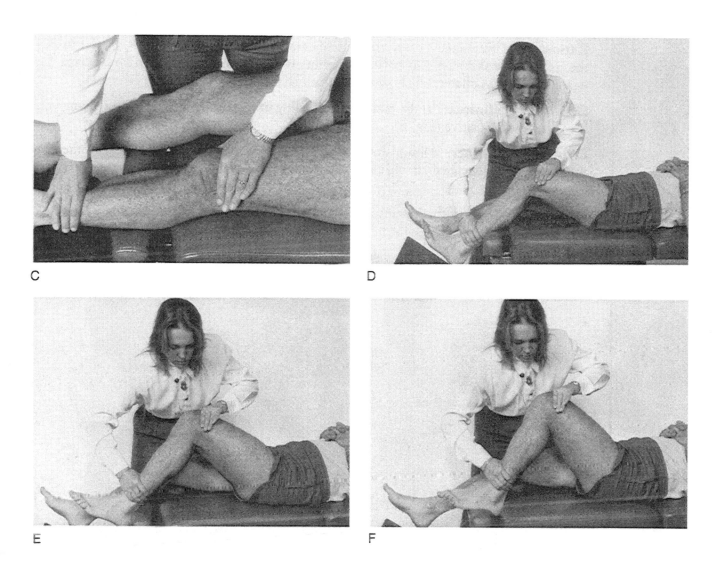

C

D

E

F

10 | *Crossover Test*

Procedure: The patient is standing upright. Ask the patient to place the unaffected foot in front of the affected one. Gently step on the affected foot to keep it planted. Then instruct the patient to rotate the torso toward the front leg 90 degrees (Figs. A–D).

Rationale: This maneuver tests the anterolateral stability of the knee joint, similar to the Helfet pivot shift test. Anterolateral stability results from an intact anterior cruciate ligament, lateral collateral ligament, and iliotibial band.

Classical Significance: If the patient has a feeling of instability or of the knee giving way, the test is positive (Fig. E).

Clinical Significance: Diminished meniscal height may result in some laxity of the supporting ligaments, which will cause instability even though the ligaments are intact (Fig. F).

Follow-up: Perform the Macintosh test, Losee's test, or the jerk test of Hughston.

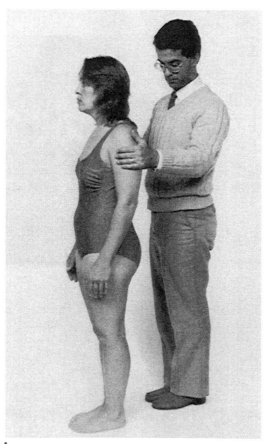

A

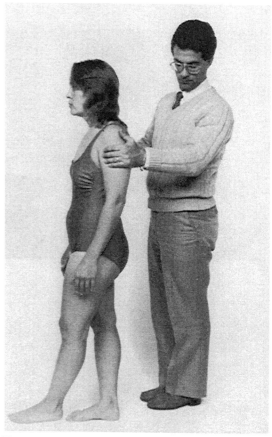

B

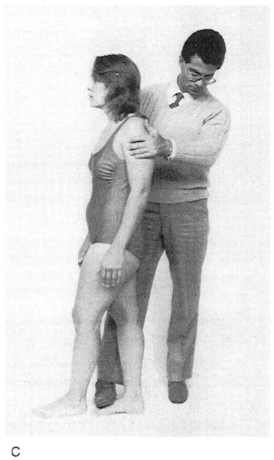

C

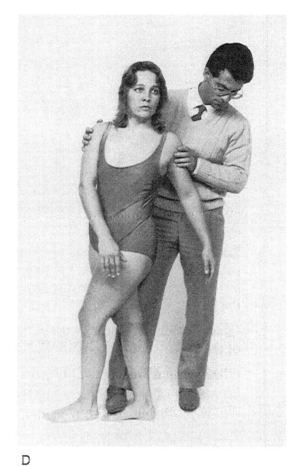

D

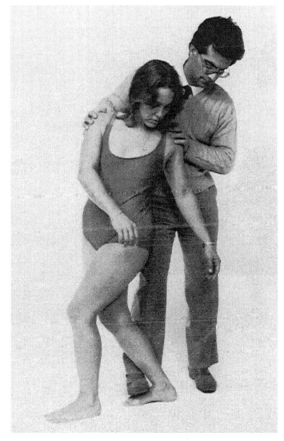

E

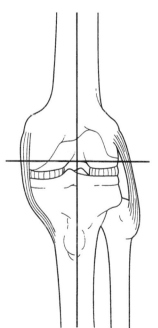

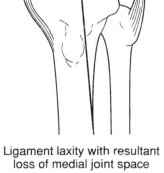

Normal

Ligament laxity with resultant
loss of medial joint space

F

11 | *Dreyer's Test*

Procedure: The patient is supine with the knees fully extended. Ask the patient to raise the leg off the table. If the patient cannot do this, stabilize the quadriceps tendon above the superior pole of the patella and ask the patient to try to raise the leg (Figs. A–D).

Rationale: In patellar fracture, contracture of the quadriceps puts extra strain on the patella, increasing the pain and the patient will be unable to perform the first part of the test. Stabilizing the quadriceps tendon removes the pressure, making it easier to raise the leg.

Classical Significance: If the patient cannot lift the leg off the table without support of the quadriceps tendon, the patient may have a fractured patella (Fig. E).

Clinical Significance: If the patient has Osgood-Schlatter disease, pain will occur on lifting the leg off the table. This test may be difficult for the patient with abdominal or hip flexor weakness.

Follow-up: Perform the Q-angle test or the tuning fork test, or refer the patient for radiography.

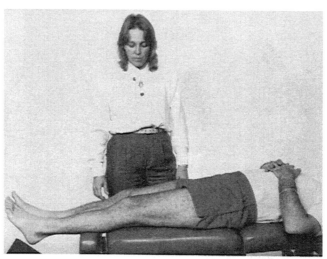

A

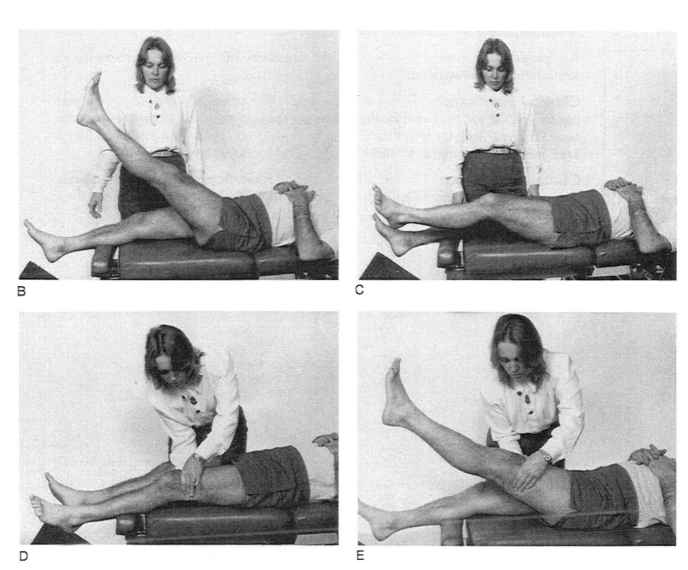

B

C

D

E

12 | *Extension Lag Test*

Procedure: The patient is seated with the lower legs dangling freely over the side of the table. Ask the patient to extend the leg slowly until parallel to the floor (full extension). Note any restriction of motion or pain, or both (Figs. A–D).

Rationale: The normal knee will be able to extend fully without pain and with a smooth motion throughout.

Classical Significance: If the patient is unable to extend the knee fully, or if pain occurs and the patient has difficulty extending the knee the final 15 degrees with the same fluidity as with the rest of the extension arc, the test is positive and indicates loss of knee joint integrity due to weakness of the vastus medialus muscle (Fig. E).

Clinical Significance: This test is classically and clinically pathognomonic for weakness of the vastus medialis muscle. However, it will also cause similar findings if the patella is dislocated.

Follow-up: Perform the Q-angle test, the patella apprehension test, or McMurray's test.

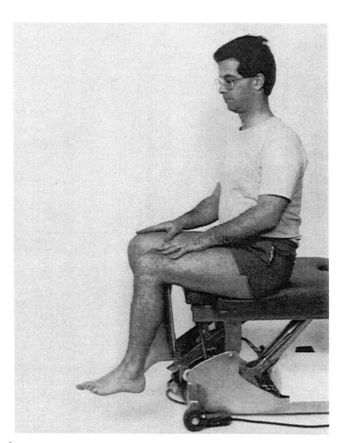

A

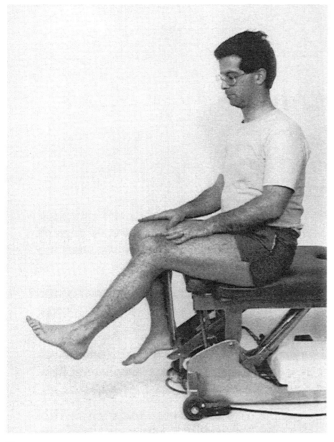

B

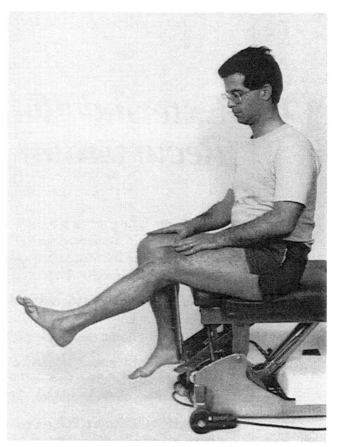

C

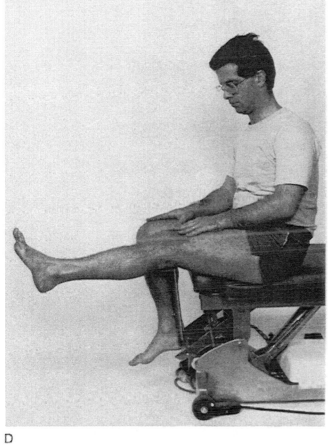

D

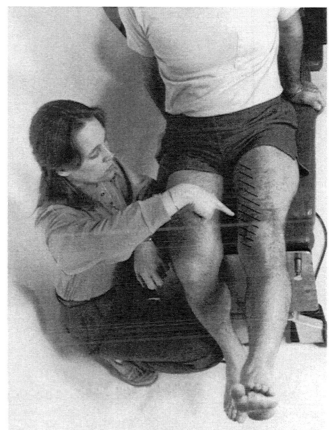

E

13 | *External Rotation Recurvatum Test*

Procedure: The patient is supine. Hold the patient's ankle with one hand and place the other behind the posterolateral aspect of the knee. Flex the knee about 40 degrees and then, feeling for relative hyperextension, extend the knee. Repeat on the other leg and compare the results (Figs. A–E).

Rationale: This test is for posterolateral rotary instability in extension. In the normal knee joint, the knee will fall to 0 degrees extension and the tibia will internally rotate into the screw home mechanism to lock the joint.

Classical Significance: If relative posterolateral hyperextension is felt on one side as compared with the other, either the posterior cruciate ligament, lateral collateral ligament, posterolateral capsule, or anterior cruciate ligament is injured.

Clinical Significance: It is normal for women to have a slight genu recurvatum. This is not a positive finding unless the hyperextension is greater that of the opposite knee.

Follow-up: Perform the anterior to posterior and posterior to anterior drawer tests, the screw home test, or the Slocum test.

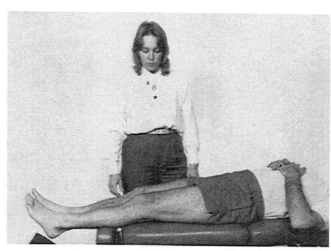

A

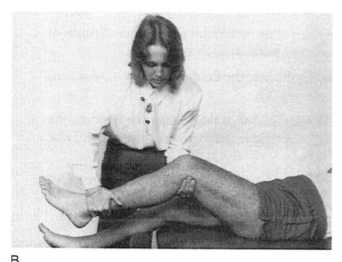

B

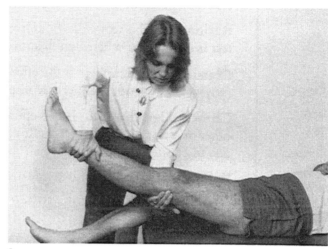

C

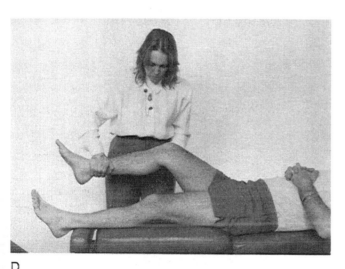

D

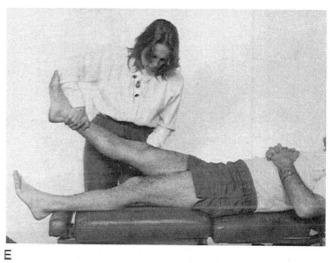

E

14 | *Fluctuation Test*

Procedure: The patient is supine with the knees locked in full extension. Place one palm over the suprapatellar pouch and the other hand over the patella itself. Then alternate pressure downward between both hands (Figs. A–E).

Rationale: This test milks fluid from one part of the knee joint to the other. A positive test is easily seen when significant retropatellar joint effusion is present.

Classical Significance: If the effusion is significant, the fluid will be felt or observed moving away from the increase in pressure (Fig. F).

Clinical Significance: If the effusion is slight, flow of fluid from one hand to the other may not be noticeable, resulting in a false-negative test. An increase in pain may be due to chondromalacia patellae.

Follow-up: Perform the brush stroke test, the patella tap, or the bounce home test.

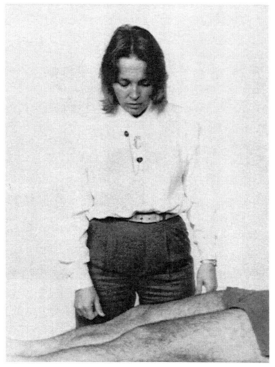

A

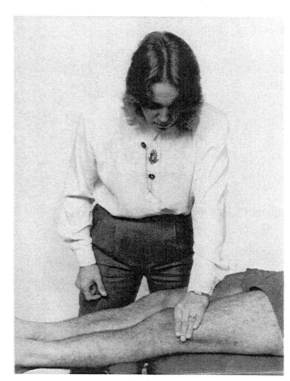

B

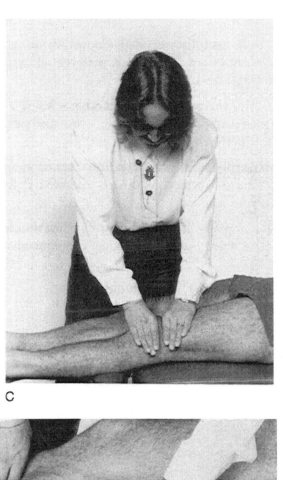

C

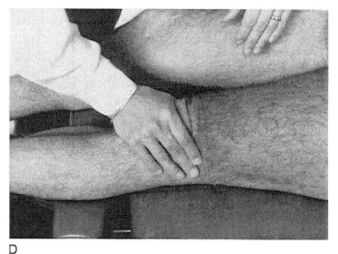

D

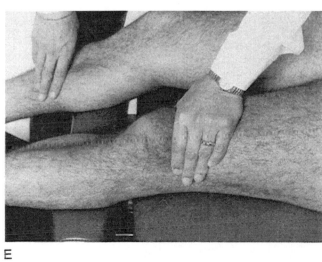

E

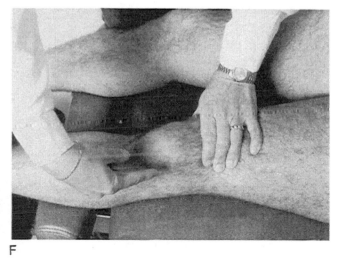

F

15 | *Fouchet's Sign*

Procedure: The patient is supine with the knees fully extended. Compress the patella at the patellofemoral groove, pushing straight down. Repeat this with the addition of medial to lateral rubbing (Perkin's sign) (Figs. A–D).

Rationale: Compression of the patella into the groove will exacerbate the patient's pain if chondromalacia patellae is present. If pain does not occur with pressure straight down, medial to lateral rubbing should be performed.

Classical Significance: An increase in retropatellar pain indicates chondromalacia patellae. Symptoms produced only with medial to lateral rubbing is a positive Perkin's sign (Fig. E).

Clinical Significance: If grating is heard or palpable grinding felt, this test should be considered positive, even in the absence of pain. Fluid in the knee can exacerbate a painful response.

Follow-up: Perform Clark's sign, the Q-angle test, or the Waldron test.

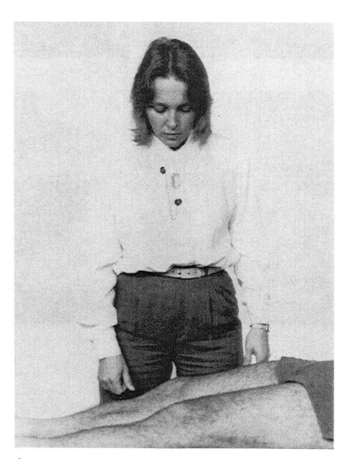

A

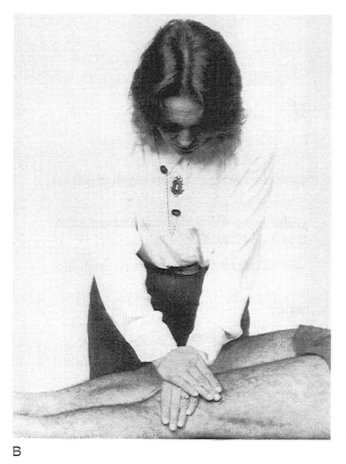

B

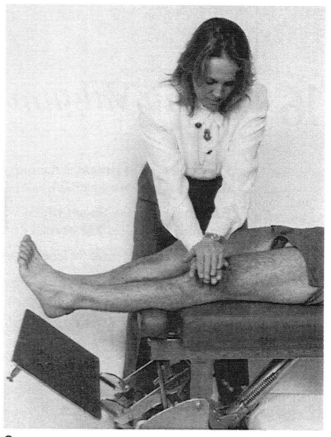

C

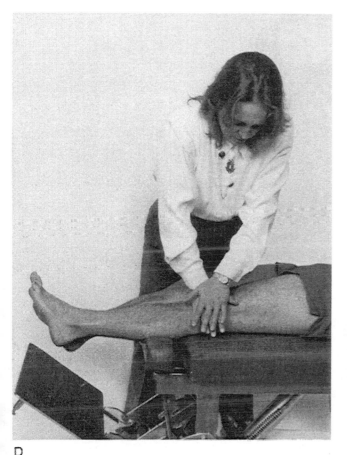

D

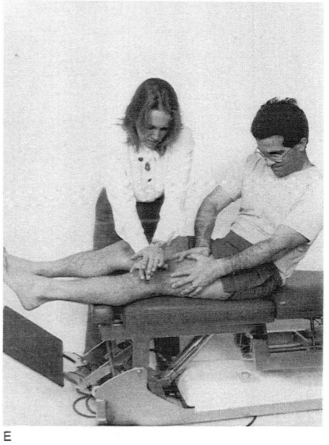

E

16 | *Genu Valgum Test*

Procedure: The patient is standing. Ask the patient to bring the feet together so that the medial malleoli touch (Figs. A–C).

Rationale: In the patient with genu valgum, the knees will touch first and not allow the ankles to touch. The normal distance is 0 to 9 or 10 cm (Fig. D).

Classical Significance: Genu valgum is present when the distance between the ankles exceeds 10 cm (Fig. E).

Clinical Significance: See Classical Significance.

Follow-up: Perform McMurray's test or the valgus stress test.

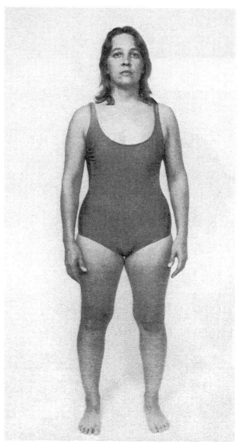

A

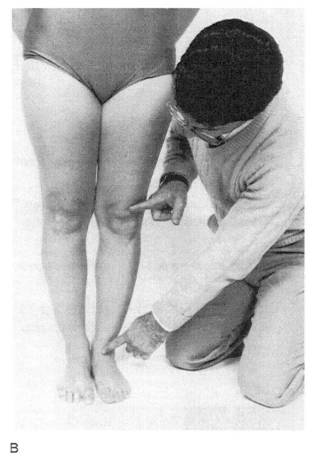

B

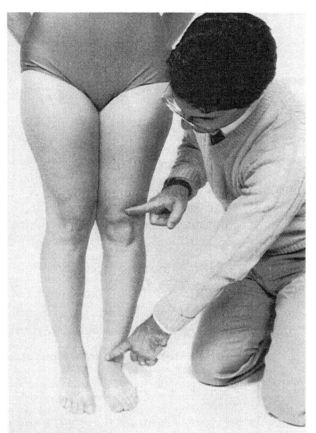

C

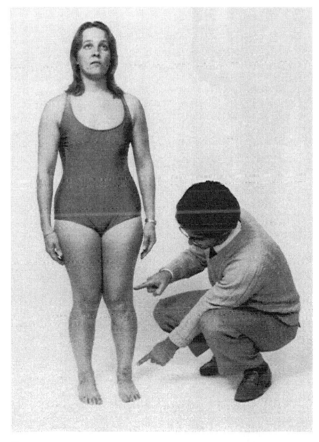

D

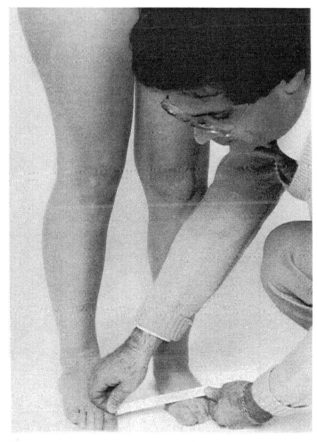

E

17 | *Genu Varum Test*

Procedure: The patient is standing. Ask the patient to bring the feet together so that the medial malleoli touch (Figs. A–C).

Rationale: In the patient with genu varum, the ankles will touch first and not allow the knees to touch. Normally, the knees abut and the ankles are no more than 9 to 10 cm apart.

Classical Significance: If the ankles touch but the knees do not the patient has genu varum (Figs. D & E).

Clinical Significance: It is normal for children younger than 3 or 4 years of age to have a genu varum position. After age 3 or 4 the legs normally begin to straighten out.

Follow-up: Perform the varus stress test or McMurray's test.

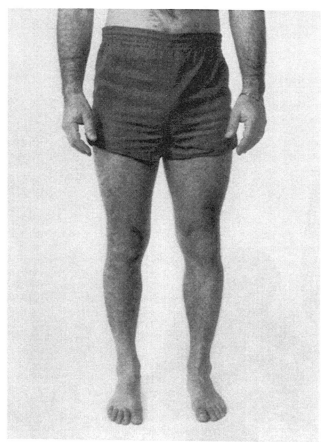

A

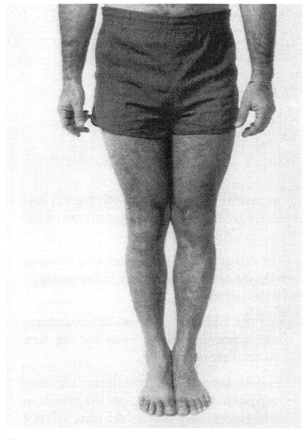

B

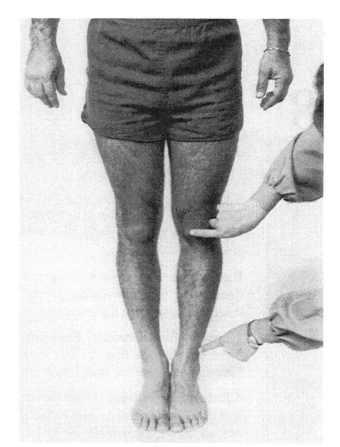

C

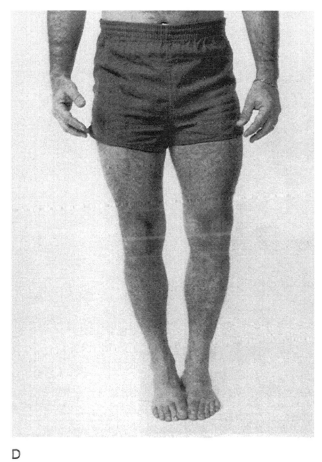

D

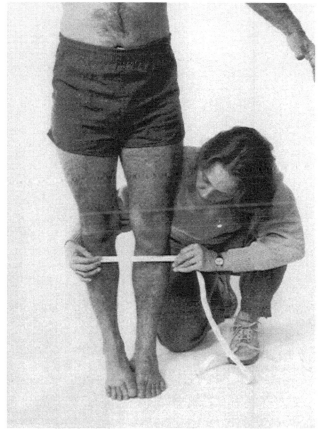

E

18 | *Godfrey's Test (Gravity Drawer Test)*

Procedure: The patient is supine. Flex the patient's knee and hip 90 degrees and support the patient's leg at the ankle or heel. Observe the patellofemoral joint (Figs. A–D).

Rationale: The tibia will sag posteriorly in this position if the posterior cruciate ligament is not functioning properly. This posterior sagging results (from gravity), since the heel is the only thing supported by the examiner.

Classical Significance: Posterior sagging of the tibia indicates posterior cruciate ligament damage (Fig. E: left, normal anatomic position; right, posterior sag sign [anterior to posterior translation secondary to cruciate laxity]).

Clinical Significance: Anterior cruciate ligament damage causes the tibia to translate forward. To confirm a positive Godfrey's test (posterior translation), ask the patient to extend the leg slightly. If the anterior cruciate ligament is damaged, the tibia will not move, whereas, if it is functional, the tibia will translate forward.

Follow-up: Perform the posterior sag sign.

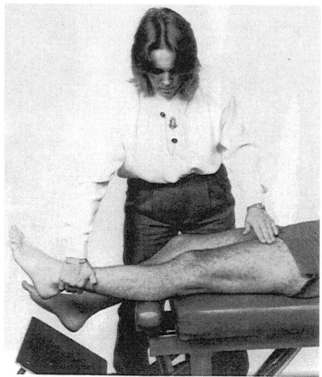

A

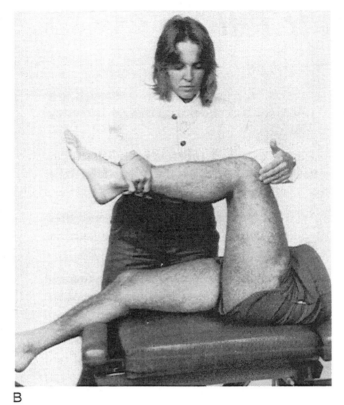

B

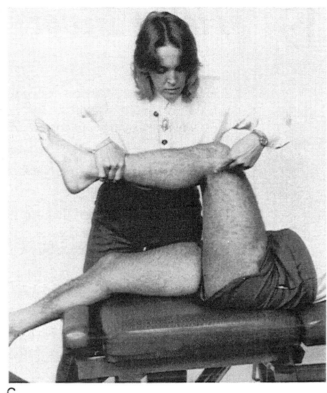

C

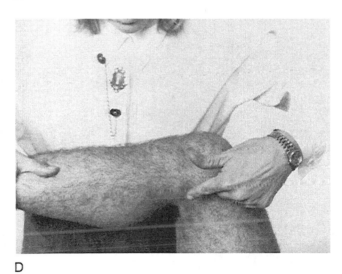

D

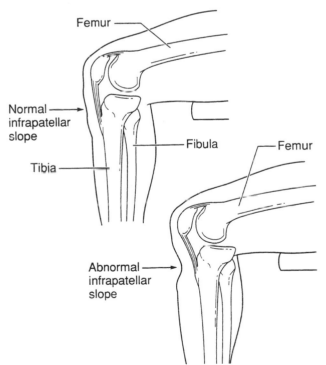

E

19 | *Helfet Pivot Shift Test*

Procedure: The patient is seated. Mark the tibial tuberosity with a grease pencil and ask the patient to extend the leg. Note the excursion of the tibial tubercle as the leg moves from flexion to extension (Figs. A–D).

Rationale: Normally, when the knee extends, the tibial tubercle rotates laterally. Remember, that at 90-degrees flexion the tibial tubercle is in the midline, considered the 0-degree mark.

Classical Significance: Failure of the tibial tubercle to rotate laterally indicates internal derangement of the knee joint itself. This failure will be more pronounced in the case of meniscus injury (Fig. E).

Clinical Significance: Posterior cruciate ligament injury or quadriceps tendon weakness will result in poor joint mechanics, which can also result in failure of the tibial tubercle to rotate laterally.

Follow-up: Perform the external rotation recurvatum test, the posterior to anterior drawer test, or Apley's compression test.

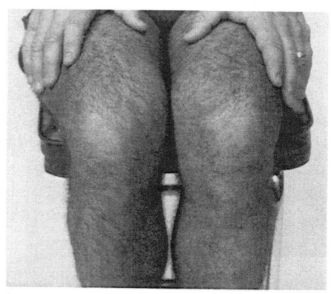

A

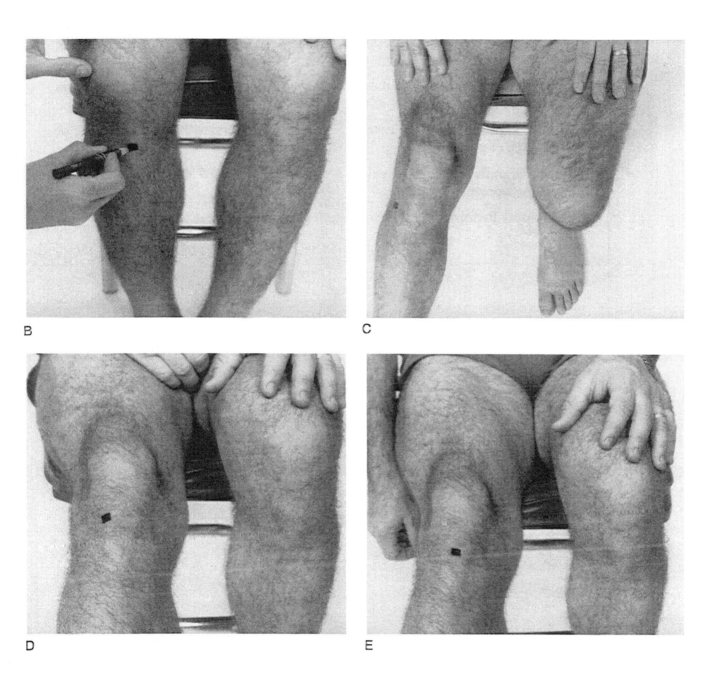

B

C

D

E

20 | *Hyperextension Test*

Procedure: The patient is supine. Grasp the legs at the ankles and lift the legs off the table, elevating them high enough to flex the hips (Figs. A–C).

Rationale: Lifting the legs off the table allows gravity to pull the knees into extension and will challenge the integrity of the cruciate complex.

Classical Significance: Evidence of hyperextension demonstrates the presence of some degree of posterior cruciate ligament laxity (Figs. D & E).

Clinical Significance: Hyperextension of no more than 5 degrees is considered normal for women.

Follow-up: Perform the external rotation recurvatum test.

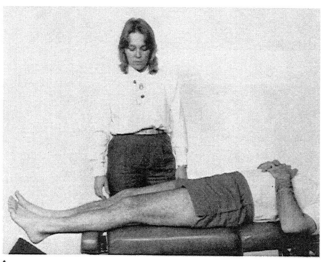

A

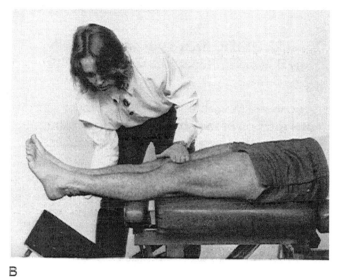

B

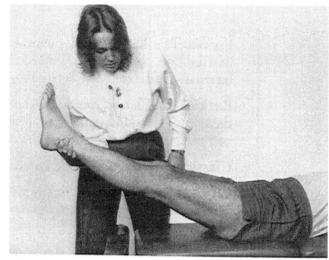

C

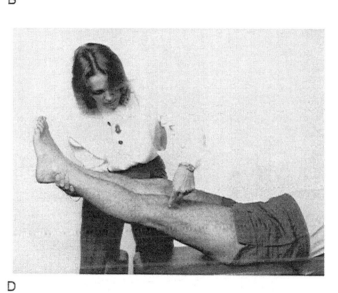

D

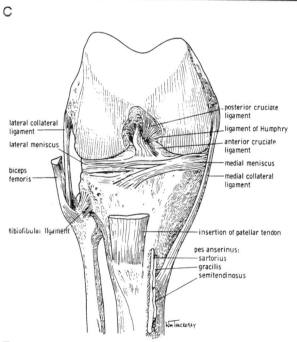

E

lateral collateral ligament

lateral meniscus

biceps femoris

tibiofibular ligament

posterior cruciate ligament

ligament of Humphry

anterior cruciate ligament

medial meniscus

medial collateral ligament

insertion of patellar tendon

pes anserinus:
sartorius
gracilis
semitendinosus

21 | *Hyperflexion Meniscus Test*

Procedure: The patient is prone. Grasp the ankle on the affected side and maximally flex the knee, bringing the heel to the ipsilateral buttock. Repeat the test with the leg internally and externally rotated (Figs. A–D).

Rationale: Flexion limitations are often encountered with internal derangement of the knee. The addition of internal and external rotation of the tiba compresses the joint and will help to determine whether the pain is from the lateral or the medial meniscus.

Classical Significance: Pain at the knee indicates a meniscal lesion.

Clinical Significance: Lateral or medial compartment strain or sprain will also cause limitation and pain, as this maneuver imposes a valgus and varus stress, respectively, on the joint (Fig. E).

Follow-up: Perform the varus and valgus stress tests or Apley's compression test.

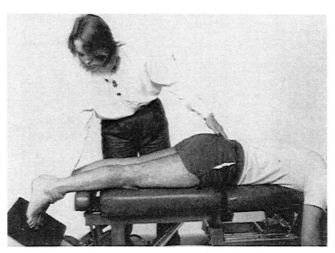

A

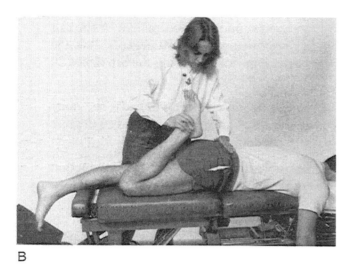

B

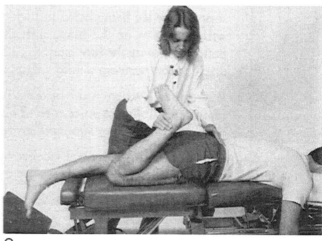

C

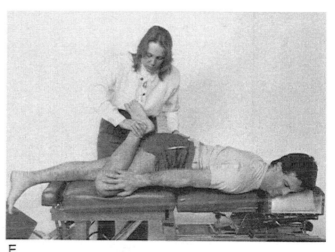

D

E

22 | *Jakob's Test (Reverse Pivot Shift Maneuver)*

Procedure: The patient is supine with the legs relaxed. Place one hand on the pelvis to support the leg being lifted and with the other hand support the lateral side of the calf with the palm on the fibula. Lift the leg, flexing the knee 70 to 80 degrees. Ask the patient to rotate the foot laterally. Then fully extend the knee keeping the hip flexed 20 degrees and perform a mild valgus stress test (Figs. A–F).

Rationale: When in the flexed position, the compromised joint will cause the tibial plateau to subluxate posteriorly. The opposing forces of knee extension and 20 degrees of hip flexion allows spontaneous reduction of the subluxation.

Classical Significance: Evidence of posterior subluxation and spontaneous reduction indicates posterolateral instability of the joint.

Clinical Significance: See Classical Significance.

Follow-up: Perform the posterior to anterior drawer test, the jerk test of Hughston, or the Macintosh test.

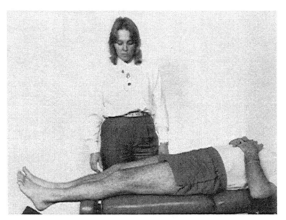

A

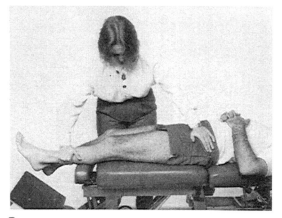

B

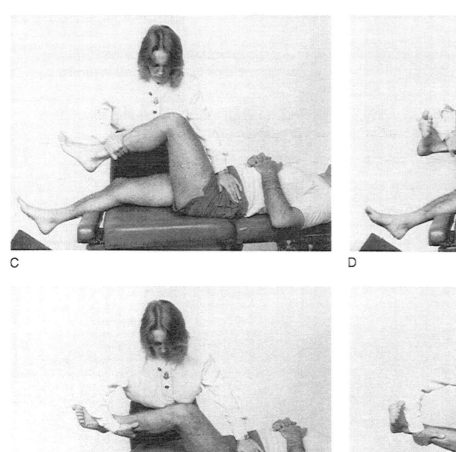

C

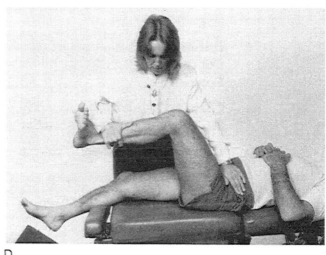

D

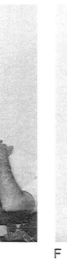

E

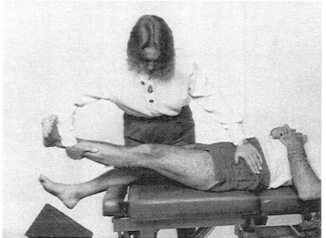

F

23 | *Jerk Test of Hughston*

Procedure: The patient is supine. Flex the hip 45 degrees and the knee 90 degrees. Then extend the leg to about 20 to 30 degrees of flexion while applying a valgus force and medially rotating the leg. Check whether a "jerk" of the lateral tibial plateau occurs (Figs. A–E).

Rationale: This procedure tests for stability of the anterolateral structures (the anterior cruciate ligaments, lateral collateral ligament, and iliotibial band) and is similar to Losee's test.

Classical Significance: A jerking of the lateral tibial plateau that occurs at about 20 to 30 degrees of flexion is a positive sign for anterolateral rotary instability.

Clinical Significance: Pain can indicate capsular insufficiency.

Follow-up: Perform Losee's test, the Macintosh test, or the Slocum test.

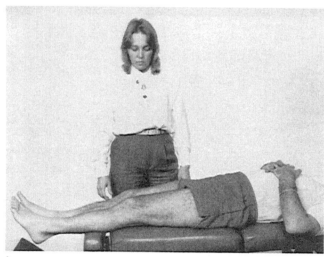

A

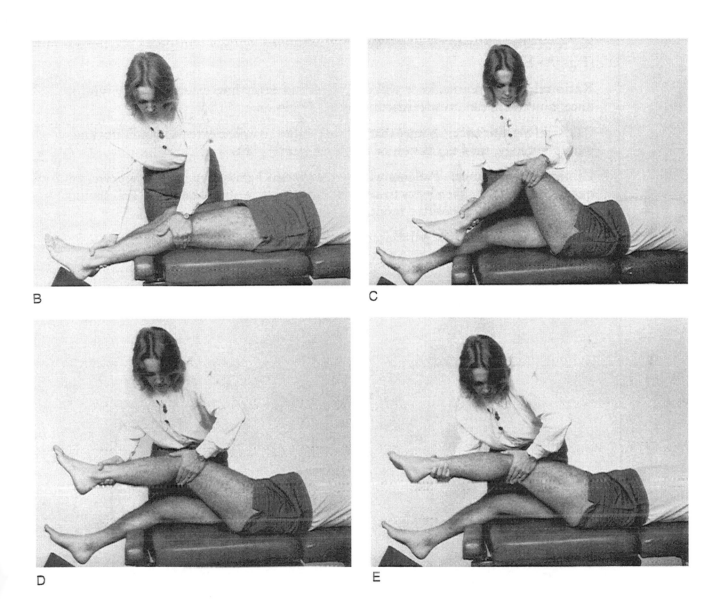

B

C

D

E

24 | *Knee Drop Test*

Procedure: The patient is prone. Place your fist under the patient's patella and flex the knee about 45 degrees with the other hand. Ask the patient to relax. When the patient has relaxed completely, drop the lower leg, allowing the knee to fall into extension (Figs. A–E).

Rationale: The normal knee will drop fully and easily into extension. Any type of knee joint lesion can cause restriction of full extension.

Classical Significance: A knee that fails to fall into complete extension indicates knee joint pathology, such as effusion or meniscus tear (Fig. F).

Clinical Significance: Patients with overexercised hamstrings and underexercised quadriceps will have a tendency to keep the knee in a state of slight flexion. This should not be mistaken for a positive result.

Follow-up: Perform the patella tap, McMurray's test, or the extension lag test.

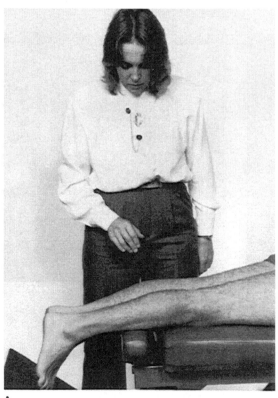

A

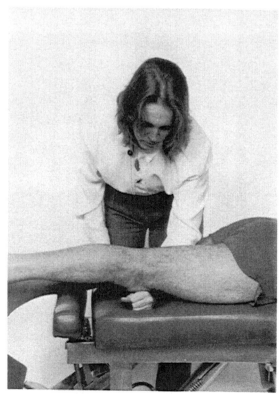

B

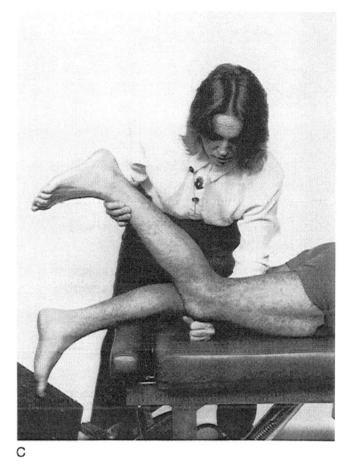

C

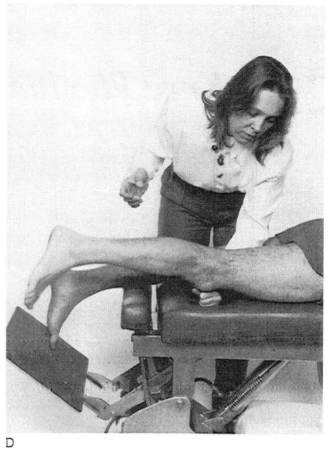

D

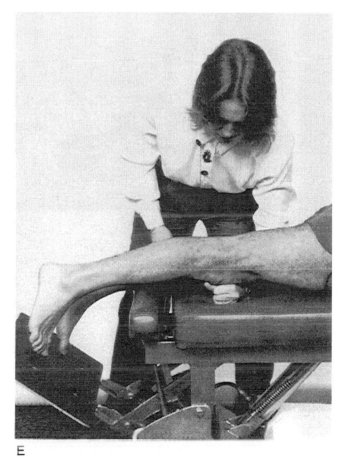

E

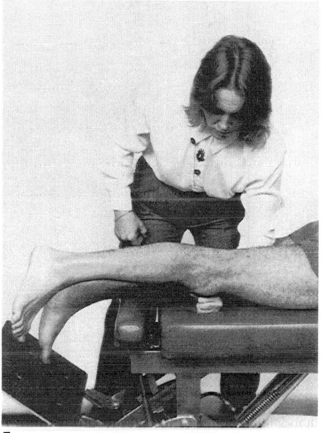

F

25 | *Knee Flexion Stress Test*

Procedure: The patient is supine. Grasp the patient's ankle and bend the knee. Then flex the knee onto the patient's chest and push the heel to the patient's buttock (Figs. A–D).

Rationale: This test places a severe amount of stress on the knee joint—all structures involved with knee flexion are stressed to the maximum.

Classical Significance: In patients with knee joint pathology, bringing the knee into full forced flexion will be restricted. This can be due to a meniscus tear or ligamentous sprain (Fig. E).

Clinical Significance: The patient with very tight quadriceps may experience a pulling sensation in the anterior thigh (Fig. F). This test may be difficult to perform if the patient's quadriceps are overdeveloped.

Follow-up: Perform McMurray's test, Apley's compression test, or Apley's distraction test.

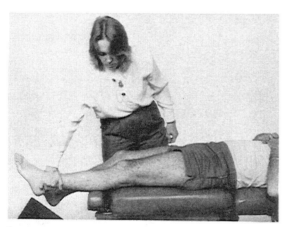

A

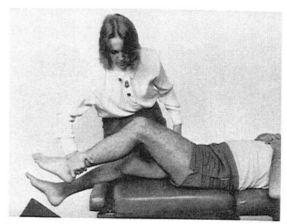

B

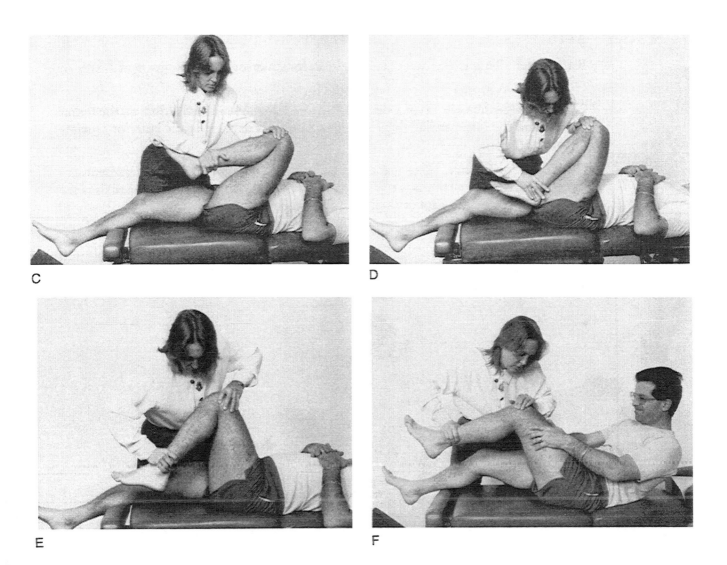

C

D

E

F

26 | *Lachman's Test*

Procedure: The patient is supine with the knee flexed about 20 to 30 degrees. Anchor the patient's foot to the examining table with your knee. Then pull the tibia forward. Note the degree, if any, of anterior translation between the tibia and the femur (Figs. A–D).

Rationale: This is the most sensitive test for anterior cruciate ligament laxity or injury.

Classical Significance: If any degree of anterior translation of the tibia on the femur occurs, and the intrapatellar slope disappears, suspect damage to the anterior cruciate ligaments (Fig. E).

Clinical Significance: The presence of a ruptured posterior cruciate ligament can sometimes result in a false-positive test. However, a clue to the correct diagnosis is the severe pain felt by the patient at the level of the rupture.

Follow-up: Perform the anterior to posterior drawer test, the screw home test, or Losee's test.

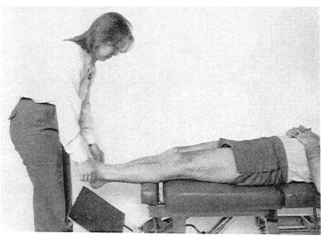

A

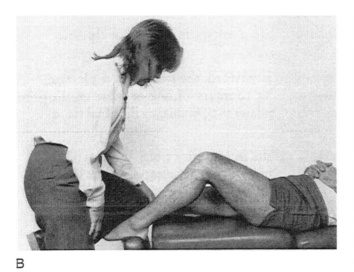

B

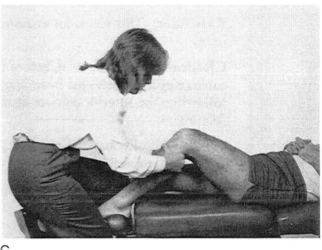

C

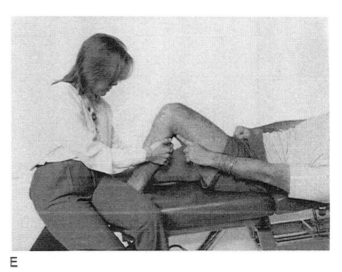

D

E

27 | *Losee's Test*

Procedure: The patient is supine. Grasp the patient's ankle, externally rotate the leg slightly, and flex the knee about 30 degrees. Then apply valgus stress and allow the knee to extend and the foot to rotate medially (Figs. A–E).

Rationale: This test is for assessment of anterolateral rotary instability of the knee joint.

Classical Significance: If, before full extension is attained, the lateral tibial plateau subluxates anteriorly, the knee joint is unstable due to injury of one or more of the following: the anterior cruciate ligament, lateral collateral ligament, or iliotibial band (Fig. F).

Clinical Significance: Knee joint instability results in posterior tibial sagging. This sag will be reduced at the beginning of the test because of external rotation of the tibia.

Follow-up: Perform the Macintosh test, the jerk test of Hughston, or the crossover test.

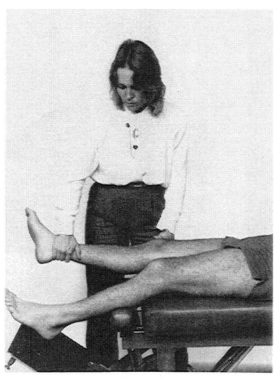

A

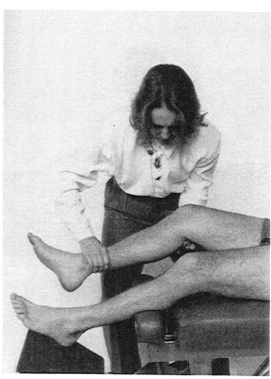

B

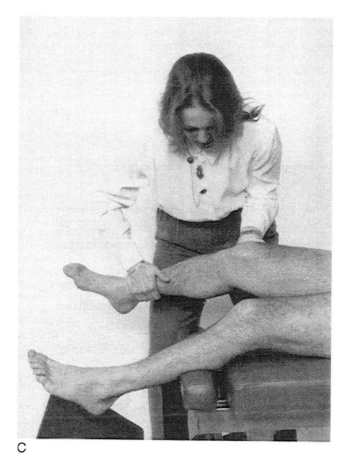

C

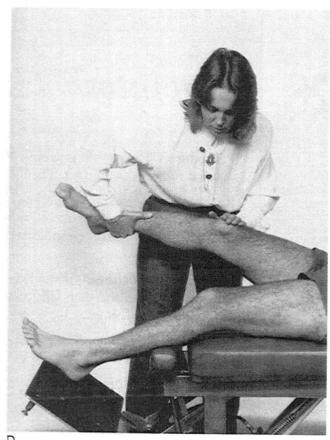

D

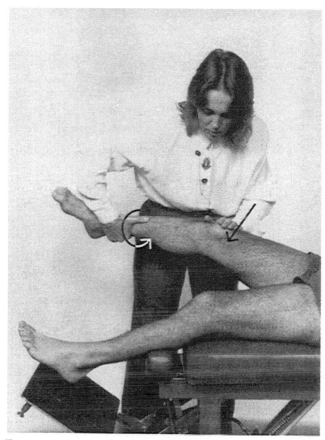

E

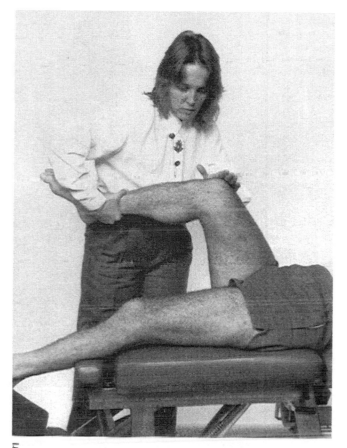

F

28 | *Macintosh Test*

Procedure: The patient is supine. Place a valgus force into the knee while applying internal rotation to the foot. Then slowly flex the knee (Figs. A–D).

Rationale: Normal knee mechanics require properly functioning synergy between the ligaments and menisci as well as between the acting and relaxing muscle groups. In this instance, a positive test indicates laxity in the structures that provide anterolateral rotatory stability.

Classical Significance: If the lateral tibial plateau subluxates forward at 20 to 40 degrees of flexion and then falls back after this point, consider anterolateral rotatory instability (Figs. E & F).

Clinical Significance: The reduction shift of the knee on the affected side is due to contraction of the iliotibial band or tensor fascia lata.

Follow-up: Perform the jerk test of Hughston, Losee's test, or the crossover test.

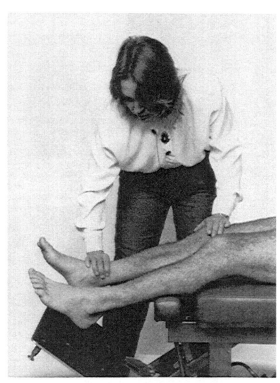

A

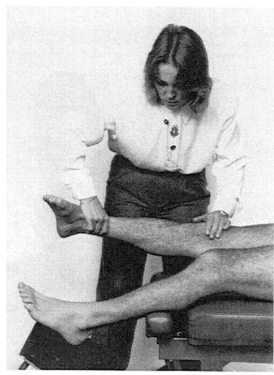

B

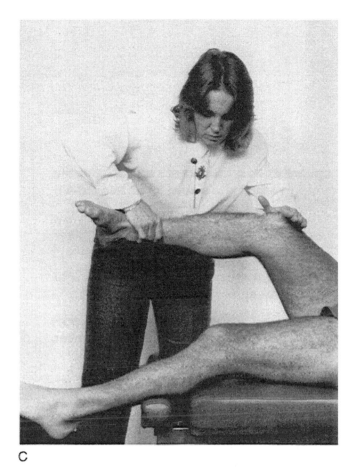

C

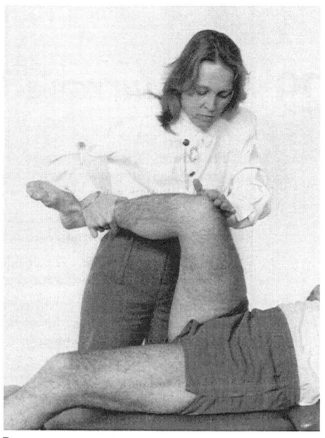

D

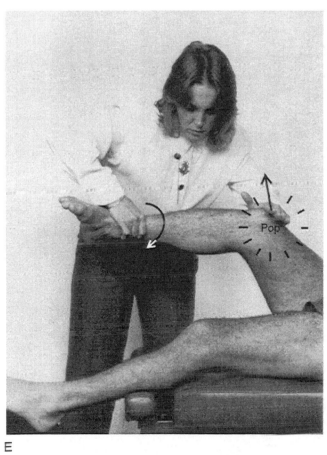

E

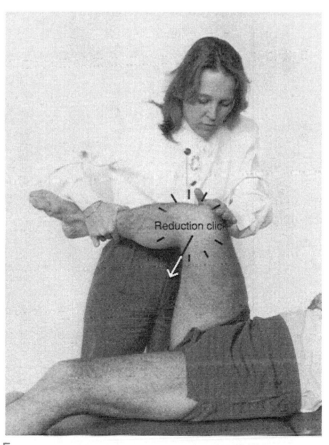

F

29 | *McMurray's Test*

Procedure: The patient is supine. Place one hand under the patient's heel and flex the knee 90 degrees with some abduction. Then apply a lateral to medial force (also known as valgus stress) to the knee while extending and adducting it (Figs. A–D).

Rationale: The valgus force on the knee stresses the medial meniscus. This test is the standard for medial meniscus evaluation.

Classical Significance: A palpable or audible click when the knee is brought into extension and adduction indicates medial meniscus injury (Fig. E).

Clinical Significance: In the patient with a medial collateral ligament injury, performance of this test may be severely limited. Therefore, medial collateral ligament damage must be ruled out before performing this test.

Follow-up: Perform Apley's compression test, the valgus stress test, or the O'Donoghues maneuver.

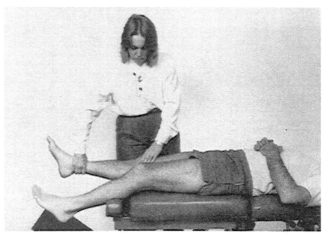

A

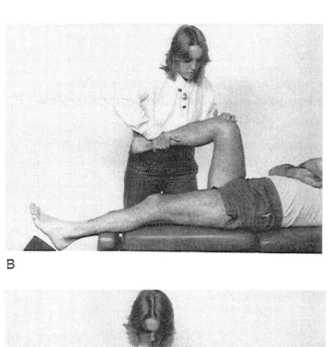

B

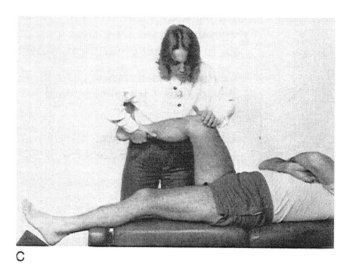

C

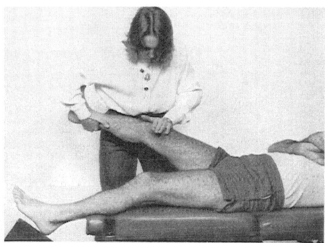

D

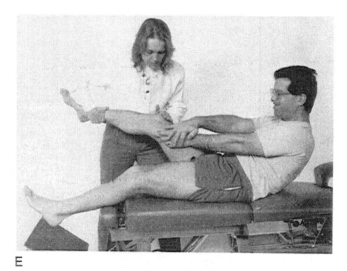

E

30 | *Mediopatella Plica Test*

Procedure: The patient is supine. Flex the affected knee 30 degrees. Then palpate and push the patella medially (Figs. A–D).

Rationale: Mediopatella plica can mimic meniscus pathology and should always be considered with a meniscus diagnosis. This test will help to differentiate plica involvement from that of meniscal involvement.

Classical Significance: Pain in the knee when the patella is pushed medially indicates that the plica is being pinched between the patella and the medial femoral condyle (Fig. E).

Clinical Significance: Chondromalacia patellae may cause some pain as well; therefore try not to compress the patella posteriorly when doing this test (Fig. F).

Follow-up: Perform the plica stutter test.

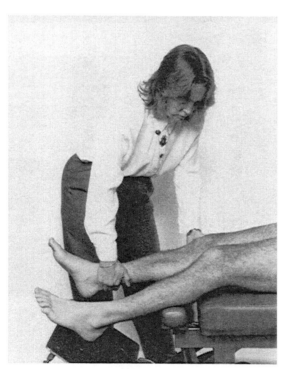

A

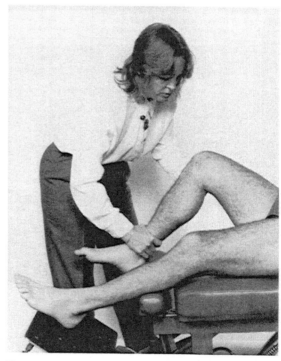

B

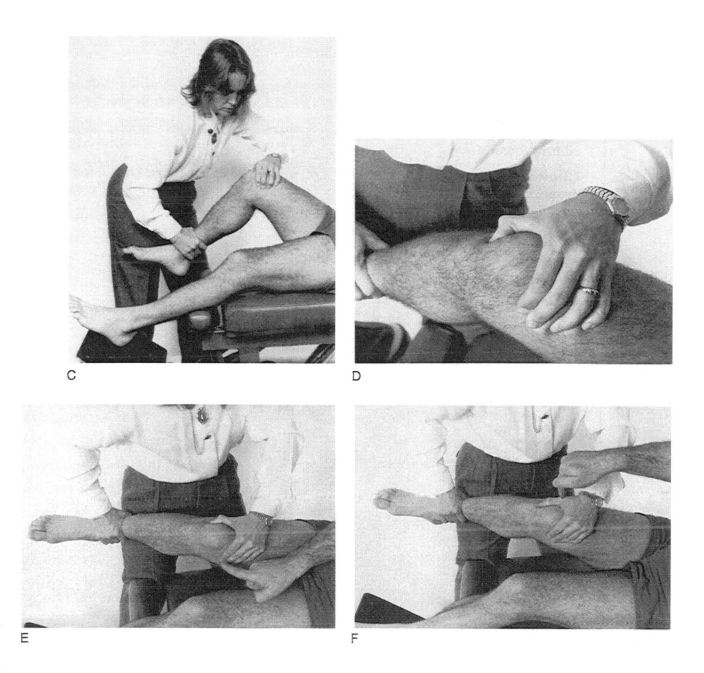

C

D

E

F

31 | *Noble's Compression Test*

Procedure: The patient is supine. Flex the patient's knee 90 degrees, apply pressure with your thumb at the lateral femoral condyle, and then passively extend the knee until flexed about 30 degrees (Figs. A–C).

Rationale: Pressing on the lateral femoral condyle puts pressure on the iliotibial band. Pressing it while extending the knee causes friction, which can result in pain.

Classical Significance: Severe pain over the lateral femoral condyle incidates iliotibial band friction (Fig. D).

Clinical Significance: The iliotibial band may be contracted; use Ober's test to determine whether this is so (Fig. E).

Follow-up: Perform Ober's test (see Ch. 10).

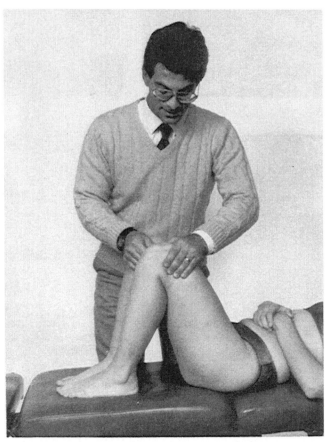

A

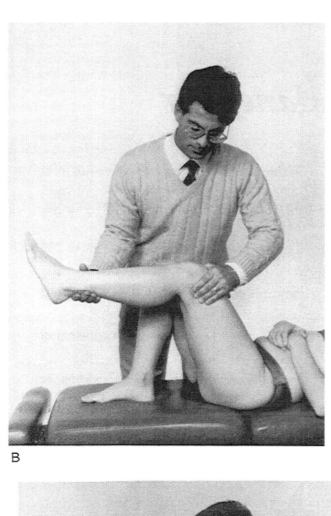

B

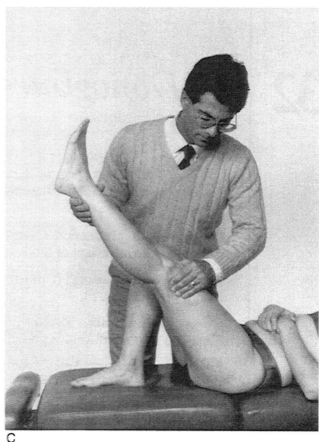

C

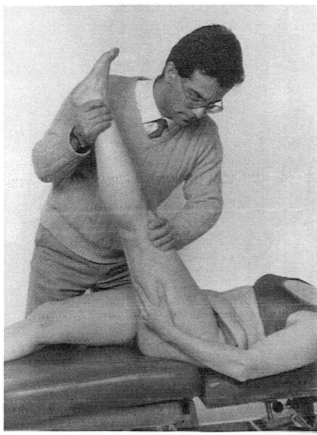

D

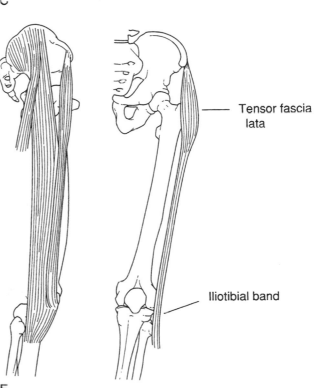

Tensor fascia
lata

Iliotibial band

E

32 | *O'Donoghues Maneuver*

Procedure: This maneuver is performed on the patient who has complained of joint line pain. The patient is supine. Flex the patient's knee 90 degrees and rotate the leg in and out twice, then fully flex the knee and again rotate the leg in and out twice (Figs. A–E).

Rationale: Reproduction or aggravation of pain with the knee flexed 90 to 135 degrees is a positive sign of knee lesion.

Classical Significance: A positive test indicates capsular irritation or a meniscal lesion, or both (Fig. F).

Clinical Significance: The knee joint will be irritated when put through the extremes of flexion if joint effusion is present.

Follow-up: Perform Apley's compression and distraction tests, McMurray's test, or the bounce home test.

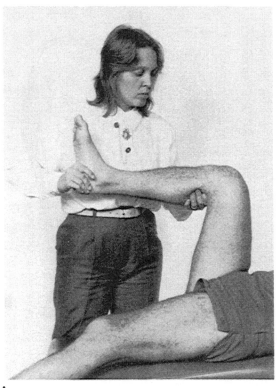

A

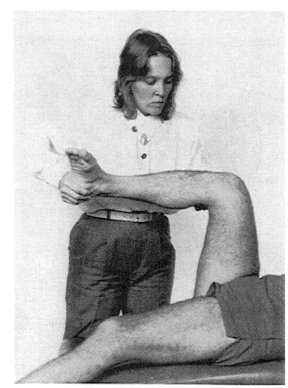

B

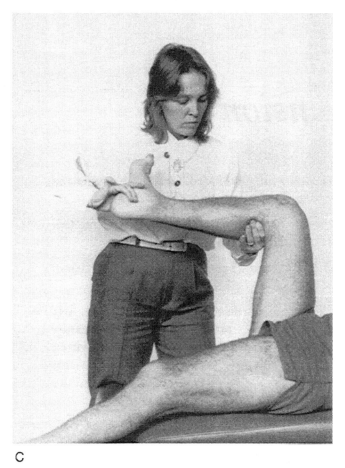

C

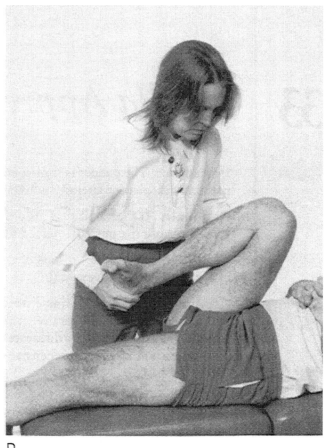

D

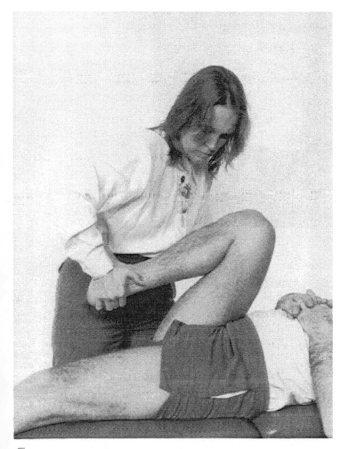

E

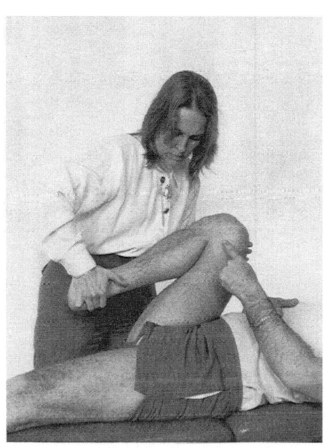

F

33 | *Patella Apprehension Test*

Procedure: The patient is supine with the knee fully extended. Grasp the patella and manually displace it laterally while observing the patient's face (Figs. A–C).

Rationale: If the patella has dislocated before or if the ligaments are lax, this maneuver may cause the unstable patella to dislocate.

Classical Significance: A look of apprehension on the patient's face because of fear of dislocation is a positive test (Fig. D).

Clinical Significance: Muscle weakness, such as of the vastus medialis muscle, may make the patella track laterally. If muscle weakness is present, then forced pressure laterally may make a patella dislocate even though it never did before (Fig. E). However, the patient will not be apprehensive.

Follow-up: Perform the Q-angle test or Dreyer's test.

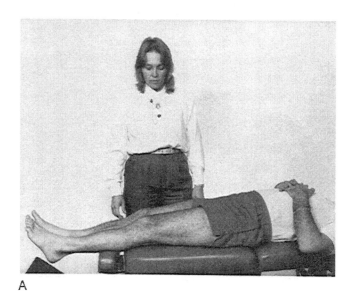

A

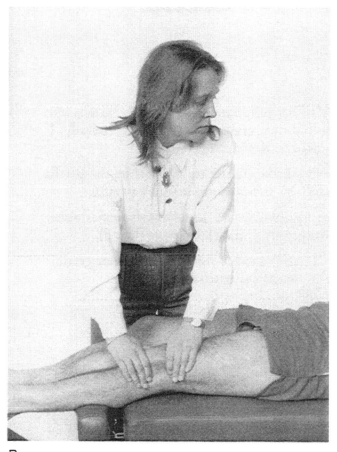

B

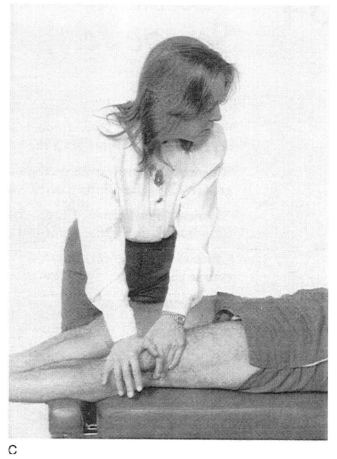

C

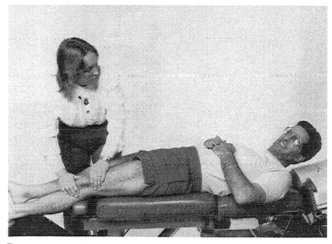

D

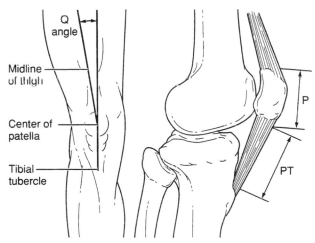

E

34 | *Patella Grind Test (Patella Scrape Test)*

Procedure: The patient is supine with the knee fully extended. Force the patella into the patellar groove with strong pressure and then grind it medially and laterally. If negative, repeat this test with the knee flexed 30 degrees (Figs. A–E).

Rationale: This test forces the underside of the patella to rub against the patella groove. Chondromalacia patellae can cause this maneuver to be quite painful.

Classical Significance: An increase in pain within the knee joint signifies either chondromalacia patellae or arthritis of the patella or patellar groove (Fig. F).

Clinical Significance: This test is similiar to Fouchet's sign. A grinding or grating, even in the absence of pain, indicates chondromalacia patellae.

Follow-up: Perform Clark's sign, Fouchet's sign, or the Q-angle test.

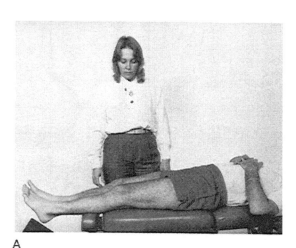

A

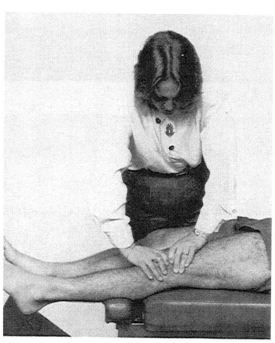

B

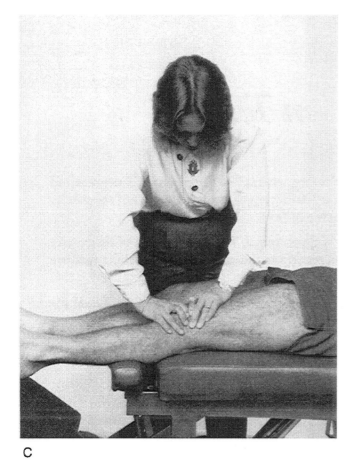

C

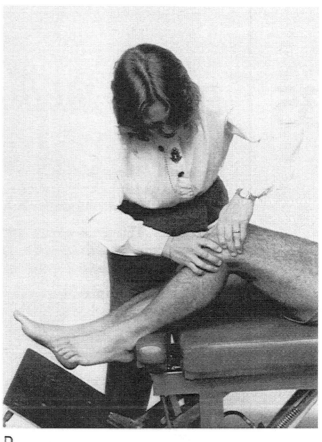

D

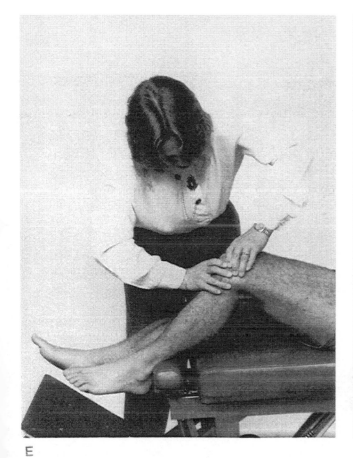

E

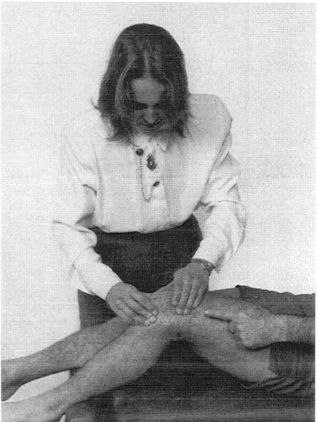

F

35 | *Patella Inhibition Test*

Procedure: The patient is supine, with the leg being tested flexed about 20 degrees and supported under the knee with a small towel roll. Cup the superior aspect of the patella and instruct the patient to fully extend the leg (Figs. A–C).

Rationale: This test is a modification of Clark's sign. The compression of the patella with the active contraction of the quadriceps forces the patella into the patellar groove and compromises the retropatellar interspace.

Classical Significance: Re-creation of pain in the retropatellar area is significant for chondromalacia patellae (Fig. D).

Clinical Significance: The inability to perform this test may be caused by quadriceps weakness or acute effusion within the knee joint (Fig. E).

Follow-up: Perform Clark's sign, the Waldron test, or Fouchet's sign.

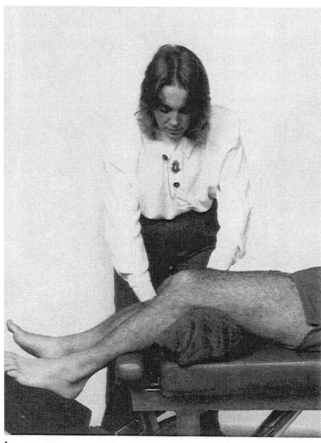

A

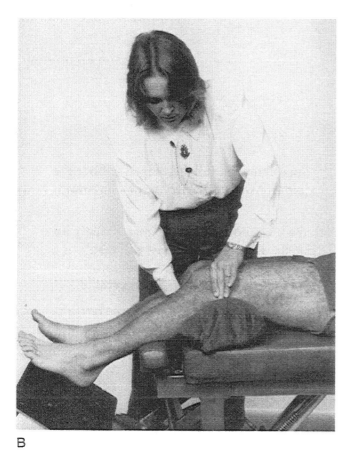

B

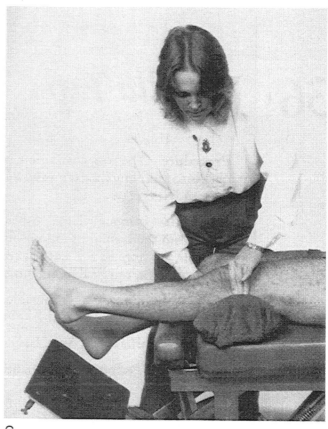

C

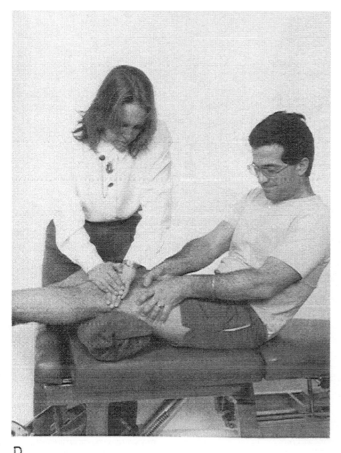

D

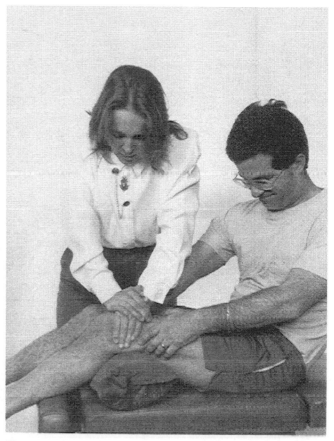

E

36 | *Patella Tap*

Procedure: The patient is supine with the knee extended fully. Compress above the patella to force any fluid down into the knee joint. Then quickly tap the patella toward the condyles (Figs. A–D).

Rationale: If enough fluid is displaced into the knee joint, the patella may actually lift away from the condyles, and pushing the patella downward quickly will result in a palpable tap (Fig. E: left, normal contour of knee is preserved when joint effusion is minimal; right, minimal joint effusion must be milked upwards to be observable).

Classical Significance: A palpable tap signifies minor joint effusion into the retropatellar space.

Clinical Significance: See Classical Significance.

Follow-up: Perform the fluctuation test or the brush stroke test.

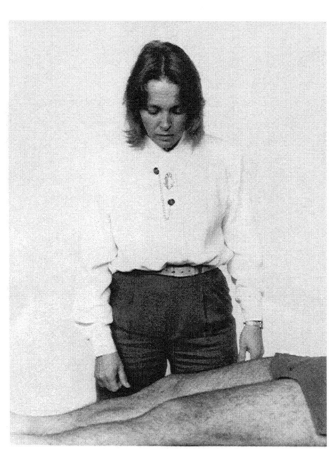

A

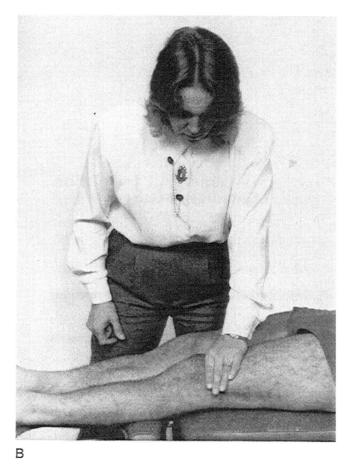

B

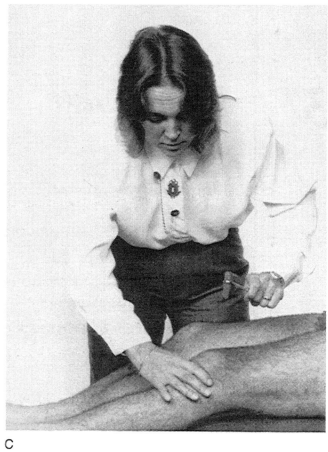

C

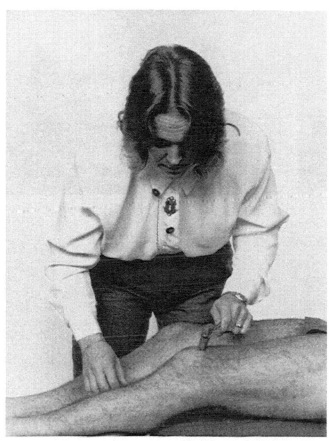

D

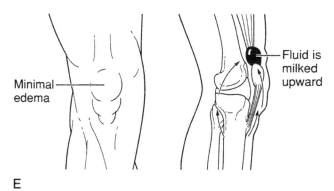

Minimal edema

Fluid is milked upward

E

37 | *Payr's Sign*

Procedure: The patient is seated. Ask the patient to sit cross-legged ("Indian" style). Then press downward on the knees (forcing the knee toward the examining table) (Figs. A–D).

Rationale: This test will aggravate a medial meniscus problem.

Classical Significance: Pain within the medial meniscus is a positive test (Fig. E).

Clinical Significance: Pain located at the lateral aspect of the knee is due to stretching of the lateral collateral ligament (Fig. F).

Follow-up: Perform the varus stress test, Apley's compression test, or McMurray's test.

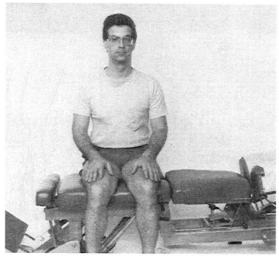

A

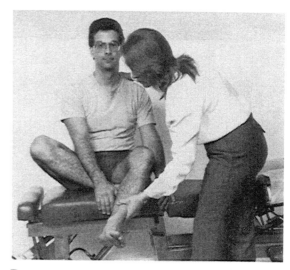

B

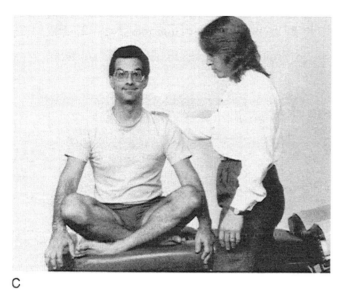

C

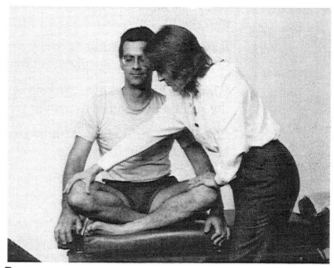

D

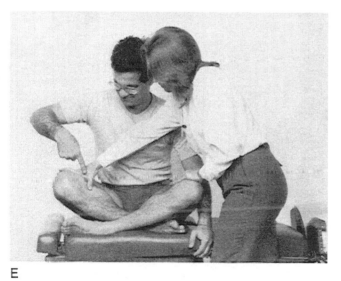

E

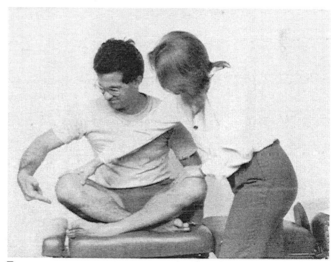

F

38 | *Plica Stutter Test*

Procedure: The patient is seated at the edge of the table with the knees flexed 90 degrees. Palpate the patella while the patient slowly extends the leg fully. Observe the movement, especially between the angles of 60 to 45 degrees of flexion (Figs. A–E).

Rationale: Palpation of the normal patella should demonstrate a smooth arc from flexion to extension without jerkiness.

Classical Significance: Stuttering or otherwise irregular restriction of movement of the patella during full extension is significant for plica entrapment (Fig. F).

Clinical Significance: Swelling in the joint will impede the normal mechanics of the knee and invalidate this test.

Follow-up: Perform the extension lag test or the jerk test of Hughston.

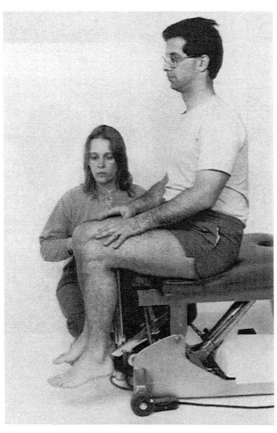

A

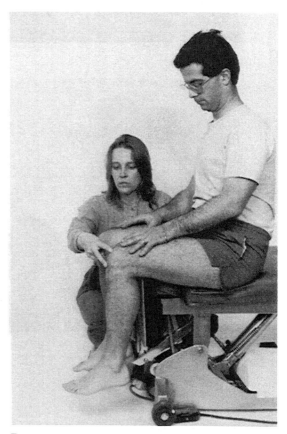

B

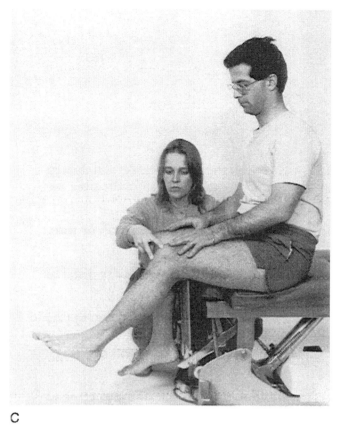

C

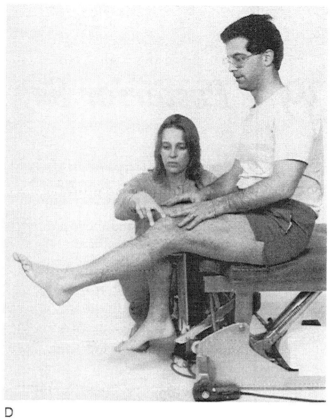

D

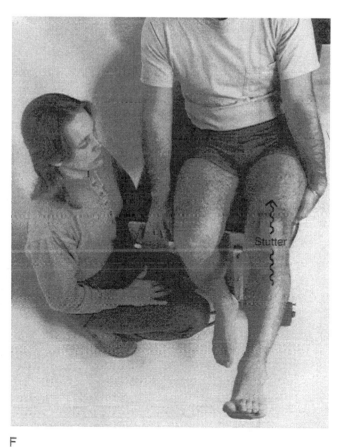

E

F

39 | *Posterior Sag Sign*

Procedure: The patient is supine. Ask the patient to flex the hip 45 degrees and then to flex the knee 90 degrees with the heel on the examining table. Observe the tibia for posterior translation in relation to the femur (Figs. A & B).

Rationale: In the above position, if the posterior cruciate ligament is weak or torn, gravity will pull the head of the tibia posteriorly.

Classical Significance: A posterior sag of the tibia (an observable concavity distal to the patella) is positive for posterior cruciate ligament damage (Fig. C).

Clinical Significance: Ask the patient with a positive sag sign to extend the leg (the voluntary anterior drawer test). If the tibial plateau translates forward, the anterior cruciate ligament is functional, confirming posterior cruciate ligament weakness (Figs. D–E).

Follow-up: Perform Godfrey's test or the anterior to posterior and posterior to anterior drawer tests.

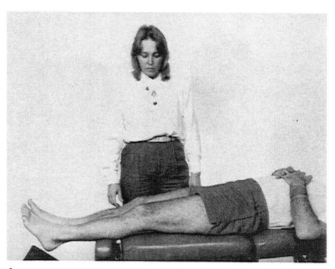

A

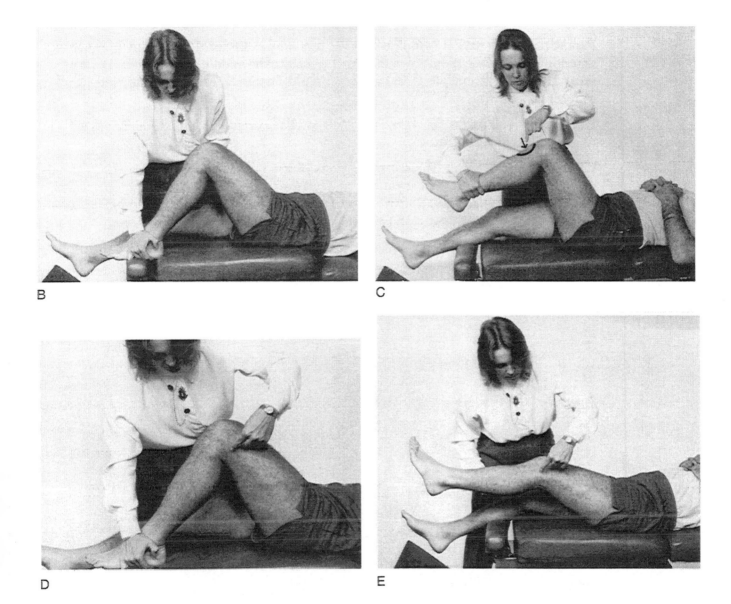

B

C

D

E

40 | *Q-Angle Test (Patellofemoral Angle Test)*

Procedure: The patient is supine with the legs fully extended. Draw a line from the anterior superior iliac spine down the femoral shaft to the middle of the patella. Draw a second line from the middle of the patella to the tibial tubercle. These two lines intersect to form an angle (Figs. A–D).

Rationale: This is a test for chondromalacia patellae, patella alta, an externally rotated tibia, and a subluxated patella.

Classical Significance: The normal angle is 10 to 13 degrees for males and 10 to 15 degrees for females. An angle greater than the normal range indicates chondromalacia patellae or a subluxated patella. An angle less than 10 degrees indicates chondromalacia patellae or patella alta (Fig. E and see Test 33, Fig. E).

Clinical Significance: If this test is positive, repeat the procedure with the patient's knee flexed and the patient seated. The normal measurement in this position is zero degrees, anything else signifies a subluxated patella.

Follow-up: Perform Clark's sign, Fouchet's sign, or the patella apprehension test.

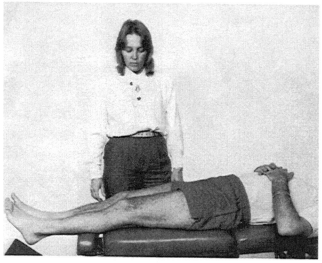

A

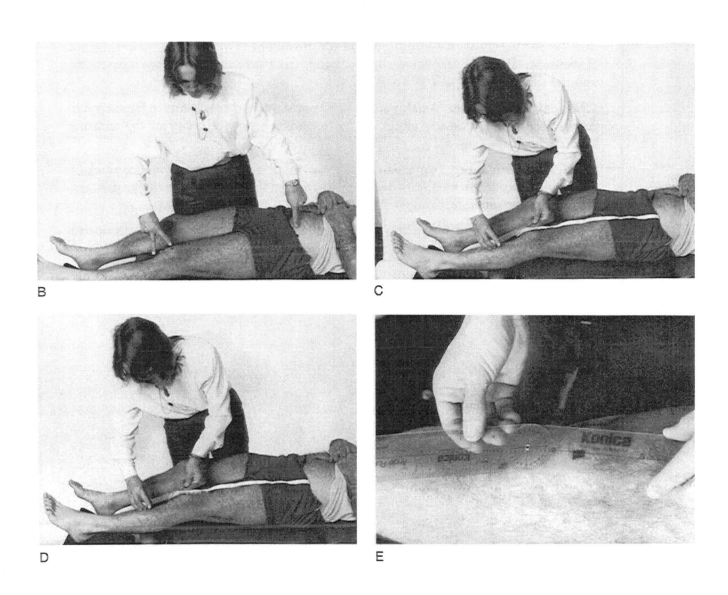

B

C

D

E

41 | *Screw Home Test*

Procedure: The patient is seated. Place one hand under the patient's heel and the index finger of the other hand on the tibial tuberosity. Then slowly extend the knee while observing the movement of the tibial tuberosity (Figs. A–D).

Rationale: In the normal knee, the tibia will rotate externally as the knee is extended and the tibial tubercle will move laterally.

Classical Significance: An alteration in the normal movement is due to ligamentous or meniscus injury, usually either medial meniscus injury or laxity of the anterior cruciate ligament (Fig. E).

Clinical Significance: Damage to, or the removal of, a meniscus may induce a lack of synergy between the meniscus and the supporting ligaments. Ultimately, this can sprain the ligaments, resulting in an improper screw home mechanism.

Follow-up: Perform McMurray's test, the anterior to posterior and posterior to anterior drawer tests, or the valgus and varus stress tests.

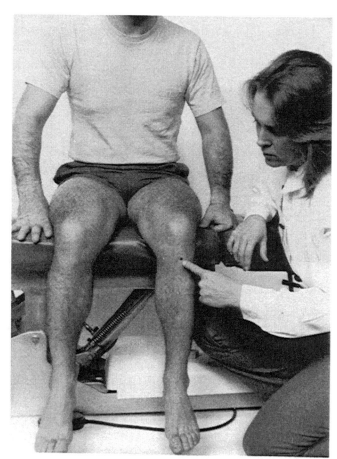

A

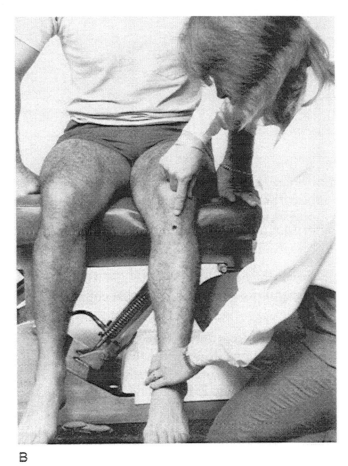

B

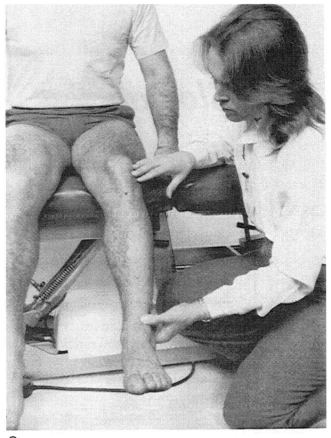

C

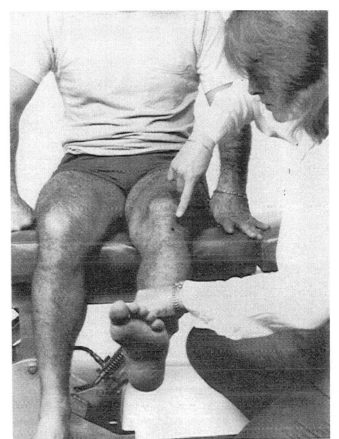

D

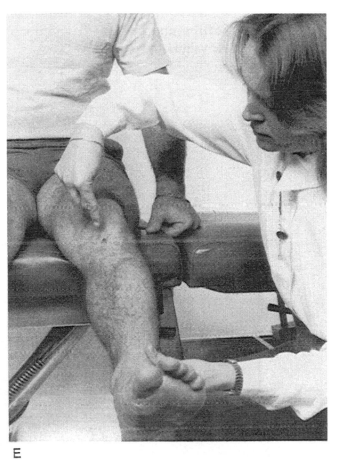

E

42 | *Slocum Test*

Procedure: The patient is supine with the knee flexed 80 to 90 degrees and the hip flexed about 45 degrees. First, rotate the foot of the flexed leg 30 degrees medially and then hold the foot in this position and pull the tibia forward. Repeat the test with the foot laterally rotated 15 degrees (Figs. A–D). Perform the test on both legs for comparison.

Rationale: This test stresses the anterior cruciate ligament and then the lateral collateral ligament. The lateral rotation stresses the anterior cruciate and medial collateral ligaments.

Classical Significance: If the lateral tibial head displaces anteriorly when the foot is rotated medially, the anterior cruciate or lateral collateral ligaments may be injured; if the medial tibial head displaces anteriorly when the foot is rotated laterally, the medial collateral or anterior cruciate ligaments may be injured (Fig. E: P–A glide, posterior to anterior glide).

Clinical Significance: This test must be performed at the degrees mentioned, because maximum rotation of the tibia will only tighten the ligaments, thereby resulting in a false-negative test.

Follow-up: Perform the anterior to posterior and posterior to anterior drawer tests or the valgus and varus stress tests.

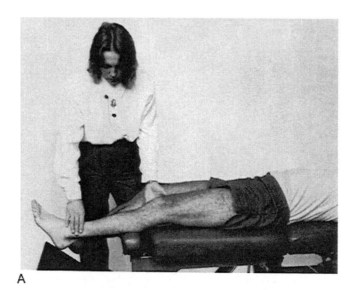

A

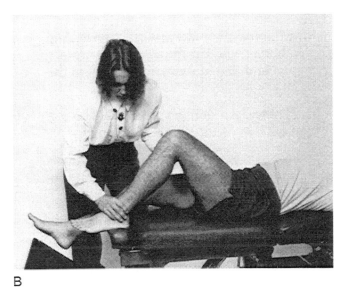

B

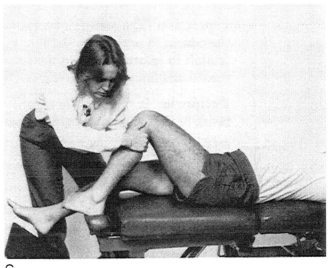

C

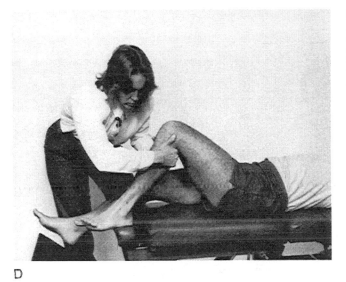

D

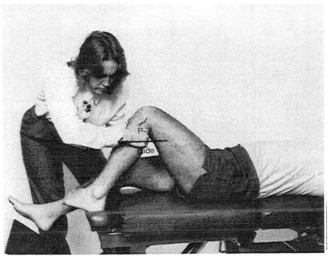

E

43 | *Steinmann's Tenderness Displacement Sign*

Procedure: The patient is seated and points to the area of tenderness in the knee. Ask the patient to actively extend and flex the knee, noting whether the tenderness appears to shift in location. Repeat the test with internal and external rotation to isolate the medial and lateral menisci (Figs. A–D).

Rationale: In meniscal injury, the patient will describe a shift in tenderness. This is a result of the changes in stress placed on the menisci by flexion and extension.

Classical Significance: The sign is present if the pain seems to move anteriorly when the knee is extended and posteriorly when the knee is flexed. Suspect a meniscal tear (Figs. E & F).

Clinical Significance: The site of tenderness will not shift if degenerative osteoarthritis of the knee is the cause of the pain.

Follow-up: Perform McMurray's test, Apley's compression test, or the screw home test.

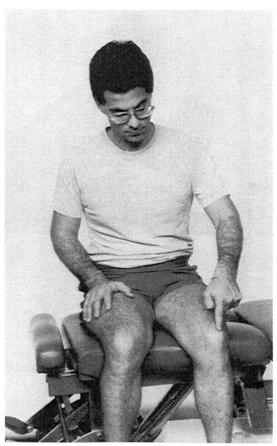

A

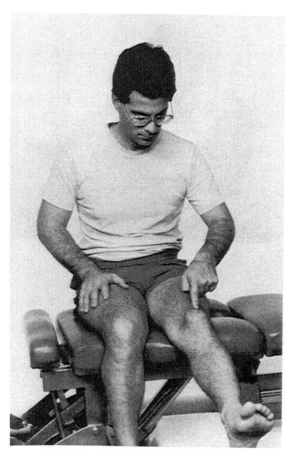

B

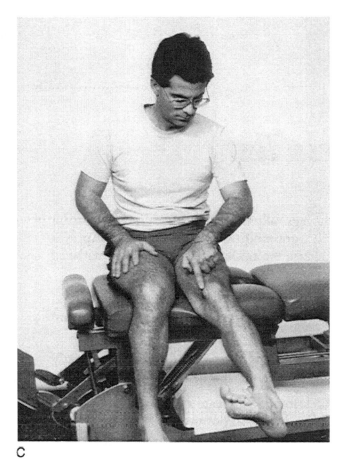

C

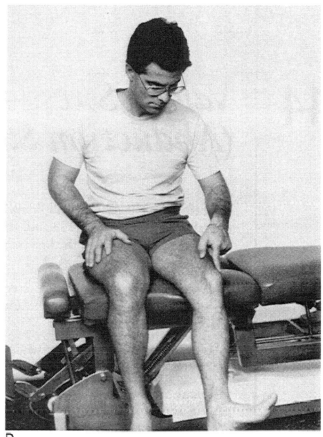

D

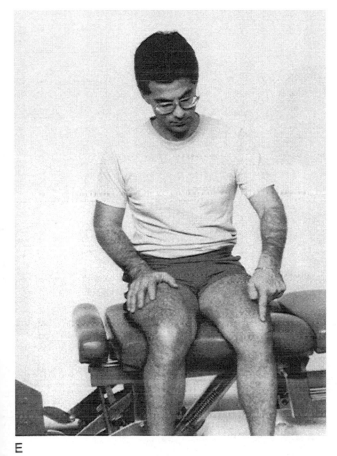

E

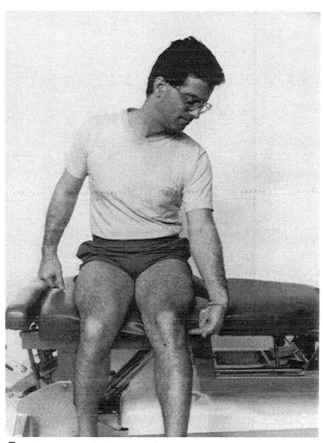

F

44 Valgus Stress Test (Abduction Stress Test)

Procedure: The patient is supine with the legs fully extended. Place one hand on the lateral knee and the other around the ankle, grasping the medial malleolus. Apply a lateral to medial force to the knee while pulling the ankle outwardly. Repeat with the knee flexed 30 degrees (Figs. A–D).

Rationale: The forces applied create maximum stress at the medial collateral ligament. At 30 degrees of flexion the test allows the capsular elements to be lax, which are not involved if pain persists.

Classical Significance: Pain that is increased at the medial side of the knee, especially when the knee is fully extended, indicates medial collateral ligament sprain (Fig. E).

Clinical Significance: Applying too much force will create a false-positive test. Be careful and compare one side with the other. Pain will occur on valgus stress if the anterior cruciate ligament is damaged.

Follow-up: Perform McMurray's test, the varus stress test, or Apley's distraction test.

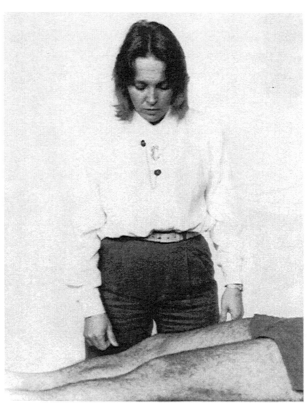

A

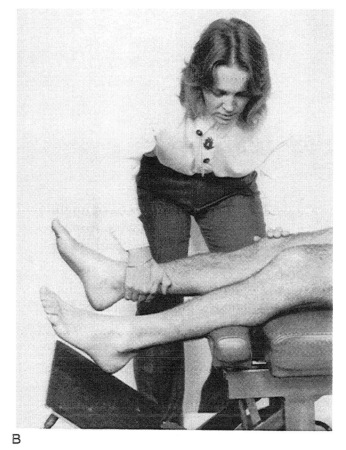

B

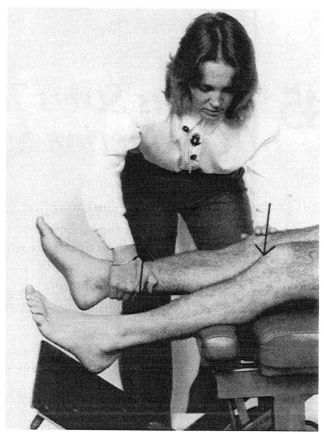

C

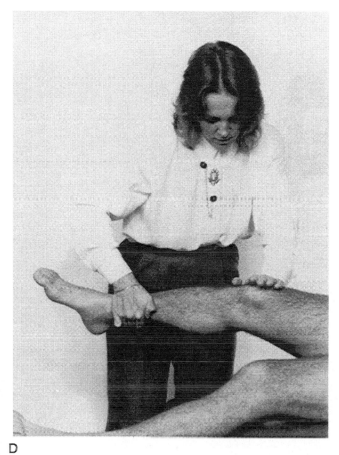

D

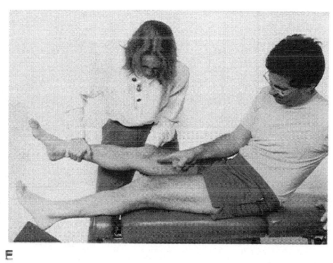

E

45 | *Varus Stress Test (Adduction Stress Test)*

Procedure: The patient is supine with the legs fully extended. Place one hand on the medial knee and the other around the ankle, grasping the lateral malleolus. Apply a medial to lateral force to the knee while pushing the ankle inwardly. Repeat with the leg flexed 30 degrees (Figs. A–D).

Rationale: The forces applied create maximum stress at the lateral collateral ligament. The 30 degrees of flexion allows the capsular elements to be lax, which are not involved if the pain persists.

Classical Significance: Pain that is increased at the lateral side of the knee, especially when the knee is fully extended, indicates lateral collateral ligament sprain (Fig. E).

Clinical Significance: Too much force can result in a false-positive test. Be careful and compare one side with the other.

Follow-up: Perform McMurray's test, the valgus stress test, or Apley's distraction test.

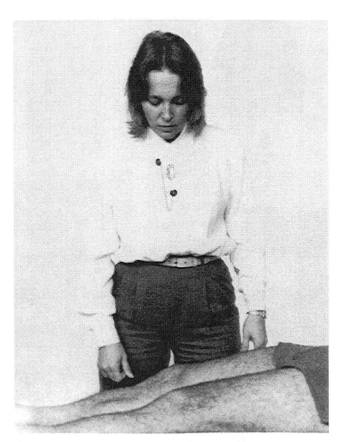

A

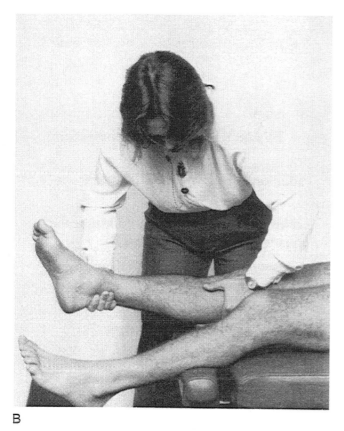

B

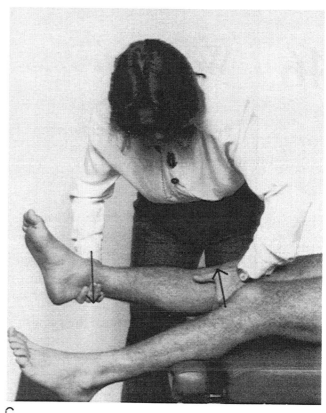

C

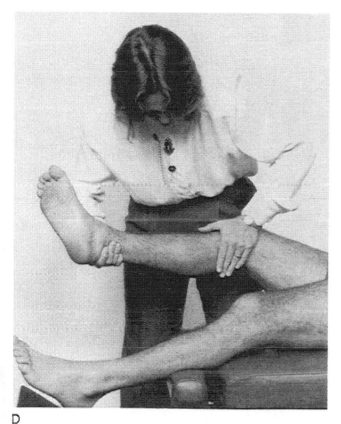

D

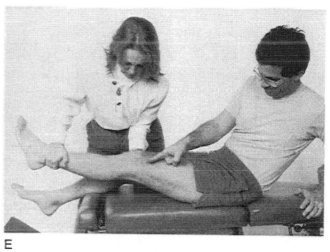

E

46 | *Waldron Test*

Procedure: The patient is standing upright. Palpate the patella while the patient performs a few deep knee bends (Figs. A–C).

Rationale: As the knee flexes and extends additional stress is placed on the retropatellar space.

Classical Significance: A palpable amount of crepitus along with pain at the time the crepitus is felt is a positive sign, indicating chondromalacia patellae (Fig. D).

Clinical Significance: The presence of crepitus without pain may indicate some degree of degenerative osteoarthritis that is not yet symptomatic (Fig. E: osteochondritis dissecans; 1, healed marginal defect; 2, joint mice; 3, perichondrial sclerosis).

Follow-up: Perform the patella grind test, Clark's sign, or Fouchet's sign.

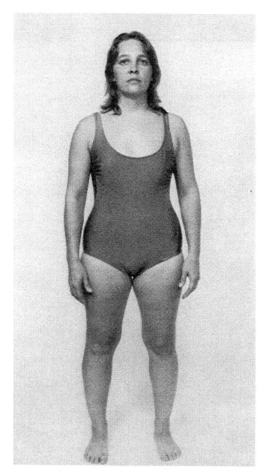

A

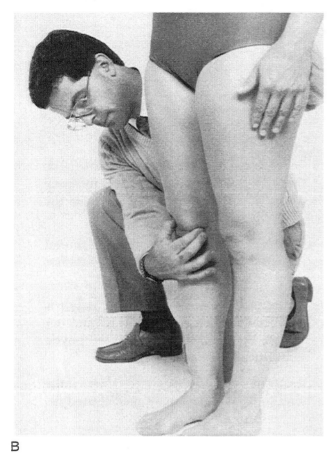

B

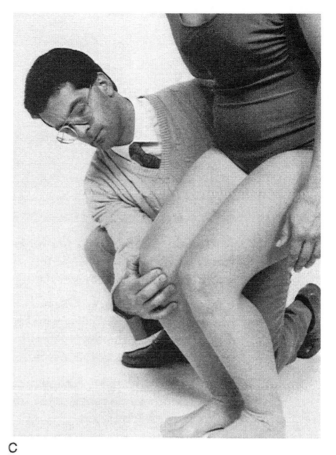

C

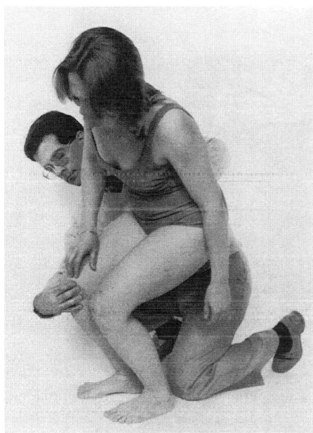

D

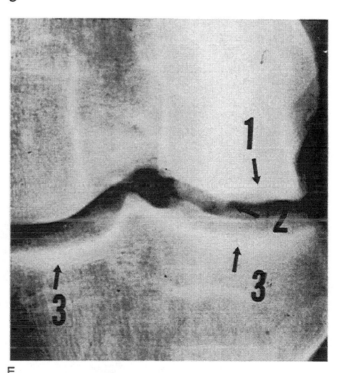

E

47 | *Wilson's Test*

Procedure: The patient is seated with the knees flexed over the examining table. Ask the patient to actively extend the knees to about 30 degrees of flexion while medially rotating the tibias. If pain is noted at this point, have the patient laterally rotate the tibias, keeping the knees flexed 30 degrees (Figs. A–D).

Rationale: The normal site for osteochondritis dissecans is at the medial femoral condyle. The first part of the test will aggravate this lesion. Lateral rotation does not stress the lesion, thereby alleviating the pain.

Classical Significance: Osteochondritis dissecans at the medial femoral condyle is present, if pain occurs when, with knee flexed 30 degrees, the leg is medially rotated, but dissapears when the leg is laterally rotated (Figs. C–E [E: arthrosis; 1, osteophytic changes; 2, joint mouse; 3, ossification of medial meniscus]).

Clinical Significance: Although rare, the test results will be opposite the above, if the osteochondritis dissecans is at the lateral femoral condyle instead of the medial condyle. Rule out plica syndrome.

Follow-up: Perform the patella grind test, the screw home test, the plica stutter test, or the mediopatella plica test.

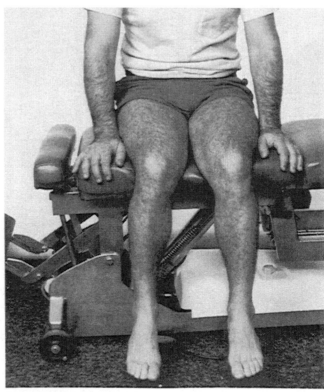

A

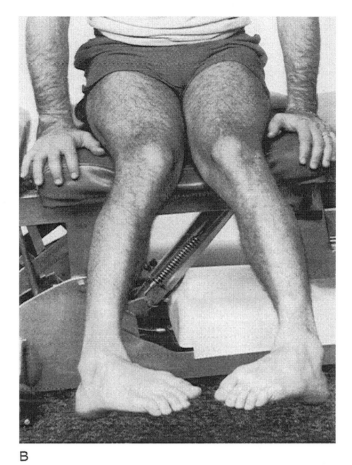

B

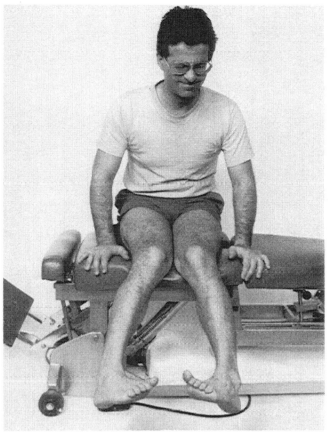

C

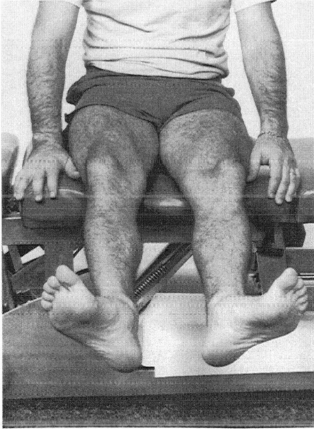

D

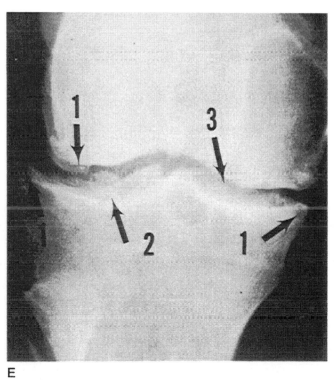

E

CHAPTER

12

Ankle and Feet Testing

1. Range of Motion Studies
2. Achilles Tap
3. Foot Drawer Test
4. Forefoot Adduction Correction Test
5. Forefoot Neuroma Squeeze Test
6. Hoffa's Sign
7. Kleiger Test
8. Lateral Stability Test
9. Medial Stability Test
10. Metatarsal Test
11. Side to Side Talar Test
12. Simmond's Test
13. Strunsky's Test
14. Talar Tilt Test
15. Test for Rigid or Supple Flatfeet
16. Tinel's Foot Test
17. Tourniquet Test

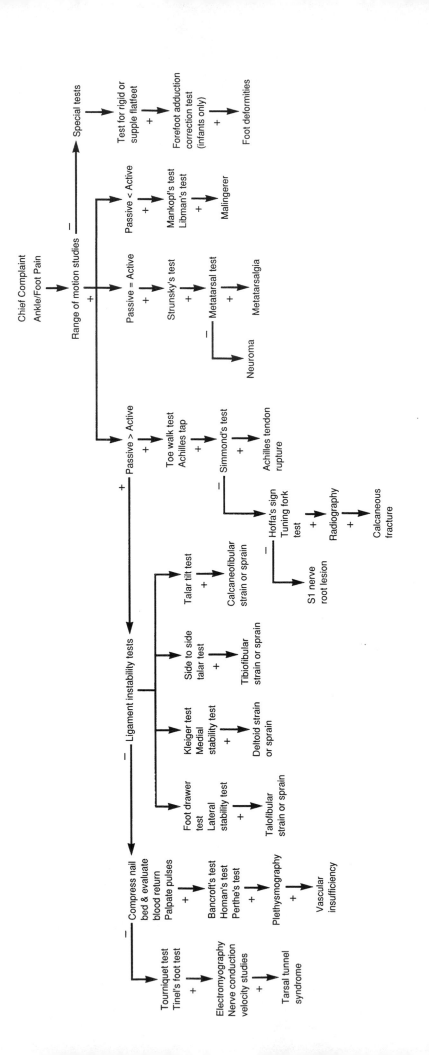

Chief Complaint
Ankle/Foot Pain

Range of motion studies

— → Special tests

+ → Test for rigid or supple flatfeet
+ → Forefoot adduction correction test (infants only)
+ → Foot deformities

+

Passive < Active
+ → Mankopf's test Libman's test
+ → Malingerer

Passive = Active
+ → Strunsky's test
+ → Metatarsal test
+ → Metatarsalgia
— → Neuroma

Passive > Active
+ → Toe walk test Achilles tap
+ → Simmond's test
+ → Achilles tendon rupture
— → Hoffa's sign Tuning fork test
+ → Radiography
+ → Calcaneous fracture
— → S1 nerve root lesion

+ Ligament instability tests

Foot drawer test Lateral stability test
+ → Talofibular strain or sprain

Kleiger test Medial stability test
+ → Deltoid strain or sprain

Side to side talar test
+ → Tibiofibular strain or sprain

Talar tilt test
+ → Calcaneofibular strain or sprain

— Compress nail bed & evaluate blood return Palpate pulses

Bancroft's test Homan's test Perthe's test
+ → Plethysmography
+ → Vascular insufficiency

Tourniquet test Tinel's foot test
+ → Electromyography Nerve conduction velocity studies
+ → Tarsal tunnel syndrome

1 Range of Motion Studies

When performing range of motion studies, it is important to use either an arthrodial protractor or an inclinometer. The *American Medical Association Guides for Impairment Ratings* now recommend the use of the inclinometer exclusively.

Dorsiflexion: The patient is supine with the ankles off the end of the examining table. Ask the patient to flex the foot upward as far as possible. Normal dorsiflexion is 20 degrees.

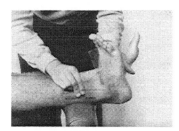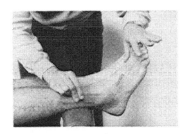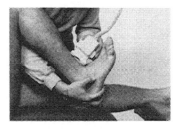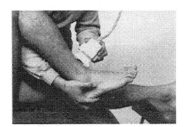

Plantar Flexion: The patient is supine with the ankles off the end of the examining table. Ask the patient to flex the foot downward as far as possible. Normal plantar flexion is 50 degrees.

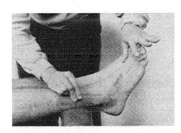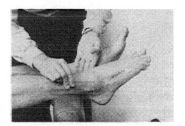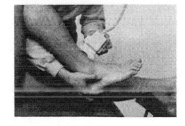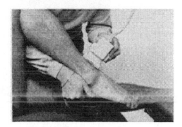

Inversion: The patient is supine with the ankles off the end of the examining table. Ask the patient to bend the feet medially so that the bottoms of the feet face each other. This is also known as supination. Normal inversion is 5 degrees.

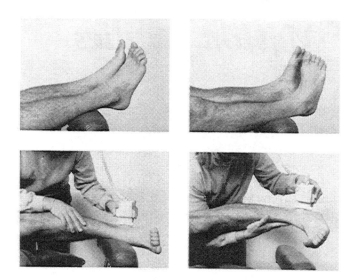

Eversion: The patient is supine with the ankles off the end of the examining table. Ask the patient to bend the feet laterally so that the bottoms of the feet face away from each other. This is also known as pronation. Normal eversion is 5 degrees.

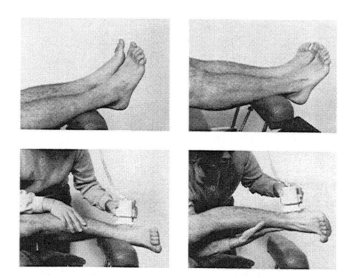

Quick Test: As a quick reference for proper functioning of the ankle and foot have the patient do the following. For plantar flexion and toe motion, ask the patient to walk on the toes. For dorsiflexion and toe motion, ask the patient to walk on the heels. For inversion, ask the patient to walk on the lateral borders of the feet. For eversion, ask the patient to walk on the medial borders of the feet. If the patient is unable to perform any of these quick tests, perform the passive ranges of motion to help determine the nature of the restriction.

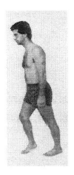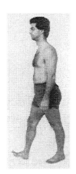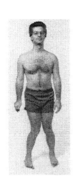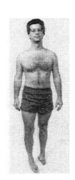

2 | *Achilles Tap*

Procedure: The patient is prone. Flex the patient's knee 90 degrees and force the ankle into dorsiflexion. Then strike the Achilles tendon with a percussion hammer (Figs. A–D).

Rationale: This test is similar to testing the S1 nerve root reflex. By dorsiflexing the ankle before striking the tendon, the tension in the tendon is increased, making any subtle plantar flexion more visible.

Classical Significance: Normally plantar flexion should occur when the tendon is hit. If this does not happen even with forced dorsiflexion, suspect an Achilles tendon rupture (Fig. E).

Clinical Significance: A positive test could also indicate neuropathy of another origin that is affecting the S1 nerve root.

Follow-up: Perform Simmond's test.

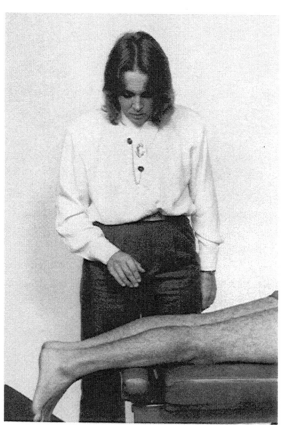

A

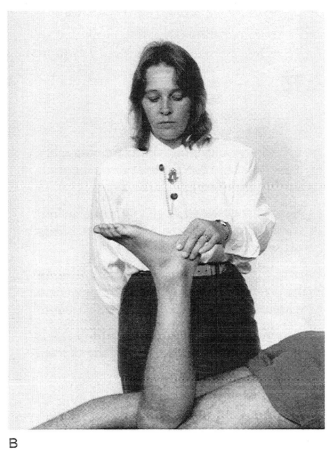

B

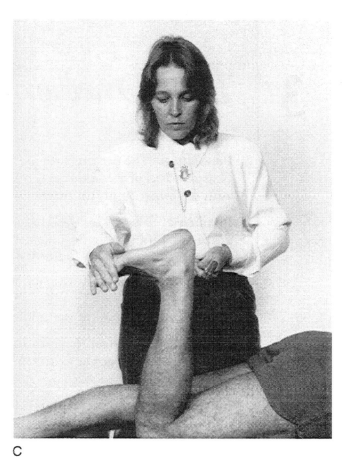

C

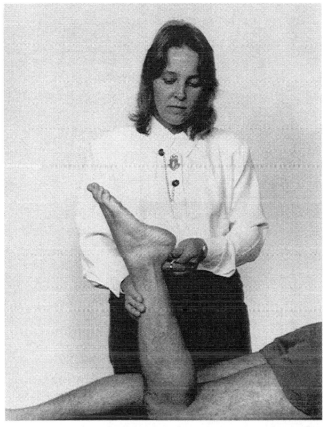

D

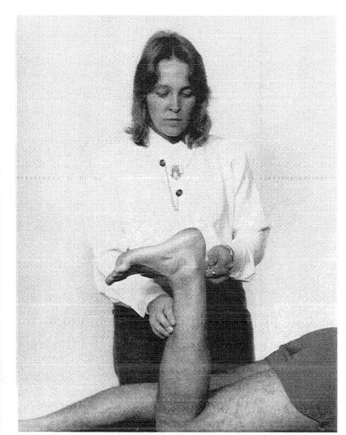

E

3 | Foot Drawer Test

Procedure: The patient is supine with the ankles off the end of the examining table. Grasp the heel of the ankle being tested with one hand and the tibia just above the ankle with the other. Apply an anterior and then a posterior force (Figs. A–D).

Rationale: The ankle is held together by ligaments designed to give support, including the anterior talofibular, calcaneofibular, and posterior talofibular ligaments. Laxity or damage to any of the ligaments will result in excessive ankle play (Fig. E).

Classical Significance: Excessive anterior movement of the talus in relation to the ankle mortise indicates an anterior talofibular problem. Excessive posterior movement of the talus in relation to the ankle mortise indicates a posterior talofibular problem.

Clinical Significance: In infants and young children, extra movement in the ankle is normal and should not be mistaken for ligament damage. Always compare the affected side to the unaffected side.

Follow-up: Perform the lateral stability test or the medial stability test.

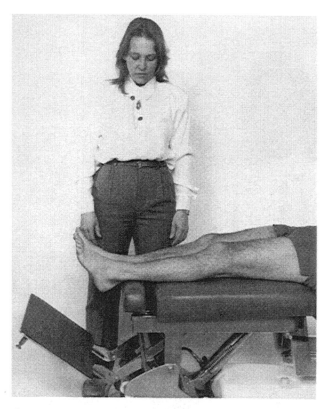

A

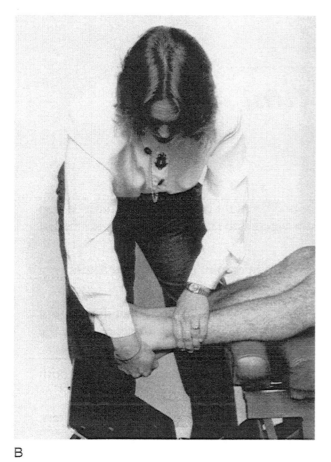

B

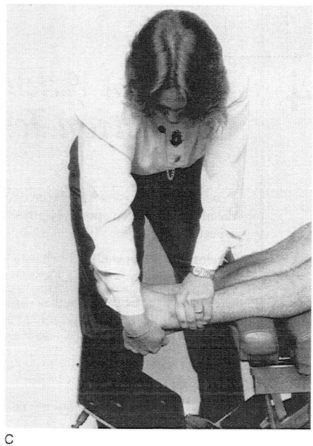

C

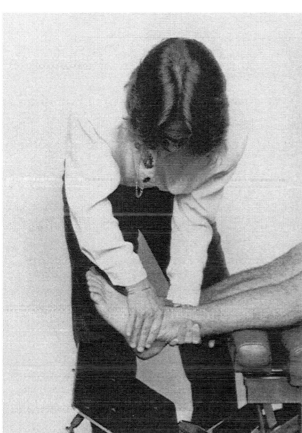

D

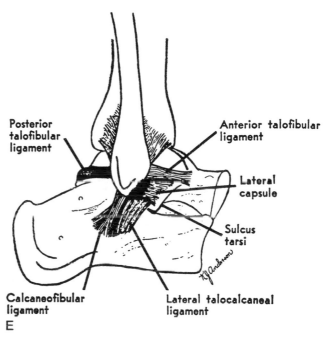

Posterior talofibular ligament

Anterior talofibular ligament

Lateral capsule

Sulcus tarsi

Calcaneofibular ligament

Lateral talocalcaneal ligament

E

4 | *Forefoot Adduction Correction Test*

Procedure: This test is performed on infants. The infant is supine on the table. Grasp the heel to support it and apply pressure from a medial to lateral direction on the medial aspect of the forefoot (Figs. A–E).

Rationale: Infants normally have a greater amount of joint play. Restricted joint play in what normally would be increased indicates an abnormality.

Classical Significance: In the normal infant, it will be possible to abduct the forefoot past the midline. If the forefoot cannot be abducted beyond the midline, evaluate the infant for orthopaedic appliances required to prevent permanent deformity.

Clinical Significance: This problem can be bilateral; therefore, be sure to check both sides when performing this test.

Follow-up: Perform the lateral stability test, medial stability test, or foot drawer test.

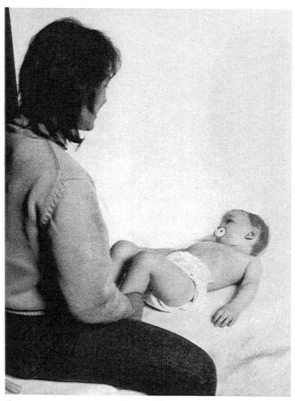

A

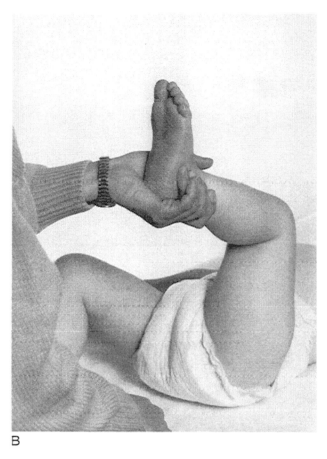

B

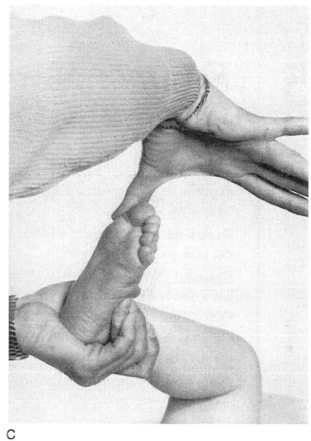

C

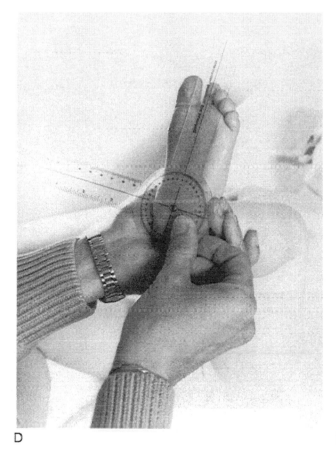

D

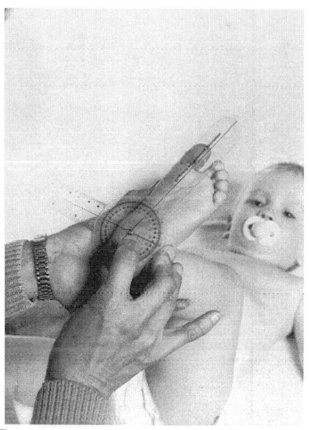

E

5 | *Forefoot Neuroma Squeeze Test*

Procedure: The patient is supine. Grasp the forefoot of the patient and squeeze the metatarsal area (Figs. A–C).

Rationale: In the patient who has metatarsalgia associated with a neuroma, lancinating pain will be reproduced.

Classical Significance: Reproduction of lancinating pain or an increase of pain that has a needle-like quality is positive for neuroma (Fig. D: inset, growth on neuron with cystic swelling).

Clinical Significance: Although uncommon in the metatarsal area, arthritis within the metatarsus can become symptomatic when the foot is squeezed (Fig. E).

Follow-up: Perform Strunsky's test or Tinel's foot test.

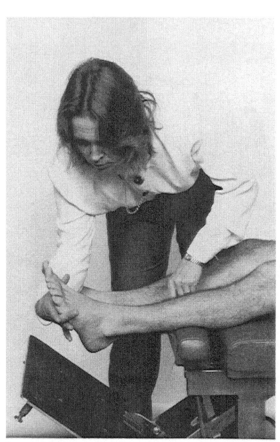

A

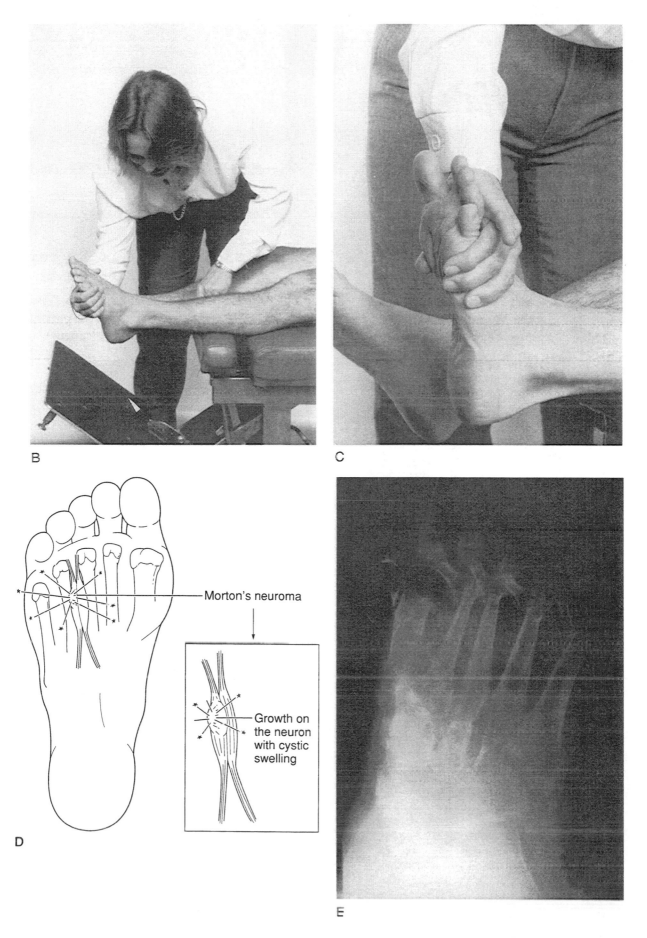

B

C

Morton's neuroma

Growth on
the neuron
with cystic
swelling

D

E

6 | *Hoffa's Sign*

Procedure: The patient is prone with the legs off the end of the examining table. Place your hands on the bottom of the feet and move the ankles (Figs. A–D).

Rationale: In calcaneal avulsion fracture, the Achilles tendon may pull away, causing it to be less tense.

Classical Significance: A decrease in tension of the Achilles tendon or a slightly more dorsiflexed ankle on the affected side signifies a calcaneal avulsion fracture (Fig. E).

Clinical Significance: A good, simple method to test whether the sign is positive is to ask the patient to walk on the toes. If a calcaneal avulsion fracture is present, the patient will not be able to do this (Fig. F: arrows, multiple fracture lines in the calcaneus).

Follow-up: Perform Simmond's test or the Achilles tap.

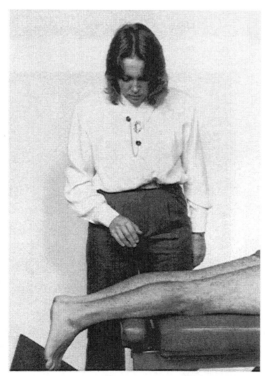

A

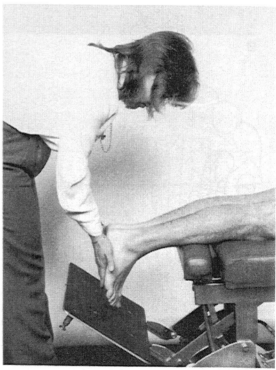

B

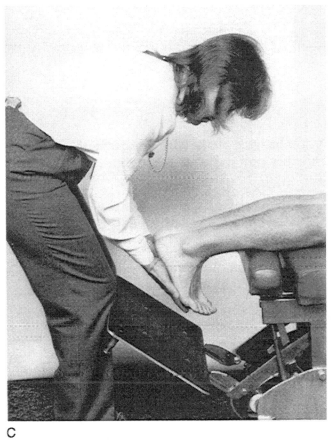

C

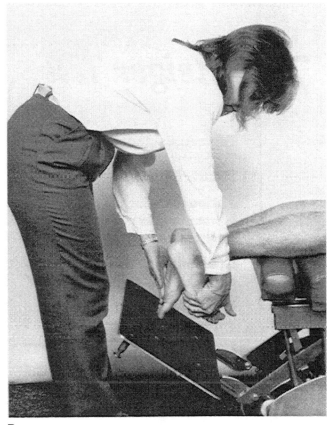

D

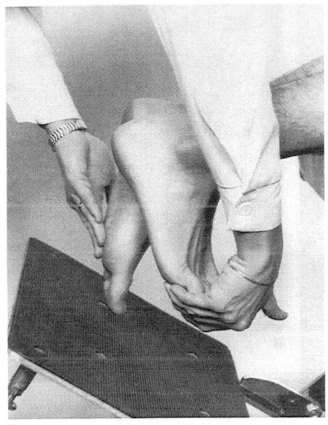

E

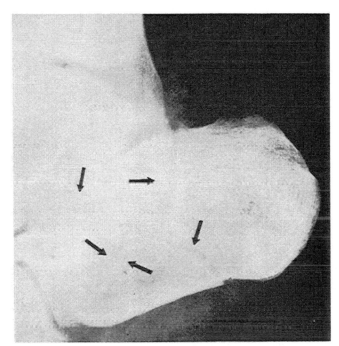

7 | *Kleiger Test*

Procedure: The patient is seated with the feet hanging off the edge of the table. Grasp the patient's foot and, while stabilizing the tibia with the other hand, rotate the foot laterally (Figs. A–D).

Rationale: The deltoid ligament of the ankle provides support when the ankle is everted, thereby preventing injury. In the above test, when lateral rotation is performed, an element of eversion is present as well.

Classical Significance: Pain medially in the ankle joint and extra play in the talus as it displaces from the medial malleolus indicates a deltoid ligament problem (Fig. E).

Clinical Significance: Some people have extra laxity in their ankles, dancers for example. To determine whether a problem exists, compare bilaterally; if only laxity exists, this may be normal for that patient (Fig. F).

Follow-up: Perform the lateral stability test or the medial stability test.

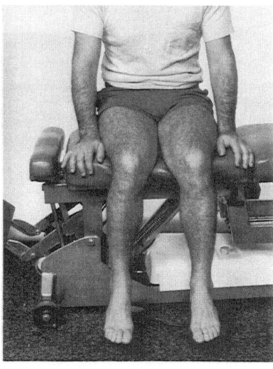

A

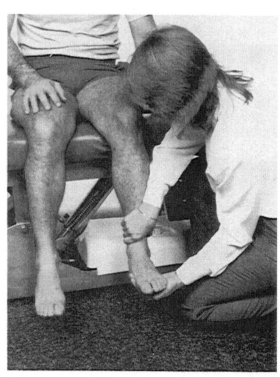

B

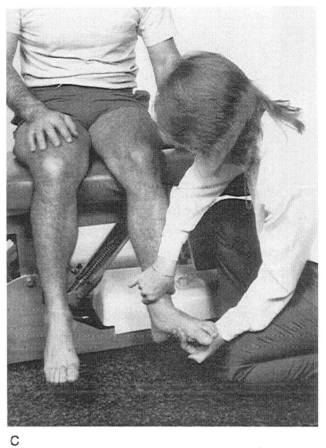

C

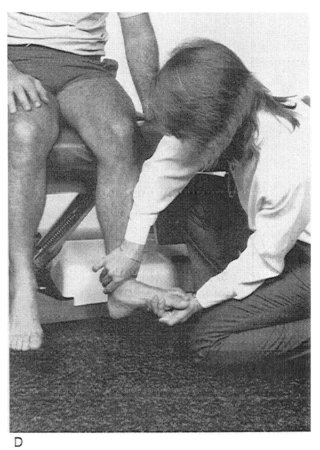

D

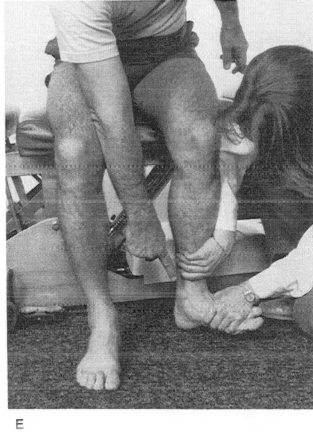

E

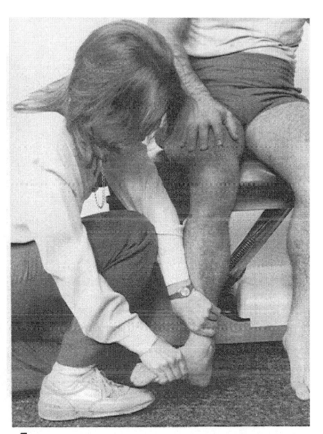

F

8 | *Lateral Stability Test (Inversion Test)*

Procedure: The patient is supine. Grasp behind the ankle with one hand and the bottom of the foot with the other. Then passively rotate the foot into inversion (Figs. A–C).

Rationale: The normal ranges of motion for eversion and inversion are contained by functioning ligaments. Injury to any of these ligaments results in excessive play in the joint (Fig. D).

Classical Significance: If excessive inversion occurs, consider anterior talofibular injury or calcaneofibular injury. Inversion sprains are the most common ankle injury and almost always involve the anterior talofibular ligament (Fig. E).

Clinical Significance: Infants and young children normally have extra movement in the ankle, which should not be mistaken for ligament damage. Always compare the affected side to the unaffected side.

Follow-up: Perform the foot drawer test or the medial stability test.

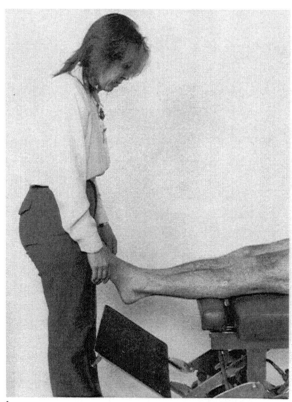

A

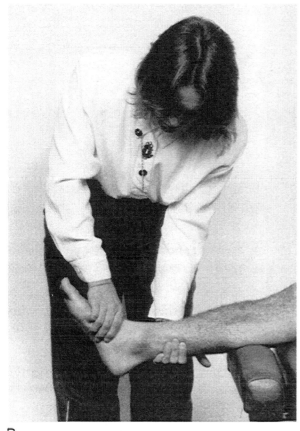

B

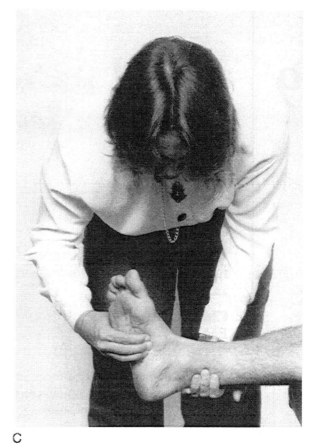

C

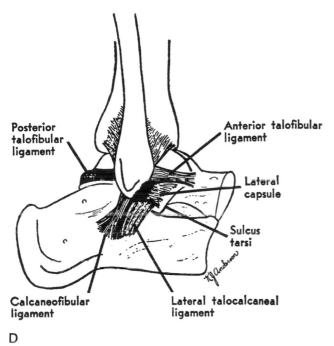

Posterior
talofibular
ligament

Anterior talofibular
ligament

Lateral
capsule

Sulcus
tarsi

Calcaneofibular
ligament

Lateral talocalcaneal
ligament

D

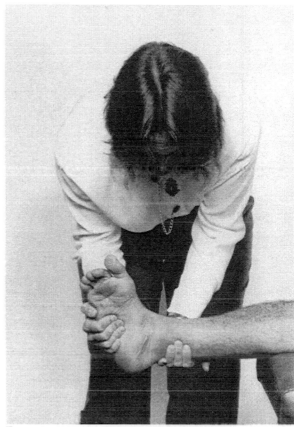

E

9 | *Medial Stability Test (Eversion Test)*

Procedure: The patient is supine. Grasp behind the ankle with one hand and the bottom of the foot with the other. Then passively rotate the foot into eversion (Figs. A–C).

Rationale: The normal ranges of motion for eversion and inversion are contained by functioning ligaments. Injury to any of these ligaments results in excessive play in the ankle (Fig. D).

Classical Significance: If excessive eversion occurs, consider deltoid ligament injury. Eversion sprains are not nearly as common as inversion sprains. People who have a fallen medial longitudinal arch are more susceptible to eversion sprains (Fig. E).

Clinical Significance: Infants and young children normally have extra movement in the ankle; this should not be mistaken for ligament damage. Always compare the affected side to the unaffected side.

Follow-up: Perform the foot drawer test or the lateral stability test.

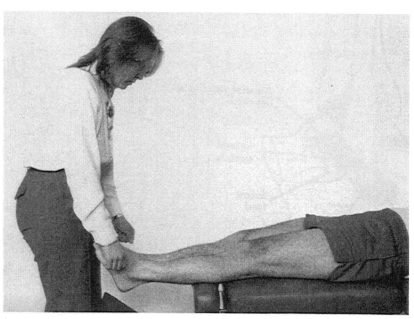

A

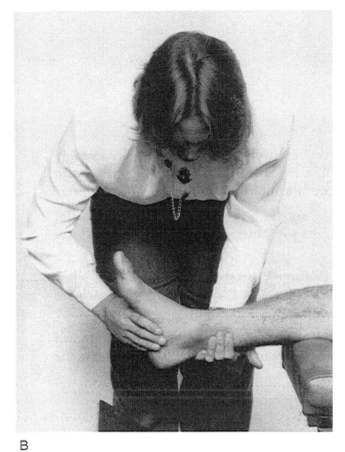

B

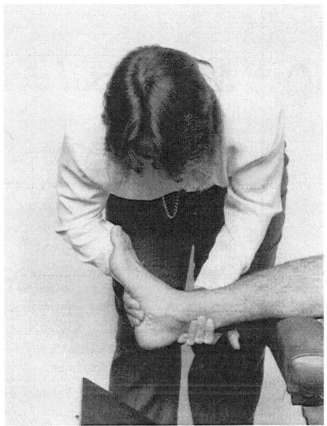

C

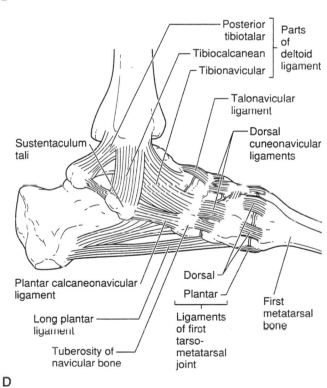

Posterior tibiotalar ⎤ Parts
Tibiocalcanean ⎥ of deltoid
Tibionavicular ⎦ ligament

Talonavicular ligament

Dorsal cuneonavicular ligaments

Sustentaculum tali

Plantar calcaneonavicular ligament

Long plantar ligament

Dorsal
Plantar
Ligaments of first tarso-metatarsal joint

First metatarsal bone

Tuberosity of navicular bone

D

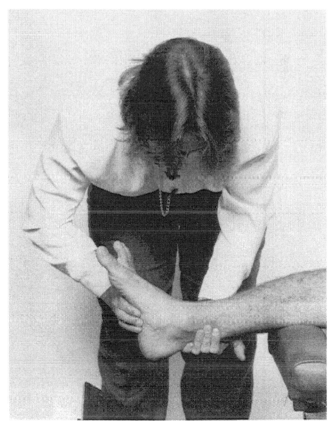

E

10 | *Metatarsal Test*

Procedure: The patient is supine with the feet over the edge of the table. Strongly dorsiflex the toes so that the ball of the foot is prominent. Then, using a percussion hammer, strike each protruding metatarsophalangeal joint (Figs. A–D).

Rationale: When the metatarsal translates anteriorly, inflammation within the joint occurs. Tapping the ball of the foot in patients with anterior metatarsalgia will increase the pain over the sites being tested.

Classical Significance: Pain over the inflamed metatarsophalangeal joint when struck with a percussion hammer is a positive test (Fig. E: nonspecific origin includes mechanical stresses and degenerative changes).

Clinical Significance: Morton's neuroma can cause pain under the third to fourth metatarsophalangeal joint as well; therefore, check a positive result by performing the forefoot neuroma squeeze test.

Follow-up: Perform the forefoot neuroma squeeze test or Strunsky's test.

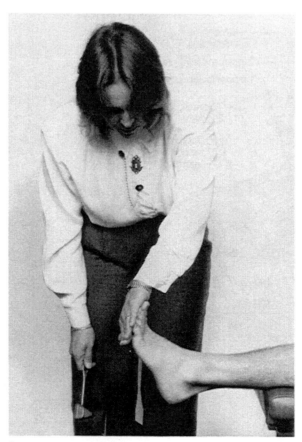

A

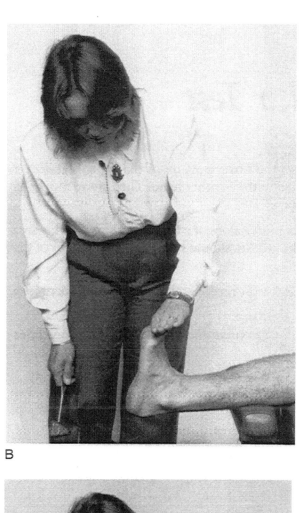

B

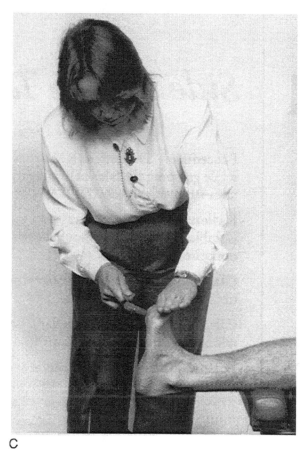

C

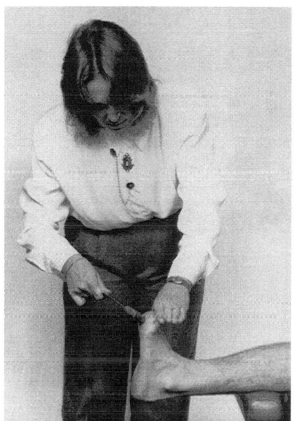

D

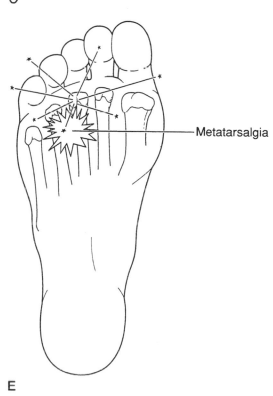

Metatarsalgia

E

11 | *Side to Side Talar Test*

Procedure: The patient is seated. Grasp the lower portion of the leg to stabilize it while grasping the talus below the malleoli with the other hand. Then try to move the talus from side to side (Figs. A–D).

Rationale: This motion causes a sheering force along the talofibular joint. If this area is stable, no movement should be felt. The motion should be comparable to that of the opposite talus (Fig. E).

Classical Significance: Excessive motion or the reproduction of pain indicates a torn tibiofibular ligament.

Clinical Significance: The injury may be extensive enough to involve the posterior talofibular and talotibial ligaments.

Follow-up: Perform the medial and lateral stability tests.

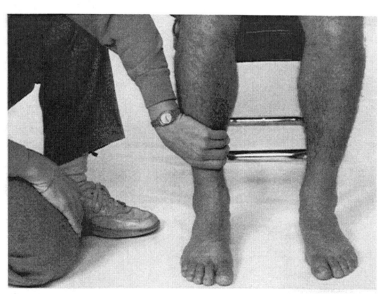

A

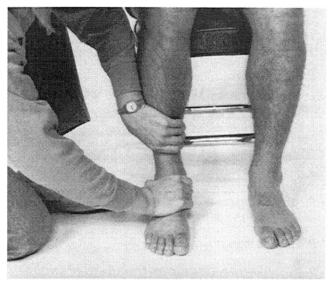

B

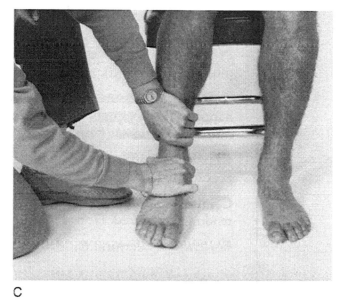

C

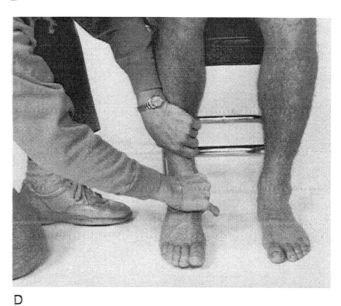

D

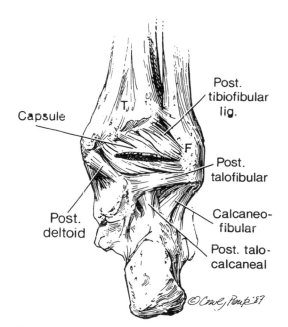

Capsule

Post.
deltoid

Post.
tibiofibular
lig.

Post.
talofibular

Calcaneo-
fibular

Post. talo-
calcaneal

T

F

©Craig Roup '87

E

12 | *Simmond's Test (Thompson Test)*

Procedure: The patient is prone. Flex the knee 90 degrees and then squeeze the calf muscles (Figs. A–C).

Rationale: Pressure into the calf muscles causes the muscles to shorten. When this happens, their common tendon (the Achilles) pulls on the calcaneus, forcing the foot into a slight plantar flexion.

Classical Significance: If plantar flexion does not occur, suspect an Achilles tendon rupture (Fig. D).

Clinical Significance: In deep thrombophlebitis, pain will result when the Achilles tendon is squeezed. However, normal plantar flexion will still occur (Fig. E).

Follow-up: Perform the Achilles tap or Hoffa's sign.

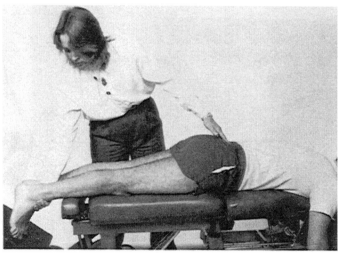

A

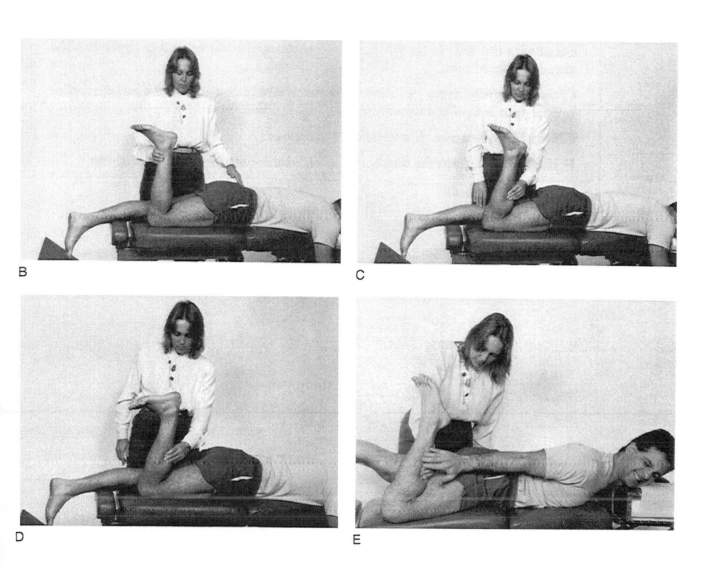

B

C

D

E

13 | *Strunsky's Test*

Procedure: The patient is supine with the feet straight out and extending off the table. Forcibly grasp the patient's toes and quickly flex them downward (Figs. A–C).

Rationale: In the normal patient without metatarsalgia, no discomfort will be associated with this test. In the patient with metatarsalgia, this maneuver aggravates the already inflamed joint.

Classical Significance: An increase in sharp pain in and around the metatarsophalangeal joint is significant for metatarsalgia (Figs. D & E).

Clinical Significance: See Classical Significance.

Follow-up: Perform the forefoot neuroma squeeze test or the metatarsal test.

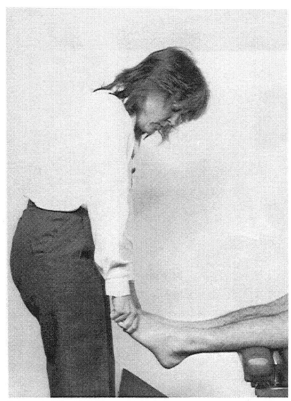

A

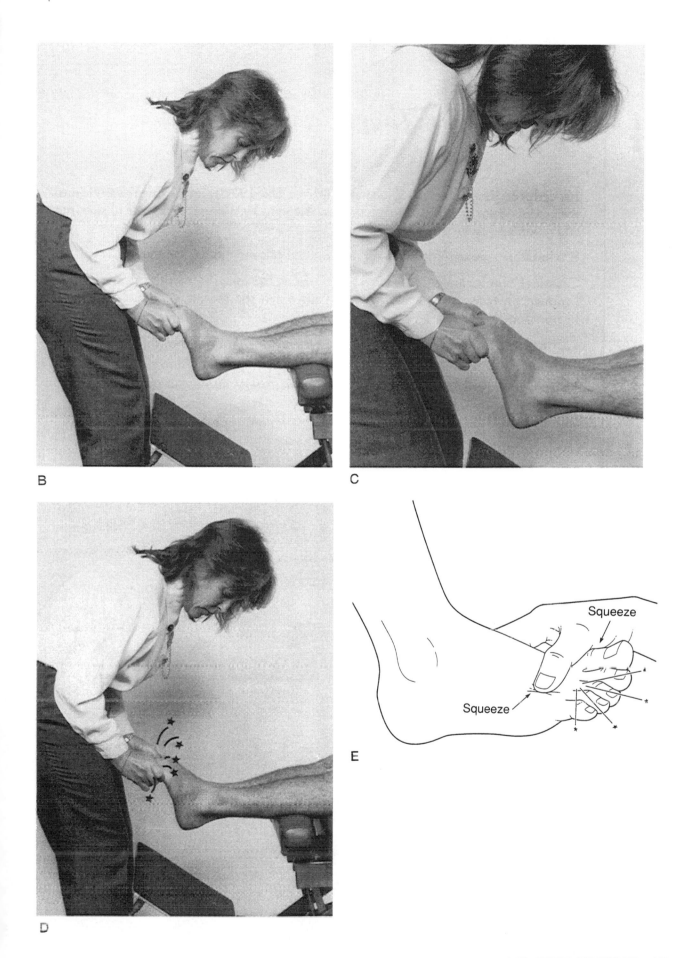

B

C

D

E

Squeeze

Squeeze

14 | *Talar Tilt Test*

Procedure: The patient is supine with the knee flexed 90 degrees. Bring the ankle into the anatomic position and then stress the ankle joint by tilting it from side to side into adduction and abduction (Figs. A–E).

Rationale: Adduction of the talus stresses the calcaneofibular ligament.

Classical Significance: An increase in pain at the location of the calcaneofibular ligament or excessive inversion of the talus when the foot is adducted signifies a ligamentous lesion.

Clinical Significance: Damage to the calcaneofibular ligament due to inversion sprain usually occurs after the anterior talofibular has been damaged.

Follow-up: Perform the foot drawer test or the lateral and medial stability tests.

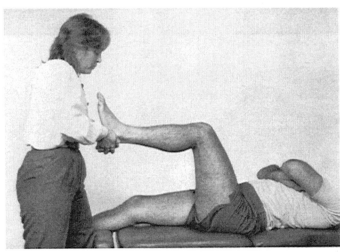

A

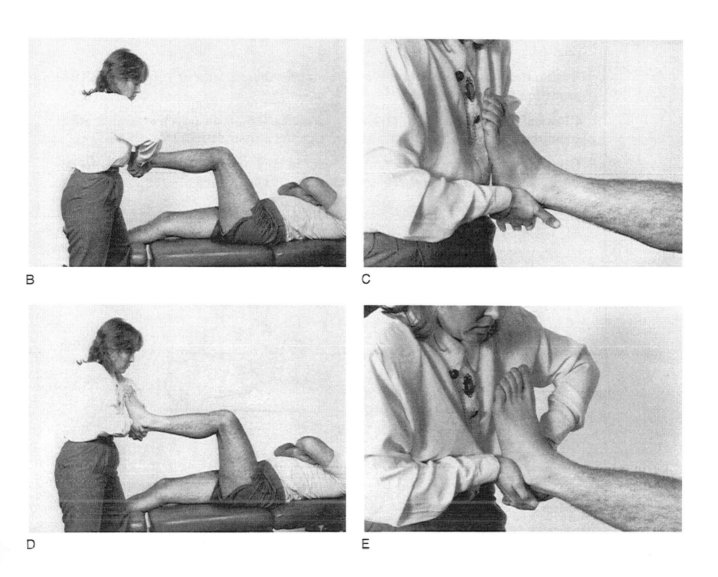

B

C

D

E

15 | *Test for Rigid or Supple Flatfeet*

Procedure: Observe the feet as the patient stands on the toes and on the complete foot (Fig. A).

Rationale: Observation of the medial arch in these positions reveals correctable pronation faults of the longitudinal arch.

Classical Significance: The absence of the medial longitudinal arch when the patient stands on the toes and on the whole foot signifies a rigid flatfoot (Figs. B & C).

Clinical Significance: If the arch is absent in only one of the positions, the foot is supple and the arch is correctable with orthoses (Figs. D & E).

Follow-up: Perform the forefoot adduction correction test.

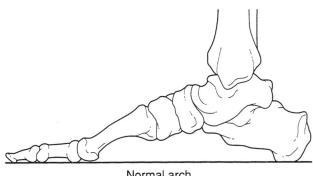

Normal arch

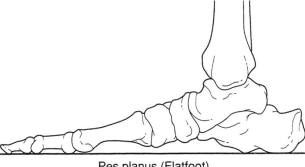

Pes planus (Flatfoot)

A

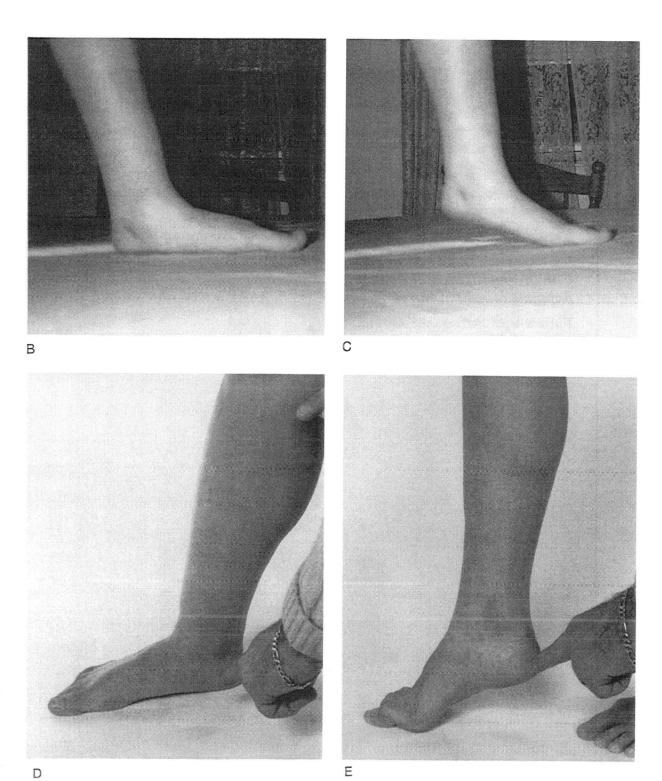

B

C

D

E

16 | *Tinel's Foot Test*

Procedure: The patient is supine with the foot and ankle off the table. Using a percussion hammer, strike the area over the posterior tibial nerve on the medial side of the ankle just posterior and superior to the malleolus (Figs. A–C).

Rationale: If nerve irritation is present, striking the area above the nerve will exacerbate the patient's symptoms of paresthesia and dysesthesia. This test is similar to Tinel's test used for carpal tunnel syndrome.

Classical Significance: An increase in dysesthesia or paresthesis in the foot is positive and indicates tarsal tunnel syndrome (Figs. D & E).

Clinical Significance: If motor weakness is seen as well as muscle atrophy, the nerve damage is considered advanced; do not expect a favorable recovery.

Follow-up: Perform the tourniquet test.

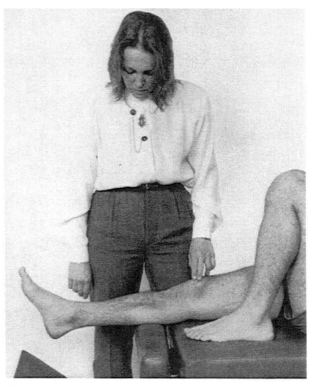

A

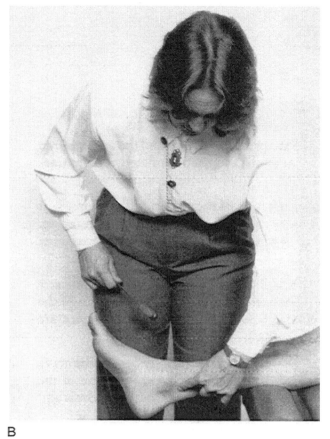

B

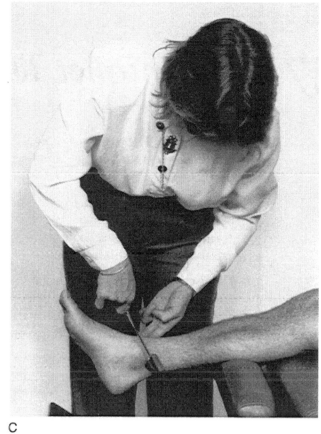

C

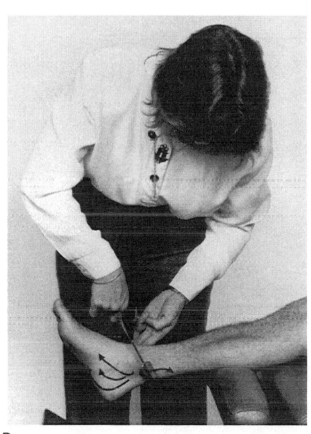

D

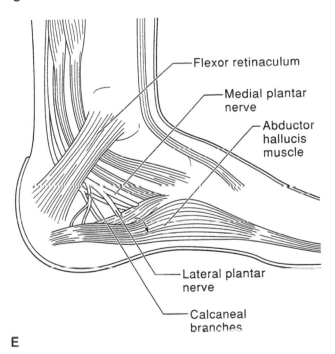

Flexor retinaculum

Medial plantar nerve

Abductor hallucis muscle

Lateral plantar nerve

Calcaneal branches

E

17 | *Tourniquet Test*

Procedure: The patient is supine. Place a blood pressure cuff around the ankle, pump it up enough to occlude the blood supply to the ankle, and keep it inflated for 2 minutes (Figs. A–C).

Rationale: Tarsal tunnel syndrome is a compression of the posterior tibial nerve as it passes through the tunnel under the flexor retinaculum on the medial side of the ankle. An increase in pressure around the retinaculum when the syndrome is symptomatic can cause a burning pain into the foot.

Classical Significance: An increase in a burning-type pain into the foot indicates compression of the posterior tibial nerve. Classically, a sensory loss in the area of the distribution of the medial and lateral plantar nerves will result. These nerves are branches of the posterior tibial nerve (Figs. D & E).

Clinical Significance: If motor weakness, as well as muscle atrophy occurs, the nerve damage is considered advanced; do not expect a favorable recovery. Inflation of the blood pressure cuff will cause extreme pain in the patient with thrombophlebitis and full inflation will not be possible.

Follow-up: Perform Tinel's foot test.

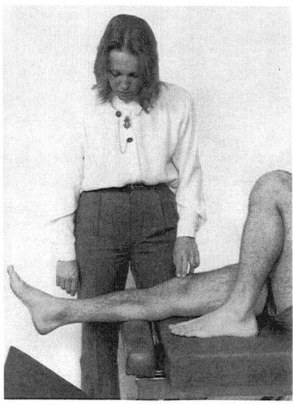

A

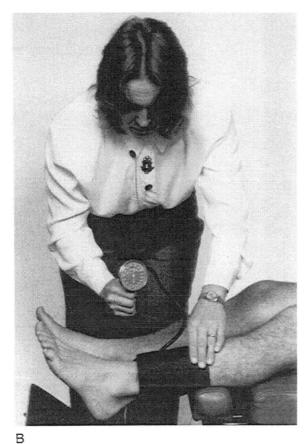

B

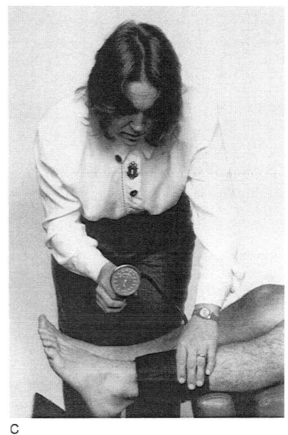

C

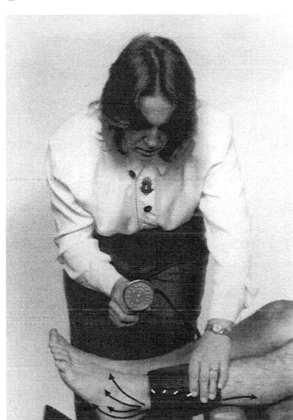

D

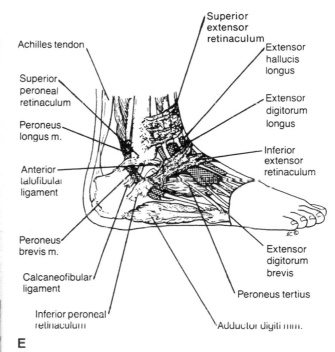

Achilles tendon

Superior
peroneal
retinaculum

Peroneus
longus m.

Anterior
talofibular
ligament

Peroneus
brevis m.

Calcaneofibular
ligament

Inferior peroneal
retinaculum

Superior
extensor
retinaculum

Extensor
hallucis
longus

Extensor
digitorum
longus

Inferior
extensor
retinaculum

Extensor
digitorum
brevis

Peroneus tertius

Adductor digiti mm.

E

1 | *Bancroft's Test (Moses' Sign)*

Procedure: The patient is prone with the legs fully extended. Compress the calf, pressing the calf muscle into the tibia. Then, grasp the calf, lifting it away from the tibia (Mose's sign). Compare the patient's responses to these maneuvers (Figs. A–C).

Rationale: If the venous system is inflamed, compression into the tibia will cause an increase in pain because of aggravation of the veins. Lifting the calf muscle off the tibia will alleviate the pain somewhat.

Classical Significance: The test is positive when more pain occurs on compression than on lifting the calf off the tibia (Fig. D). This is significant for thrombophlebitis.

Clinical Significance: Compressing the muscle onto the tibia and then lifting it off will have no effect on the pain, if lumbar radiculopathy is the cause (Figs. E & F).

Follow-up: Perform Lowenberg's sign, Homan's test, or Pratt's test.

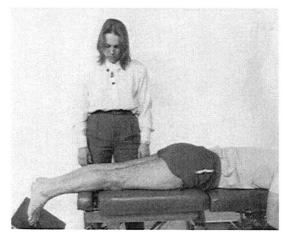

A

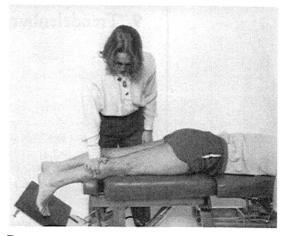

B

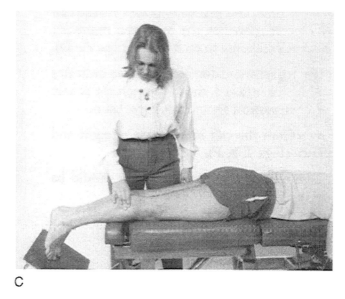

C

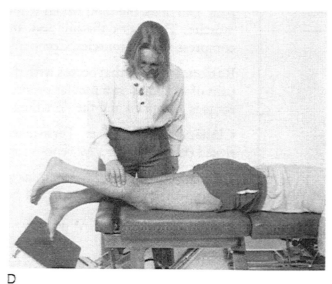

D

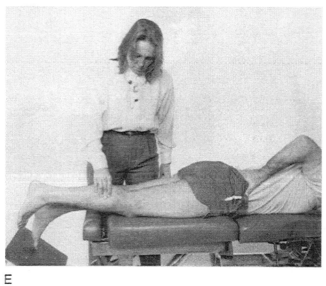

E

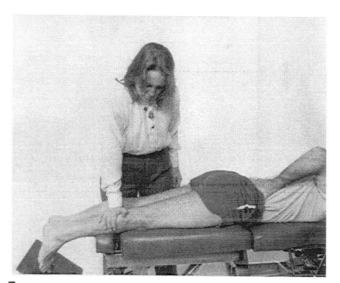

F

2 | *Homan's Test*

Procedure: The patient is supine. Raise the suspected leg off the table; this will cause pain. Dorsiflex the foot, which will cause more pain, and manually compress the calf muscles. Then, flex the hip and knee 90 degrees, dorsiflex the foot, and manually compress the calf muscles. Compare the patient's response to each phase (Figs. A–D).

Rationale: Pain that occurs with the straight leg raise and dorsiflexion often indicates pain of vertebral or muscular origin. When the leg is flexed, the tension on the sciatic roots is alleviated and the dorsiflexion and compression should not cause pain.

Classical Significance: Persistence of pain from the calf in both the straight and flexed positions indicates venous insufficiency (Figs. E & F).

Clinical Significance: Muscular pain from the gastrocnemius muscles should be reduced with the leg in the flexed position.

Follow-up: Perform the Trendelenburg test or Perthe's test.

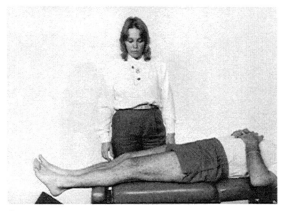

A

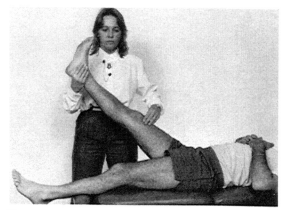

B

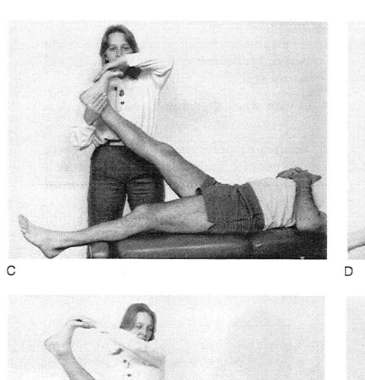

C

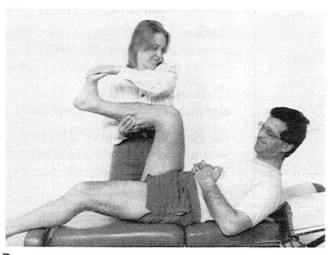

D

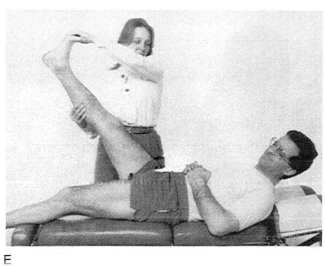

E

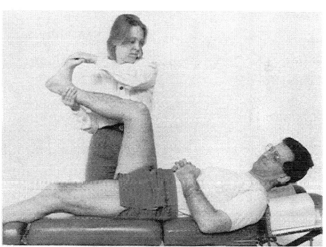

F

3 | *Louvel's Test*

Procedure: The patient is standing. Ask the patient to sneeze. If this increases the pain into the calves, apply digital pressure just proximal to the involved vein and ask the patient to sneeze again. Record the patient's responses (Figs. A–E).

Rationale: Sneezing increases venous pressure and can evoke pain at the site of the thrombophlebitis in the calves. The digital pressure alleviates the flow backward and should reduce the pain when the patient sneezes again.

Classical Significance: Alleviation of the pain when digital pressure is applied is significant for thrombophlebitis.

Clinical Significance: This test can also result in a painful response if lumbar nerve root lesions are present. However, the pain will not be relieved when digital pressure is applied if lumbar nerve root lesions are the cause of the pain. This is the differential diagnosis.

Follow-up: Perform Homan's test, Bancroft's test, or the tourniquet test (see Ch. 12).

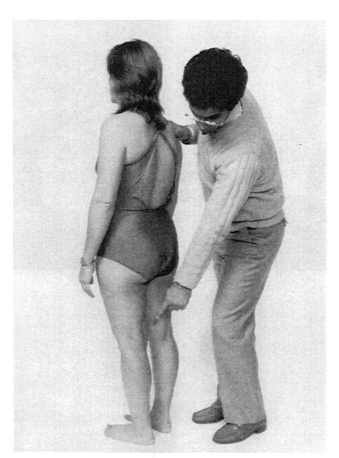

A

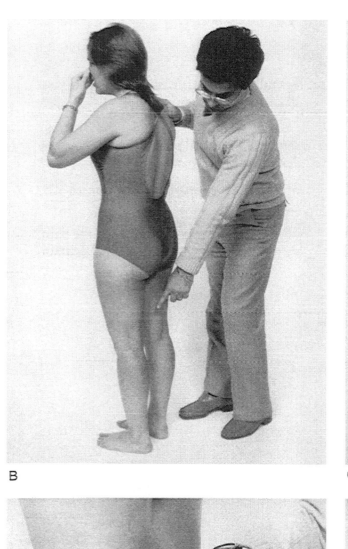

B

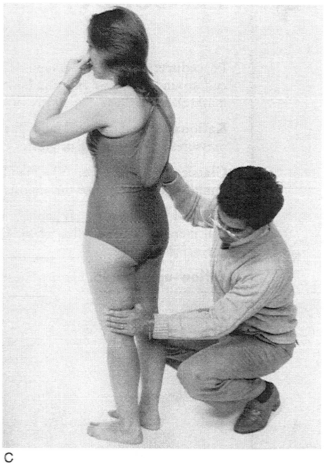

C

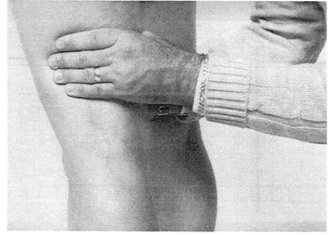

D

E

4 | *Lowenberg's Sign*

Procedure: The patient is supine with the legs fully extended. Wrap a blood pressure cuff around each calf and simultaneously inflate them (to a minimum of 175 to 180 mmHg). Record the patient's response (Figs. A–D).

Rationale: In the normal individual, the inflation of the blood pressure cuff to normal pressures of 175 mmHg or greater can be tolerated without pain.

Classical Significance: The inability to withstand the pressure of inflation to 175 mmHg is significant for thrombosis (Fig. E).

Clinical Significance: If lumbar radiculopathy is the cause of the calf pain, the pain will increase with inflation of the blood pressure cuff, but the pressure will remain normal (Fig. F).

Follow-up: Perform Homan's test, Bancroft's test, or Pratt's test.

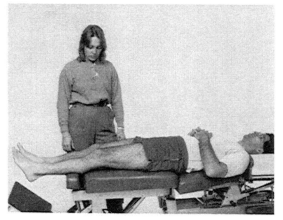

A

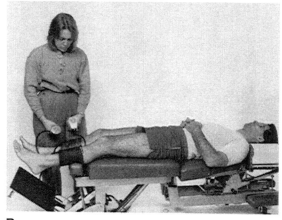

B

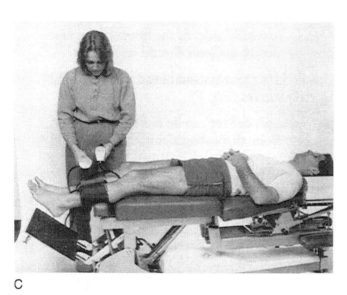

C

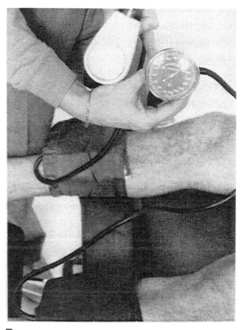

D

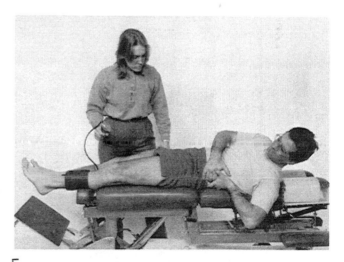

E

F

5 | *Peabody's Sign*

Procedure: The patient is supine with the legs fully extended. Place your thumbs under the second metatarsal head of each foot and apply pressure, lifting the feet 2 ft off the table. Observe the alignment of the medial malleoli as well as of the first metatarsals (Figs. A–E).

Rationale: When this position is maintained, the medial sides of the heads of the first metatarsals should be at the same level and the medial malleoli should be aligned.

Classical Significance: A difference in the levels of the metatarsal heads as the medial malleoli are aligned signifies spasm of the calf muscles (Fig. F).

Clinical Significance: Pain associated with this procedure can be due to the amount of pressure applied to the metatarsal head or from thrombophlebitis. This should reduce slightly as the leg is raised.

Follow-up: Perform Homan's test, Louvel's test, or Ramirez's test.

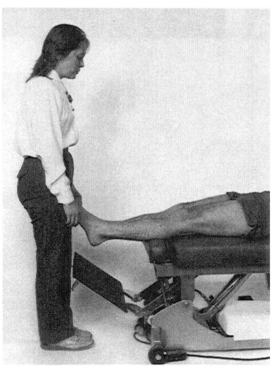

A

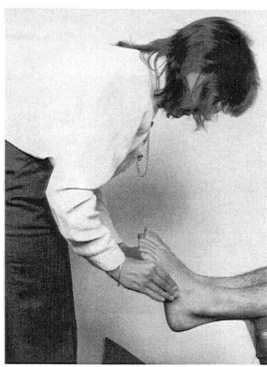

B

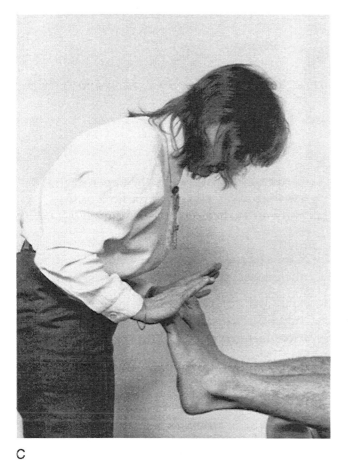

C

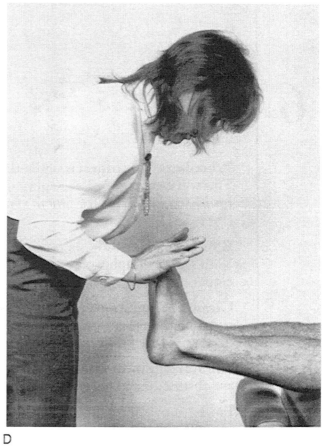

D

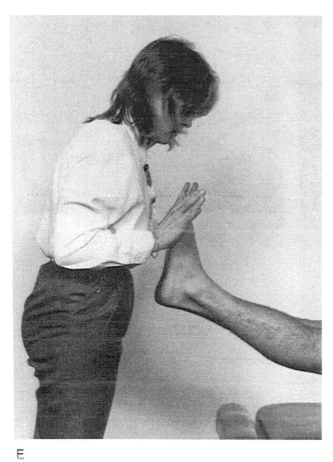

E

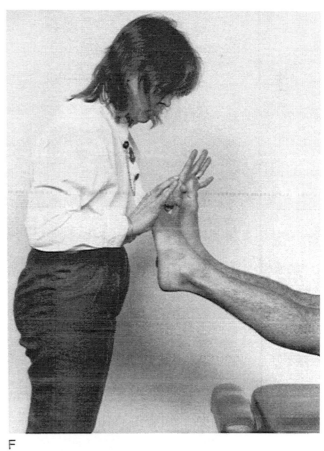

F

6 | *Perthe's Test*

Procedure: The patient is supine. Place an elastic tourniquet around the upper thigh. This will compress the long saphenous vein. Ask the patient to exercise the limb briskly for 60 seconds. Note the prominence of any varicosities before and after the exercise (Figs. A–D).

Rationale: Normally, the muscular action of the exercise will cause the veins to drain. With the long saphenous vein compressed, the deeper communicating veins should empty the area.

Classical Significance: If the superficial varicosities disappear, the valves of the communicating veins are competent. If the varicosities remain, both the superficial and deep valves are incompetent (Figs. E & F).

Clinical Significance: If the varicosities worsen and if pain develops, the deep veins are obstructed and the communicating veins are incompetent.

Follow-up: Perform the tourniquet test (see Ch. 12) or Homan's test.

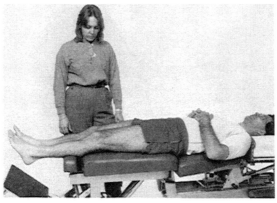

A

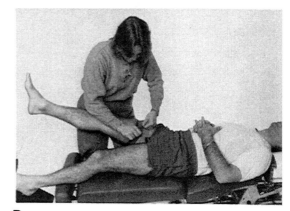

B

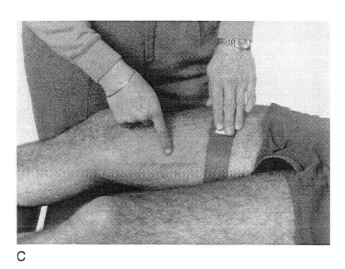

C

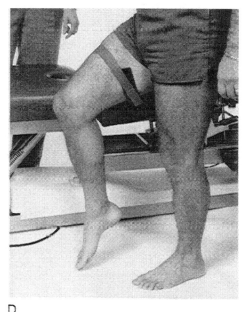

D

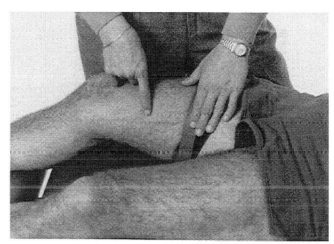

E

F

7 | *Pratt's Test*

Procedure: The patient is supine with the leg elevated onto the examiner's shoulder. Apply a tourniquet to the upper thigh to compress the long saphenous vein. Apply an elastic bandage from the toes to the tourniquet. Ask the patient to stand. Remove the bandage and look for bulging from incompetent venous drainage (Figs. A–F).

Rationale: Bulging that occurs as the bandage is removed indicates areas where the deep communicating veins are insufficient. Repeat the procedure until all areas of insufficiency are marked and identified.

Classical Significance: Any bulging areas indicate venous incompetency related to the communicating venous system.

Clinical Significance: Severe deep pain and swelling in the calf indicates occlusion in the deep veins.

Follow-up: Perform Perthe's test or Homan's test.

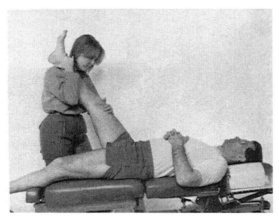

A

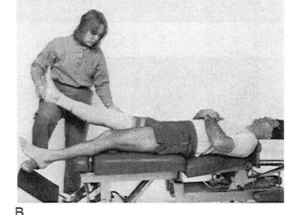

B

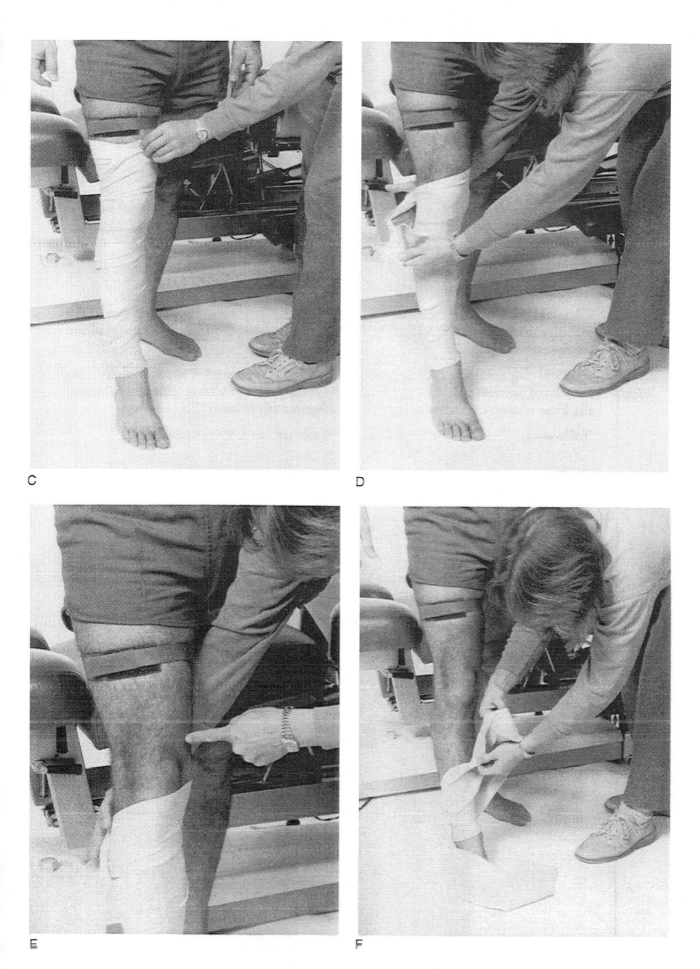

C

D

E

F

8 | Ramirez's Test

Procedure: The patient is supine with one knee slightly flexed and the foot on the table. Wrap a blood pressure cuff around the thigh and inflate it to 40 mmHg. Maintain this pressure for at least 2 minutes (Figs. A–C).

Rationale: The resulting venous pressure imposed by this modification of the tourniquet test will result in pain in the calf at the site of venous thrombosis.

Classical Significance: An increase in pain is significant for venous thrombosis. The inability to have the cuff pressure inflated and sustained for 2 minutes is also significant for thrombosis (Fig. D).

Clinical Significance: If the problem is lumbar nerve root radiculopathy, this amount of pressure will have no effect on the nerve root. In addition the slight flexion of the knee removes the tractioning from the lumbar nerve roots (Fig. E).

Follow-up: Perform Bancroft's test, Homan's test, or Louvel's test.

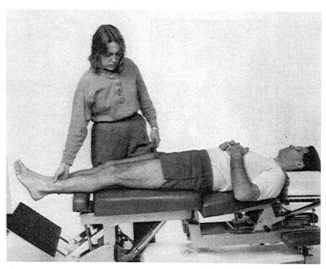

A

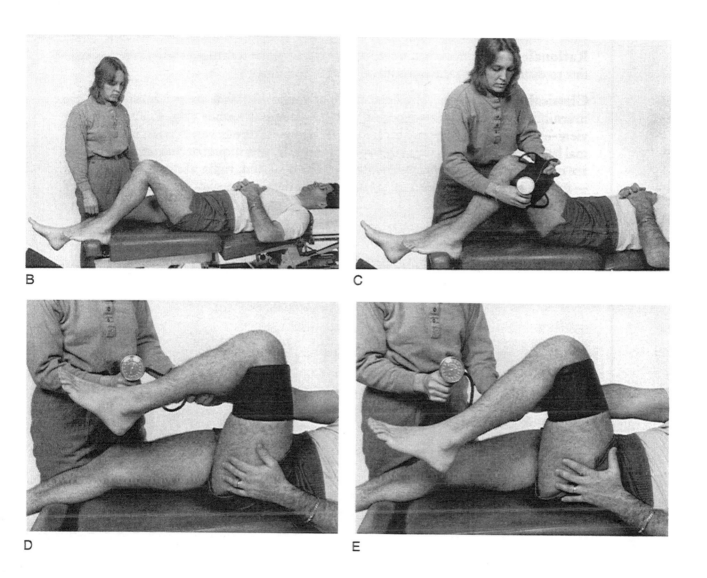

B

C

D

E

9 | *Trendelenburg Test*

Procedure: The patient is supine. Elevate the leg above heart level to empty the veins. Then apply a tourniquet to the upper thigh to occlude the superficial veins. Ask the patient to stand up; release the tourniquet (Figs. A–D).

Rationale: With incompetent veins, the release of the tourniquet will cause varicosities to distend due to the pressure of venous flooding.

Classical Significance: The appearance of varicosities that are produced when the tourniquet is released is evidence of venous valve insufficiency (Fig. E: left, posterior view—venous incompetency is often suggested by tortuous varicosities; middle, normal lateral view—venous drainage compromised by tourniquet occlusion; if deep veins are competent, no superficial varicosity will be observed; right, abnormal lateral view—incompetent venous drainage creates areas of deep venous pooling and pronounced varicosities).

Clinical Significance: For more precise localization, other tourniquet tests can be performed.

Follow-up: Perform the tourniquet test (see Ch. 12), Perthe's test, or refer the patient for venography or thermography.

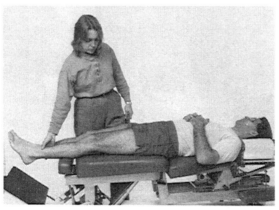

A

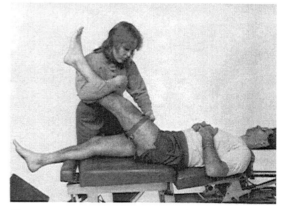

B

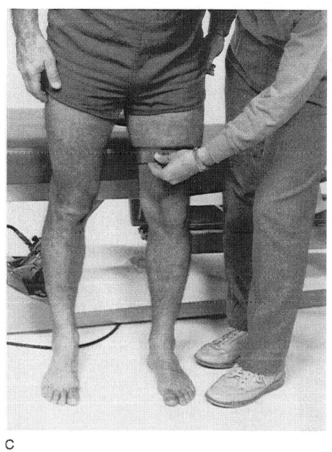

C

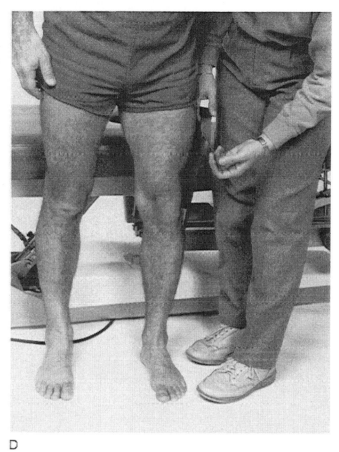

D

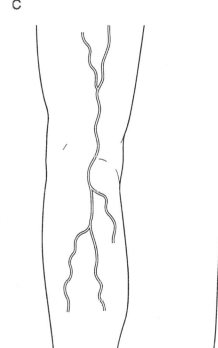

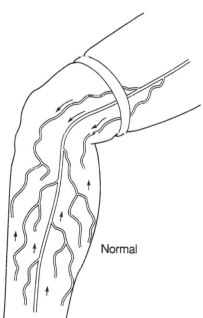

Normal

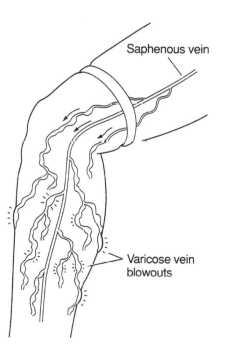

Saphenous vein

Varicose vein
blowouts

E

Malingering Tests

1. Libman's Test
2. Magnuson's Cervical Test
3. Mankopf's Cervical Test
4. O'Donoghues Cervical Maneuver
5. Magnuson's Dorsal Test
6. Mankopf's Dorsal Test
7. O'Donoghues Dorsal Maneuver
8. Burn's Bench Test (Lumbar)
9. Hoover's Test (Lumbar)
10. Magnuson's Lumbar Test
11. Mankopf's Lumbar Test
12. McBride's Test (Lumbar)
13. O'Donoghues Lumbar Maneuver
14. Sitting Lasegue Test (Lumbar)

1 | *Libman's Test*

Procedure: The patient is seated. Stand in front, facing the patient, and place your thumbs on each of the patient's mastoid processes, exerting manual pressure toward the midline (Figs. A–D).

Rationale: This test gauges the patient's pain threshold and should be performed before performing any other orthopaedic tests.

Classical Significance: The patient with an intact sensitivity to pain will complain of a mild pressure or some degree of moderate pain. Patients with a high pain threshold may not complain of anything at all. Patients with a low threshold will complain of a large amount of pain (Fig. E).

Clinical Significance: The patient with an abnormally low pain threshold should be evaluated cautiously if the response is inappropriate to the amount of digital pressure applied. Consider a suspicion of malingering (Fig. F).

Follow-up: Perform Magnuson's cervical test or Mankopf's cervical test.

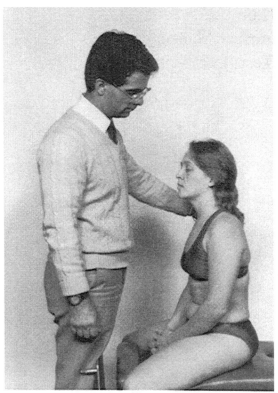

A

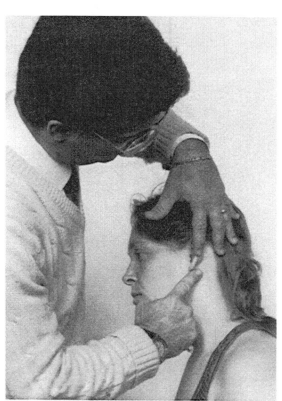

B

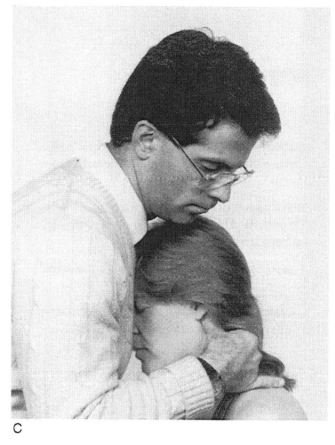

C

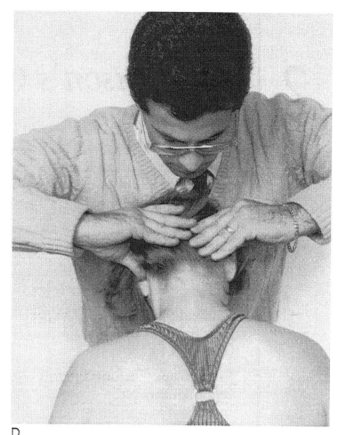

D

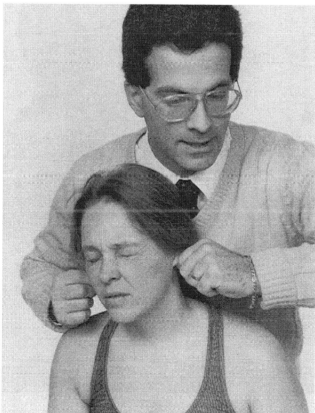

E

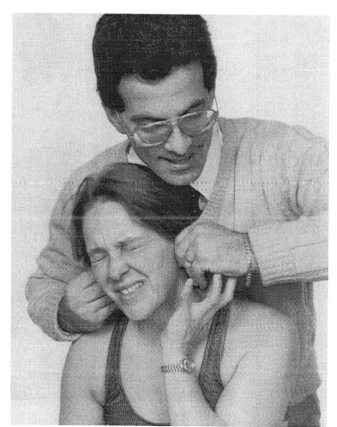

F

2 | *Magnuson's Cervical Test*

Procedure: The patient is prone. Ask the patient to point to the alleged area of pain. Mark the area with a grease pencil and then distract the patient. Later, ask the patient to point to the site of pain again (Figs. A & B).

Rationale: The patient with a true complaint of pain will be able to identify accurately the site of pain time after time. However, the patient who is feigning pain will not be able to identify the site of pain accurately on repeated tries.

Classical Significance: If the location of pain changes significantly on successive trials, suspect a malingerer (Figs. C & D).

Clinical Significance: The patient with scleratogenous, myotogenous, or dermatologic pain will always be able to identify the pain site with accuracy despite distraction (Figs. E & F).

Follow-up: Perform Libman's test, Mankopf's cervical test, or the O'Donoghues cervical maneuver.

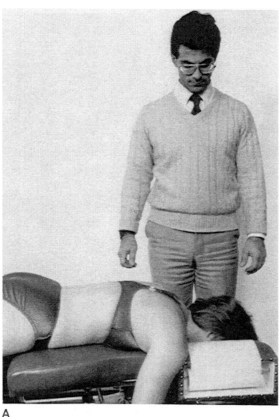

A

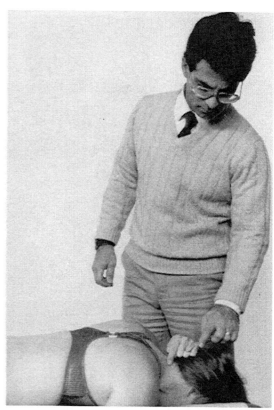

B

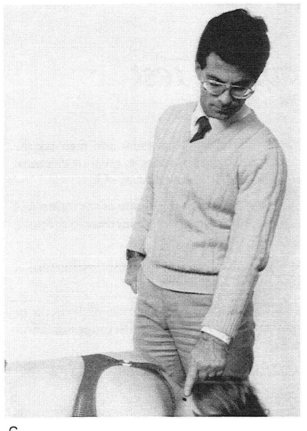

C

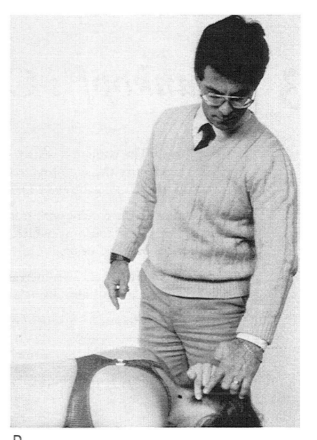

D

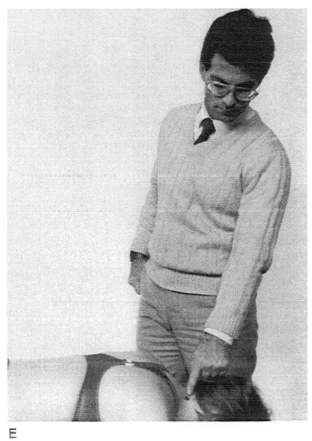

E

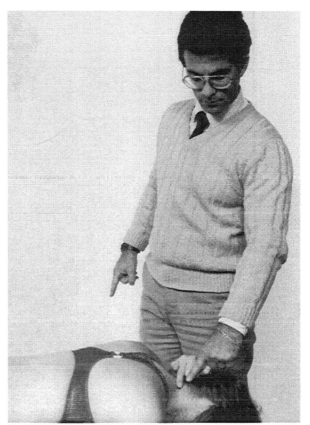

F

3 | *Mankopf's Cervical Test*

Procedure: The patient is seated. Establish a baseline radial pulse and then ask the patient to identify the site of pain. Once identified, apply either manual or electrical irritation to that site and retake and record the radial pulse (Figs. A–E).

Rationale: In the patient with true spinal pain, irritation of the site of the lesion will elicit a sympathetic response, which will be recorded as a 5 percent increase in the pulse rate over the baseline value.

Classical Significance: An increase of 5 percent or more above the baseline radial pulse is evidence of a painful spinal lesion.

Clinical Significance: Failure to create this elevation is evidence of hysteria or malingering. Be sure, however, that the patient is not medicated with drugs that affect heart rate or that dull the sensation of pain.

Follow-up: Perform Magnuson's cervical test or Libman's test.

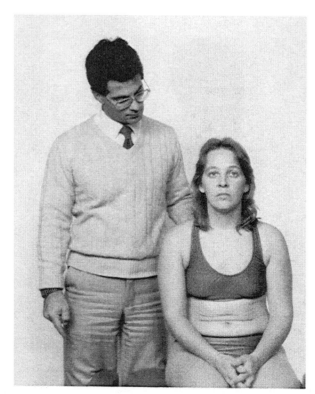

A

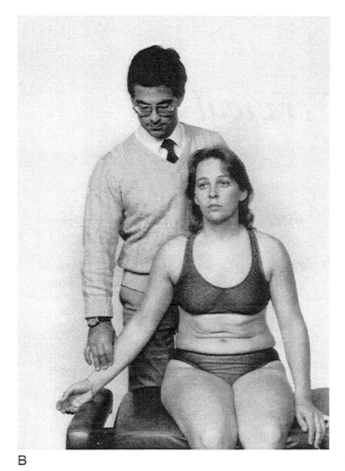

B

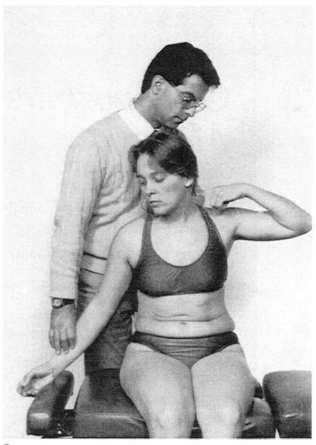

C

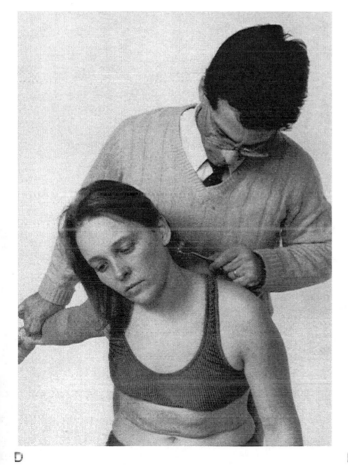

D

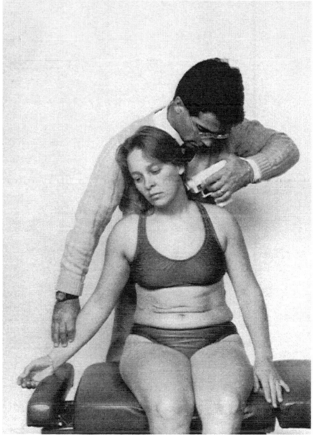

E

4 | O'Donoghues Cervical Maneuver

Procedure: The patient is seated. Put the cervical spine through its ranges of motion both actively and passively (Figs. A–C).

Rationale: Active ranges of motion will always be less than or equal to passive ranges of motion. This is because, to perform actively, the affected muscles must be used. When passively performed the muscles should not be aggravated.

Classical Significance: If the active ranges of motion are less than the passive ranges, active muscle involvement is the cause of the patient's pain.

Clinical Significance: If the active ranges of motion are greater than the passive ranges of motion, suspect a malingerer (Figs. D & E).

Follow-up: Perform Magnuson's cervical test or Mankopf's cervical test.

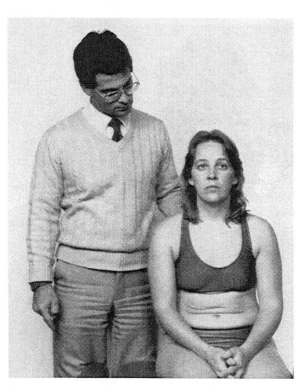

A

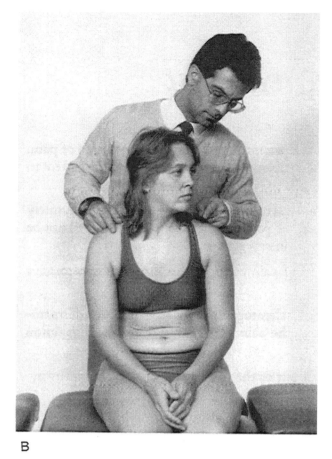

B

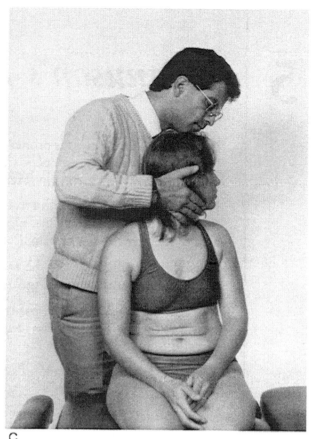

C

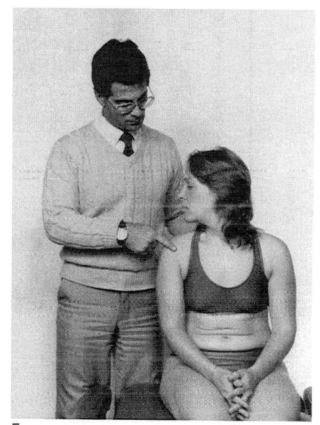

D

E

5 | *Magnuson's Dorsal Test*

Procedure: The patient is prone. Ask the patient to point to the alleged area of pain. Mark that area with a grease pencil and then distract the patient. Later, ask the patient to point to the site of pain again (Figs. A–C).

Rationale: The patient with a true complaint of pain will be able to identify accurately the site of pain time after time. However, the patient who is feigning pain will not be able to identify the site of pain accurately on repeated tries.

Classical Significance: If the location of pain changes significantly on successive trials, suspect a malingerer (Fig. D).

Clinical Significance: The patient with scleratogenous, myotogenous, or dermatologic pain will always be able to identify the pain site accurately despite distraction (Figs. E & F).

Follow-up: Perform Mankopf's dorsal test or the O'Donoghues dorsal maneuver.

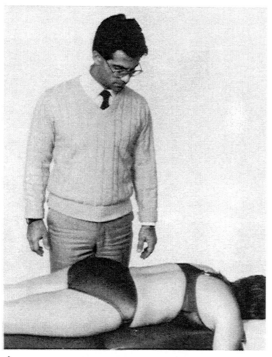

A

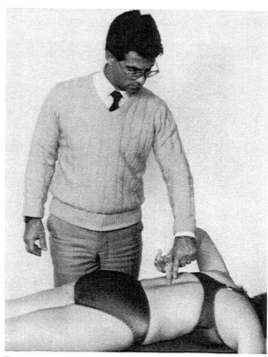

B

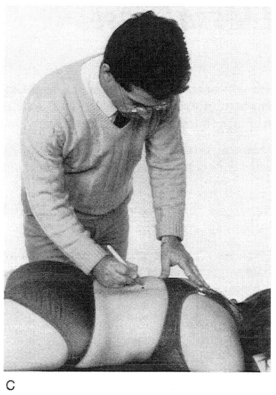

C

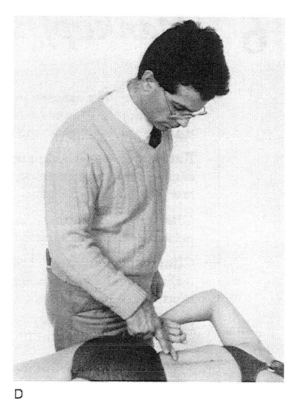

D

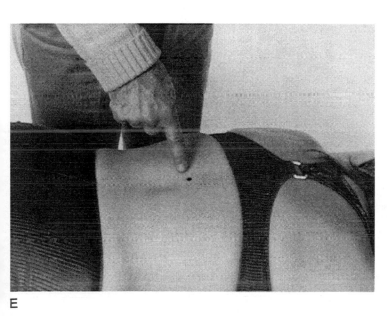

E

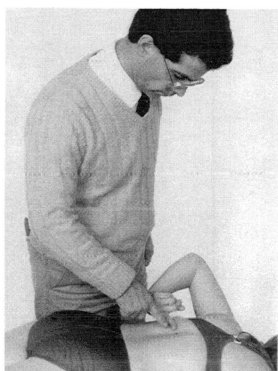

F

6 | *Mankopf's Dorsal Test*

Procedure: The patient is prone. Establish a baseline radial pulse and ask the patient to identify the site of pain. Once identified, apply either manual or electrical irritation to that site and then retake the radial pulse and record it (Figs. A–E).

Rationale: In the patient with true spinal pain, irritation of the site of the lesion will elicit a sympathetic response, which will be recorded as a 5 percent increase in the pulse rate over the baseline value.

Classical Significance: An increase of 5 percent or more above the baseline radial pulse is evidence of a painful spinal lesion.

Clinical Significance: Failure to create this elevation is evidence of hysteria or malingering. Be sure, however, that the patient is not medicated with drugs that affect heart rate or that dull the sensation of pain.

Follow-up: Perform the O'Donoghues dorsal maneuver.

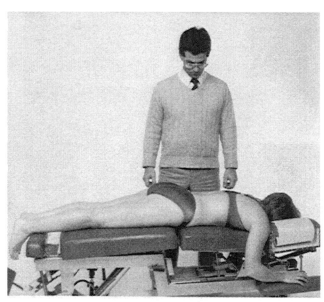

A

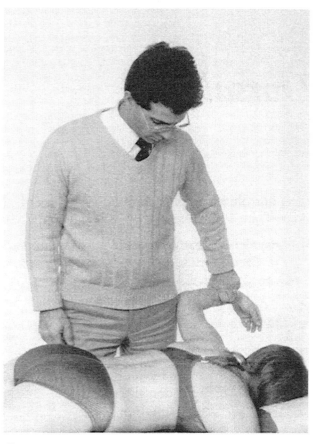

B

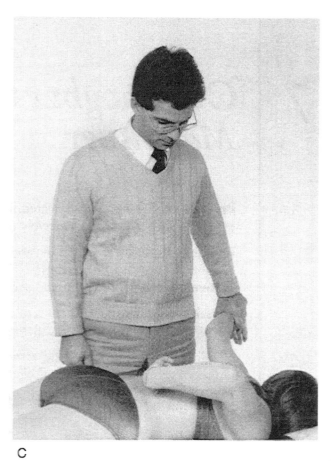

C

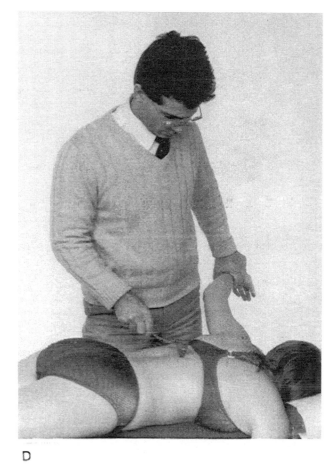

D

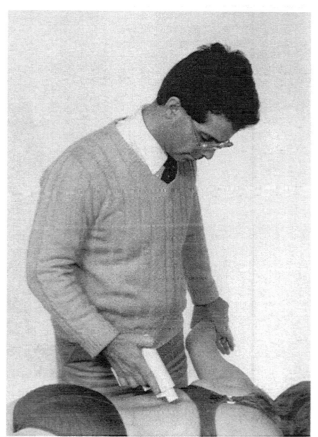

E

7 | O'Donoghues Dorsal Maneuver

Procedure: The patient is seated. Put the dorsolumbar spine through its ranges of motion both actively and passively (Figs. A–C).

Rationale: Active ranges of motion will always be less than or equal to passive ranges of motion, because, to perform actively, the affected muscles must be used. When passively performed the muscles should not be aggravated.

Classical Significance: If the active ranges of motion are less than the passive ranges, active muscle involvement is causing the patient's pain.

Clinical Significance: If the active ranges of motion are greater than the passive ranges of motion, suspect a malingerer (Figs. D & E).

Follow-up: Perform Magnuson's dorsal test or Mankopf's dorsal test.

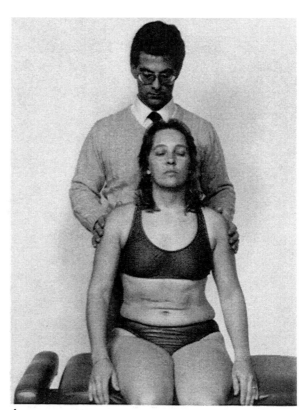

A

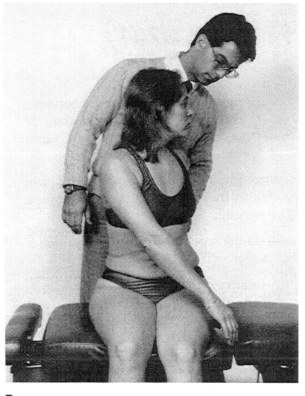

B

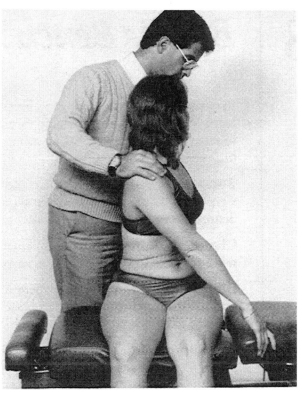

C

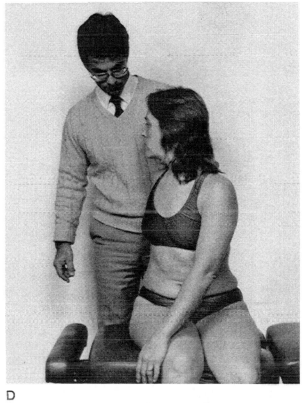

D

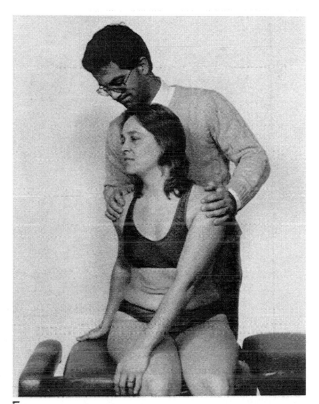

E

8 | *Burn's Bench Test (Lumbar)*

Procedure: Ask the patient to kneel on the examining stool. Stabilize the patient's ankle and ask the patient to bend forward as much as possible. The patient must be able to attempt to touch the floor from an examination stool that is a minimum of 18 inches high (Figs. A–C).

Rationale: Patients, other than those debilitated by injury or disease or who have significant knee or hip disease, should be able to perform this maneuver without distress, because the lower back is not greatly stressed.

Classical Significance: If the patient cannot do this test or refuses to try because it will make the lower back worse, suspect a malingerer (Fig. D).

Clinical Significance: The patient with knee or hip pathology may note an aggravation of pain at these sites when performing this test. However, the patient will still attempt to perform the test, even with pain, whereas the malingerer will not (Fig. E).

Follow-up: Perform Hoover's test, Magnuson's lumber test, or McBride's test.

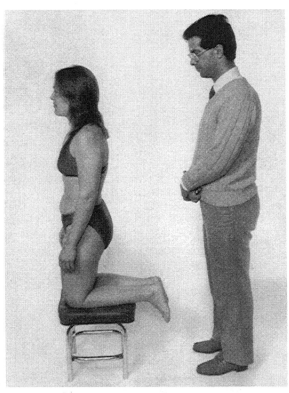

A

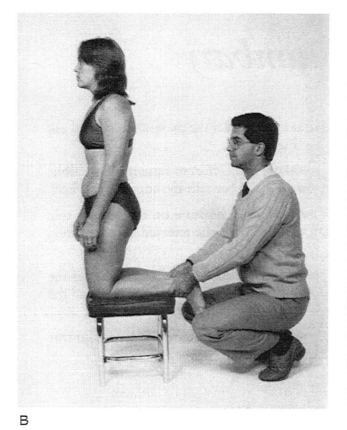

B

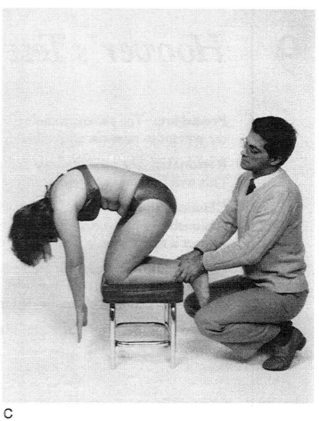

C

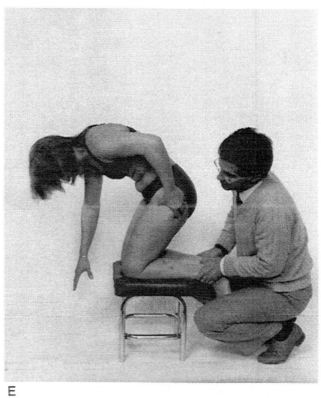

D

E

9 | *Hoover's Test (Lumbar)*

Procedure: The patient is supine. Place your hands under the patient's heels and ask the patient to raise the affected (paretic) leg (Figs. A–D).

Rationale: The patient with a paretic leg will use extra effort to raise it off the table. This will be felt as an increase in pressure on the hand beneath the contralateral heel.

Classical Significance: The absence of an increase in pressure on the healthy side demonstrates that extra effort is not being used to raise the affected leg; therefore, suspect a malingerer.

Clinical Significance: An increase in pressure under the healthy heel indicates the need for extra effort in raising the affected limb. Thus, the limb is truly paretic and the patient has a confirmed lesion affecting that extremity (Fig. E).

Follow-up: Perform Magnuson's lumbar test, McBride's test, or Mankopf's lumbar test.

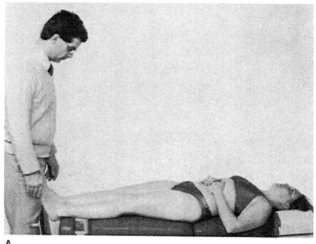

A

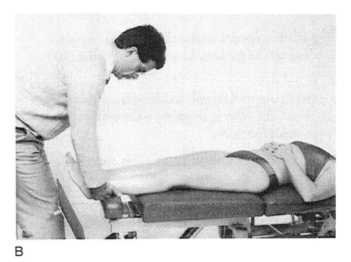

B

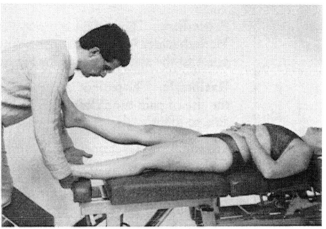

C

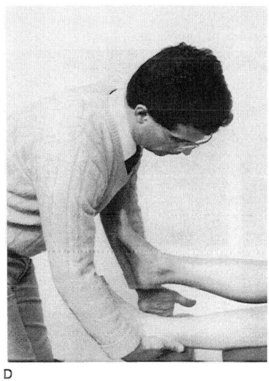

D

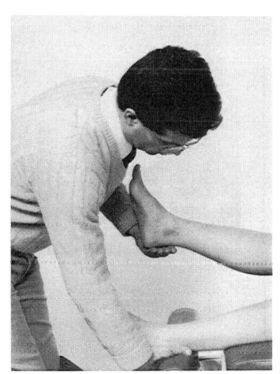

E

10 | *Magnuson's Lumbar Test*

Procedure: The patient is prone. Ask the patient to point to the alleged area of pain. Mark that area with a grease pencil and then distract the patient. Later, ask the patient to point to the site of pain again (Figs. A & B).

Rationale: The patient with a true complaint of pain will be able to identify accurately the site of pain time after time. However, the patient who is feigning pain will not be able to identify the site of pain accurately on repeated tries.

Classical Significance: If the location of pain changes significantly on successive trials, suspect a malingerer (Figs. C & D).

Clinical Significance: The patient with scleratogenous, myotogenous, or dermatologic pain will always be able to identify the pain site accurately despite distraction (Figs. E & F).

Follow-up: Perform Mankopf's lumbar test, Hoover's test, or Burn's bench test.

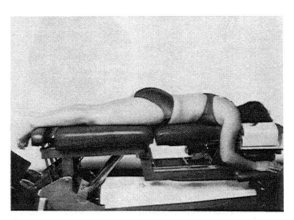

A

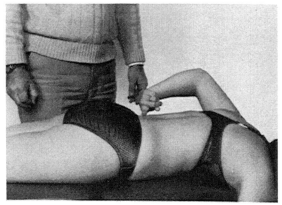

B

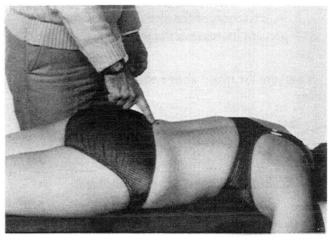

C

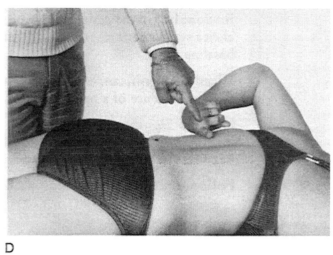

D

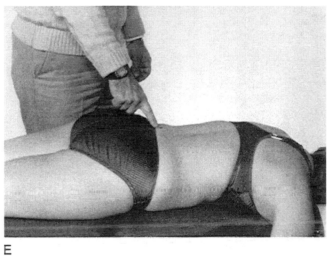

E

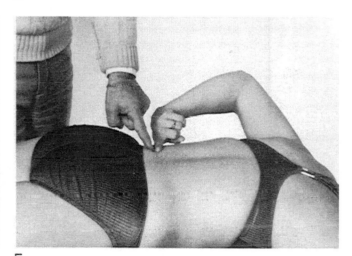

F

11 | *Mankopf's Lumbar Test*

Procedure: The patient is prone. Establish a baseline radial pulse and then ask the patient to identify the site of pain. Once identified, apply either manual or electrical irritation to that site and retake and record the radial pulse (Figs. A–E).

Rationale: In the patient with true spinal pain, irritation of the site of the lesion will elicit a sympathetic response, manifested as a 5 percent increase in the pulse rate over the baseline value.

Classical Significance: An increase of 5 percent or more above the baseline radial pulse is evidence of a painful spinal lesion.

Clinical Significance: Failure to create this elevation is evidence of hysteria or malingering. Be sure, however, that the patient is not medicated with drugs that affect heart rate or that dull the sensation of pain.

Follow-up: Perform Magnuson's lumber test, McBride's test, or Hoover's test.

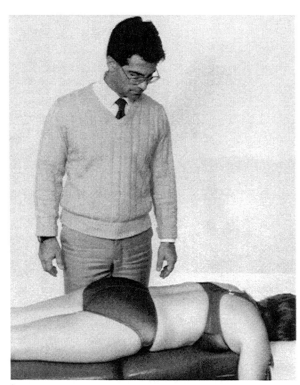

A

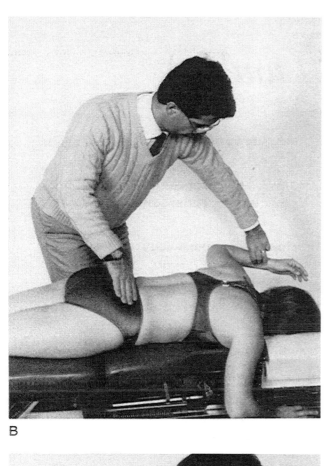

B

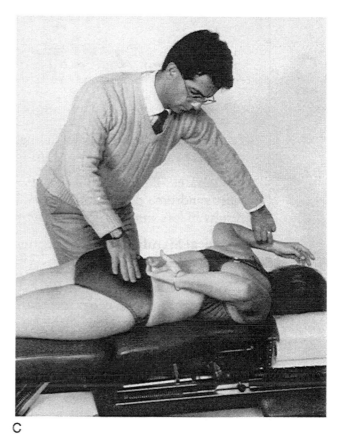

C

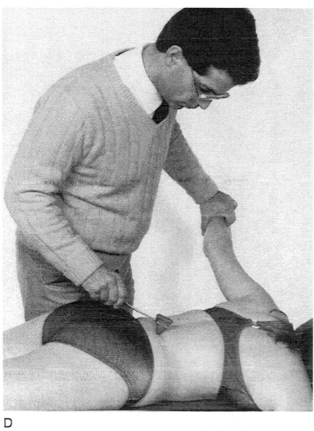

D

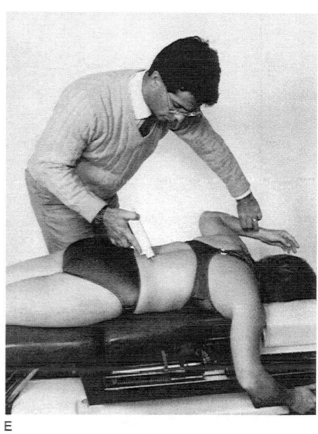

E

12 | *McBride's Test (Lumbar)*

Procedure: The patient is standing. Ask the patient to stand on one leg, bending the other knee and bringing it toward the chest (Figs. A–C).

Rationale: This procedure causes a flattening of the lumbar curve. In patients with facet syndrome or irritation of the lumbar spine from hyperlordosis, this flattening results in less strain along the facet plane.

Classical Significance: A reduction in lower back symptomatology is a positive test (Fig. D).

Clinical Significance: This test is normally used as a malingering test. If the patient with lower back pain believes the test will make the problem worse and refuses to do it, suspect a malingerer (Fig. E).

Follow-up: Perform Magnuson's lumbar test, Mankopf's lumbar test, or Hoover's test.

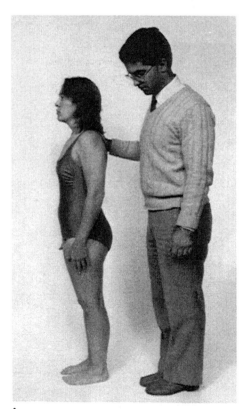

A

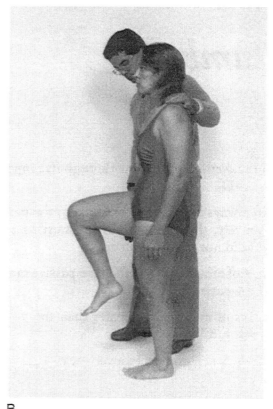

B

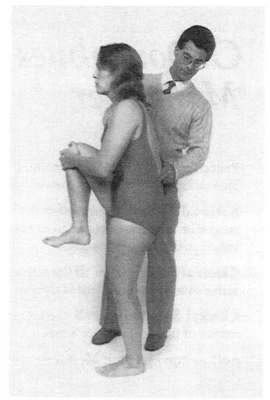

C

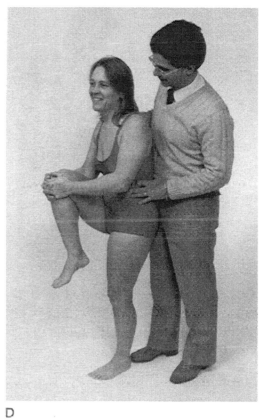

D

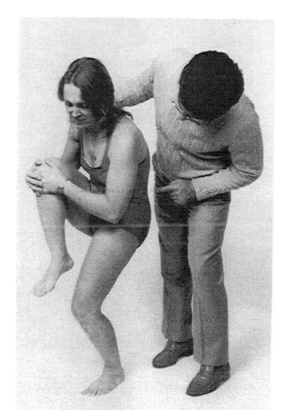

E

13 | O'Donoghues Lumbar Maneuver

Procedure: The patient is standing. Put the dorsolumbar spine through its ranges of motion both actively and passively (Figs. A–D).

Rationale: Active ranges of motion will always be less than or equal to the passive ranges of motion, because, to perform actively, the affected muscles must be used. When passively performed the muscles should not be aggravated.

Classical Significance: If the active ranges of motion are less than the passive ranges, active muscle involvement is the cause of the patient's pain.

Clinical Significance: If the active ranges of motion are greater than the passive ranges of motion, suspect a malingerer (Figs. E & F).

Follow-up: Perform McBride's test, Burn's bench test, or Hoover's test.

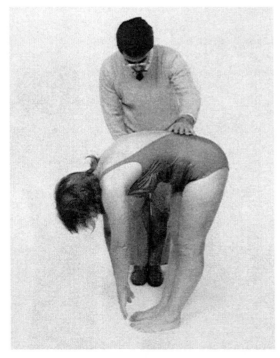

A

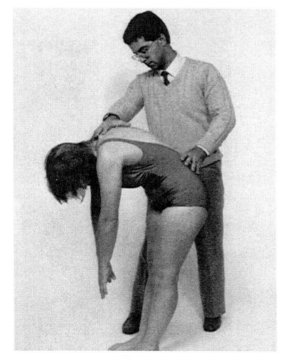

B

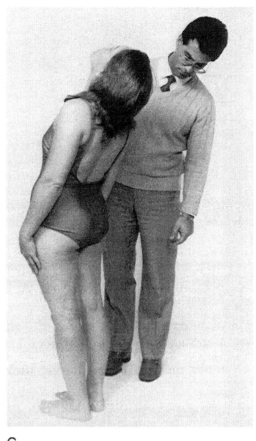

C

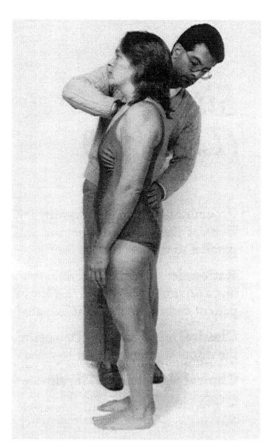

D

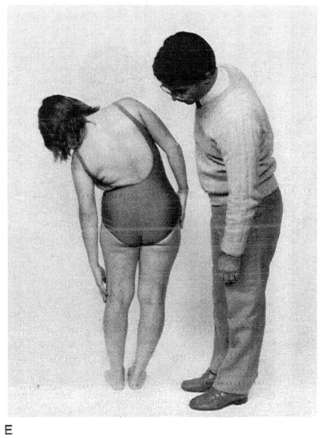

E

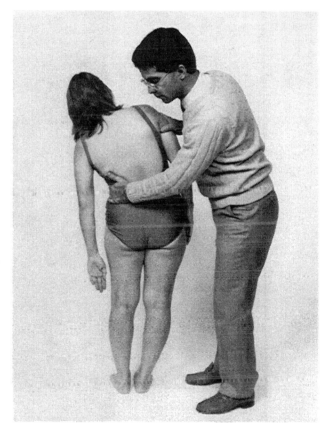

F

14 | *Sitting Lasegue Test (Lumbar)*

Procedure: The patient is seated with the legs dangling off a table without a backrest. Distract the patient's attention while extending one knee at a time until the leg is parallel to the floor (Figs. A–C).

Rationale: This test is similar to the straight leg test. However, because the patient is more secure when seated and because the patient is being tested while distracted, the patient cannot feign the anticipated painful response.

Classical Significance: Pain or the attempt of the patient to lean backward to alleviate the discomfort indicates a low back lesion or radioculopathy, or both (Figs. D & E).

Clinical Significance: If pain does not occur or if the patient does not lean backward, suspect a malingerer (Fig. F).

Follow-up: Perform McBride's test, Hoover's test, or Mankopf's lumbar test.

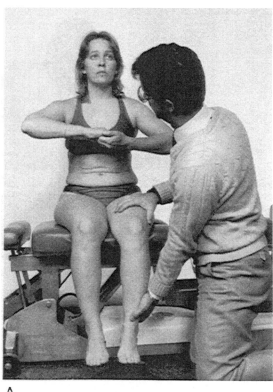

A

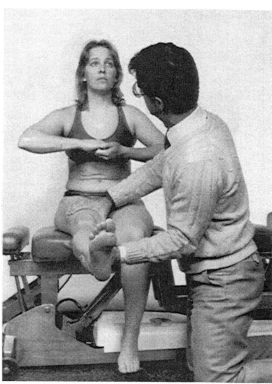

B

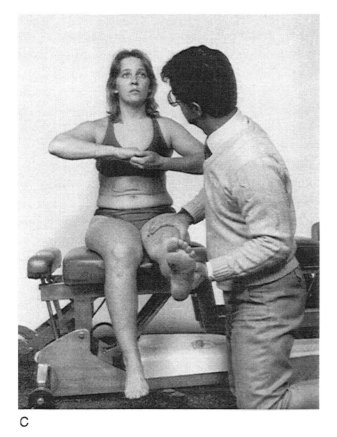

C

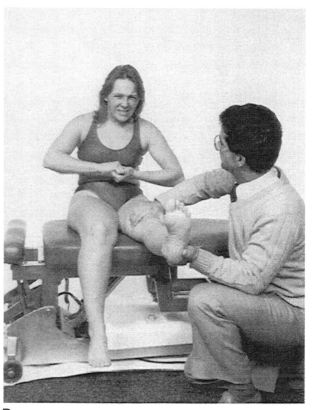

D

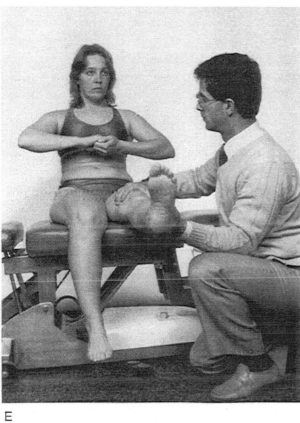

E

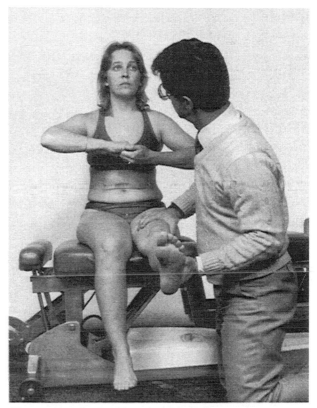

F

Bibliography

American Chiropractic Association: Basic Chiropractic Procedural Manual. 2nd Ed. American Chiropractic Association, Des Moines, 1977

American Medical Association: Guides to the Evaluation of Permanent Impairment. American Medical Association, Chicago, 1990

Blauvelt CT, Nelson F: A Manual of Orthopaedic Terminology. 3rd Ed. CV Mosby, St. Louis, MO, 1983

Caillet R: Knee Pain and Disability. 2nd Ed. FA Davis, Philadelphia, 1983

Caillet R: Low Back Pain Syndrome. 2nd Ed. FA Davis, Philadelphia, 1968

Calliet R: Neck and Arm Pain. FA Davis, Philadelphia, 1964

Calliet R: Shoulder Pain. FA Davis, Philadelphia, 1966

Christensen K: Clinical Chiropractic Orthopedics. 1st Ed. Foot Levelers, Dubuque, IA 1984

Cipriano JJ: Photographic Manual of Regional Orthopaedic Tests. Williams & Wilkins, Baltimore, 1985

Hoppenfeld S: Physical Examination of the Spine and Extremities. Appleton-Century-Crofts, E. Norwalk, CT, 1976

Magee DL: Orthopaedic Physical Assessment. WB Saunders, Philadelphia, 1982

Mazion JM: Illustrated Manual of Neurological Reflexes/Signs/Tests: Orthopedic Signs/Tests/Maneuvers For Office Procedure. Mazion, Casa Grande, AZ, 1980

Post M: Physical Examination of the Musculoskeletal System. Year Book Medical Publishers, Chicago, 1987

Schamber D: Simply Performed Tests of the Hand. Vantage Press, New York, 1984

Skogsbergh DR: The Knee. Graduate Instructional Lecture Series. Regional Orthopedics. Skogsbergh, Cincinatti, 1985

Turek SL: Orthopaedics: Principles and Their Application. 4th Ed. JB Lippincott, Philadelphia, 1984